Principles & practice of plastic surgery:
for the busy resident

MUBASHIR CHEEMA MRCS, FRCS(PLAST)

Locum consultant, Major Trauma Service,
Queen Elizabeth Hospital Birmingham

ISBN 978-0-9935699-0-6 (Hardback)
ISBN 978-0-9935699-1-3 (Paperback)
ISBN 978-0-9935699-2-0 (Kindle)
ISBN 978-0-9935699-3-7 (iBook)

Published by S&C Publishing

Disclaimer
This book is not intended for patients. Even for doctors/surgeons,this is not a gospel/prescription. No book (including this one) can take the place of your common sense and clinical experience. Always use your clinical judgment and common sense, and base your decisions on the current best practice and evidence available. If in doubt, ask for a second opinion. Approach complex cases as a multidisciplinary team.

Acknowledgment: Many thanks to Dr Wardah Bajwa for her help in writing the chapter on Topical Negative Pressure therapy and searching for the relevant references.

نگارِ من که به مکتب نرفت و خط ننوشت

به غمزه مسئله آموز صد مدرس شد

Hafez Shirazi** (c. 1325-1389)

Dedicated

To my teachers...

for their time, kindness and patience

To my patients...

for making this a worthwhile journey

...and to my long suffering family & friends*

*Aisha, Hiba, Mom & Zed

Preface

There is an old Punjabi anecdote that an emperor hired the best brain in all the lands and required of him to teach a young prince in all the known sciences, as well as common sense. The wise man pleaded that while sciences may be taught, common sense cannot be imparted readily. The king relented and the teaching began. Once the wise man declared the prince ready, the king improvised a test with a round mint coin hidden in his fist and challenged the prince to an educated guess. The prince analysed the anatomy of the regent's closed fist and concluded that it contained a round object [The hand surgeon in me _so_ hopes that he compared it with the other side!]. The king, duly impressed, decided to test his common sense and asked, "what could it be?". With the briefest of thoughts the prince replied, "It can be a milling stone".

"What could it be?" is an innocuous looking question often asked in ward, in clinics and the FRCS(Plast) examination. How you answer it determines if you will sail well with the wind in your sails, or bump down the stairs as in the famous introduction of A.A.Milne's Winnie the Pooh. In all honesty, I've seen it happen as a junior, have bumped down the stairs myself and now warn all my colleagues to stay clear of the bumpy road. The exam is less taxing if you have a systematic mode of thinking and a methodical pattern of approaching each situation.

This book started out when I began preparing for the FRCS(Plast). I could not find any book or any person who can guide preparation in a way that was directly applicable to how the exam proceeds. Algorithm for breast cancer recon, marking or choosing a pedicle for BBR, choosing an implant, marking a cleft lip repair are some of the examples where most books are either silent or dish out one surgeon's view although it may not what is commonly used in practice. I found a generic pool of notes akin to a pot of broth with variably "cooked" fragments. The oft quoted "concise" books give fragments of information but not a systematic order. The reference books put various degrees of emphasis on various topics. Every now and again, review articles get published in leading journals but consolidating them by topic is a tall order and while they may serve very well for CME purposes can be insufficient for the exit exam. The end result for me was to read a large body of information (especially original papers and review/CME articles in PRS, as you'll notice in the references), weed it out, align it with my thought process and re-write it all for ease of reference.

The organisation of this book is different from any other. I have not tried to make it an encyclopaedia and instead focussed on clinical approach and identifying points that change management. Where possible I've either summarised the key findings from key papers or quoted a direct reference. So do not take this book as an all encompassing prescription. There are some excellent review articles out there e.g. by Al Aly, Phillip Blondeel, Kevin Chung, Bahman Guyron, Dai Davis, Rod Rohrich, Julia Tertzis (& many more) that I will strongly recommend that you read. It is not possible for me to summarise these any further than the excellent language with which these have already been written. Of these, I've only quoted the sources that I have read in depth. I have tried to reference all sources as accurately as possible and will only be too happy to rectify any omissions.

The sections are organised as per FRCS(Plast) vivas. Additional topics are covered at the very end. There is a core knowledge base that is needed for each topic, which broadly conforms to the ISCP syllabus (but is less boring;). Approach to a clinical scenario varies widely amongst surgeons, but there are common themes that need to be addressed. The depth to which a given element of history, or examination is explored in exam will vary with the clinical situations and will reflect your experience and training. Similarly, choice of treatment given here are either based on broad consensus (e.g. skin cancer or lower limb trauma guidelines) or widely known safe middle ground practices (e.g. cleft lip or hypospadias repair). I (or any one else) cannot give you a solution that will fit every case you will ever encounter. Please also note that the "Expected clinical questions" list is indicative at best and cannot be exhaustive.

The following piece of advice helped me considerably:
1. Define things. Have a one line definition of common conditions (e.g. skin cancers, Dupuytren's, rheumatoid hand). A succinct definition gets the message across that you know what you are saying.
2. Have an opening gambit i.e. a few introductory sentences about some common conditions. It gives you time to think ahead in what is a stressful situation during the exam.
3. "Big box, little box, little box!" Make a broad statement first before engaging in specifics i.e. introduce the breadth of a topic before diving in to the nitty gritty. Remember that the examiner is seeing you probably for the first time and have 30 minutes to decide whether you are consultant quality material. Give them an opportunity to know your train of thoughts and do not ignore intervening steps.
4. Make conversation as you would with a senior colleague. Polite, rational and not rushed.

Remember your immediate goal is to save life, and in long term to return the patient to premorbid level of function and appearance within a reasonable length of time. Its a very useful to consider that your "management depends upon" x, y & z i.e. take into account patient specific factors and individualise the management decision to that patient

A very useful yardstick for decision making in a challenging situation is to imagine what your expectations would be if one of your dear ones was there instead of the patient. Think what will *you* expect of another professional to do for your loved one, and just do the same for your patient too - you will always make correct decisions.

If your practice differs in any respect from the content of this book please use your experience, judgement and common sense to make clinically relevant, safe and evidence based decisions for your patients. Remember, safety first!

Mubashir Cheema, FRCS(Plast)

Glossary of terms

ABG	Arterial blood gas
ADL	Activities of daily living
ADM	Acellular dermal matrix
AROM	Active range of movement
BA	Breast augmentation
BAHA	Bone anchored hearing aid
BM	Blood sugar (actually an acronym for Bohringer Medical whose portable blood sugar machine was the first such instrument to be used widely in UK)
BNF	British National Formulary (or equivalent)
BOT	Base of tongue
BT	Breslow thickness
BW	Breast width
CE	Completely excised / complete excision
CMAP	Combined Motor Action Potential
CO	Cardiac output, Carbon monoxide (depending on context)
CFNG	Cross facial nerve grafting
D5W	5% dextrose saline
D/C	Direct closure
DD	deep dermal (burn)
DIO	Dorsal Interosseus (interossei)
EBRT	External beam radiation therapy
FOM	Florr of mouth
FNA	Fine needle aspiration
FT	Full thickness (burn)
HT	Hypertrophic (scar)
IMF	Infra-mammary fold

IPPV	Intermittent Positive Pressure Ventilation
LA	Local anaesthetic
LCFA	Lateral circumflex femoral artery
LR	Local recurrence
LLC	Lower lateral cartilage (of nose)
LSMDT	Local skin multidisciplinary meeting
LVP	Levator veli palatini (= Levator palati)
LMWH	Low molecular weight heparin
MEP	Motor end plate
MMP	Matrix metalloproteinase
MMS	Mohs' micrographic surgery
MRI	Magnetic resonance imaging
MRA	Magnetic resonance angiogram (also called 'MR Angio')
MSKCC	Memorial Sloan Kettering Cancer Centre
MWL	Massive weight loss
NCS	Nerve conduction studies
NPA	NasoPharyngeal Airway
OPG	Orthopantomogram
PIA	Posterior interosseous artery (flap)
PIN	Posterior interosseous nerve
PIO	Palmar Interosseus (interossei)
PMHx	Past medical (*and* surgical) history
PROM	Passive range of movement
pt	patient
PT	partial thickness (burn)
r/o	risk of', or 'rule out' depending on context
RMT	Retromolar trigone
RT	Radiotherapy
RTA	Road Traffic Accident

SCIA/V	Superficial circumflex iliac artery/vein
SCM	Sternocleidomastoid muscle
SIEA/V	Superficial inferior epigastric artery/vein
SNAP	Sensory Nerve Action Potential
TBSA	total body surface area (burnt)
TE	Tissue expander/expansion
TNP	Topical Negative Pressure Therapy (generic term)
TPF	Temporo-parietal fascial flap
TVP	Tensor veli palatini
ULC	Upper lateral cartilage (of nose)
UO	Urinary output
VAC™	Vacuum Assisted Closure (trademark of KCI Ltd)
VRAM	Vertical Rectus Abdominis Muscle flap
WLE	Wide local excisiony
[…]	Author's opinion given within square brackets so as not to interrupt the flow

Contents

Cleft lip & palate 245

Craniofacial 261

Classifications of craniofacial deformities 266

Cranio-synostosis 266

Craniofacial clefts 271

Hypospadias 280

Congenital - Hands 289

Syndactyly 291

Apert hand 295

Basic Science   421

Basic science   423

Assessment of adverse scar   427

Management of HT / keloid scar   431

General & Misc. topics   433

General & Miscellaneous   435

Extravasation injury   436

Necrotising fasciitis   438

Perineal recon.   440

Pressure sores   444

LASER   449

Topical negative pressure therapy (TNP)   455

Workhorse Flaps   459

RFFF: Radial forearm free flap   461

Definitions 473

Sources used in this book

GRABB & SMITH

I think it is an absolute must read at a junior trainee level as it gives many great insights. I didn't read it for my exit exam.

MICHIGAN MANUAL (1ST ED.)

Great concise book that gives you a lot of information. Very good for fact checking while on the run. Given the choice, this is the only book I'd carry in my pocket.

JANIS (2ND ED.)

Detailed book with a lot of information. I read very little of it (<5 chapters) but found it well written and detailed. Given that the authors of each chapter are usually a specialist in their field it can be too detailed without addressing "why" a particular management is favored.

WEINZWEIG'S SECRETS PLUS (2ND ED.)

A very good book to read with detailed information but can be a daunting task. Its written in Q&A format which makes it both easy to locate information and difficult to grasp the bigger picture. A third of the book is dedicated to head & neck (some of it very specialised, even for me who worked in a craniofacial centre), a third is for hand surgery & a third for the rest of plastic surgery. I read it cover to cover, more than once and gained many a concepts from there.

HELLMAN & DEVITA

I've read this book since my elective in medical oncology, years ago. Since a lot of my plastics training has involved cancer resection & reconstruction, I often find it useful to see the world from an oncologist's perspective. Information on obscure cancers comes predominantly from this source.

REVIEW ARTICLES IN PRS, JHS & OTHER JOURNALS

These have been the major source of knowledge for me. I found them either in hospital library or by searching PubMed for specific topics, key authors and article types. Not all review articles are suitable for exam prep and some were clearly written as short CME topics. You'll need to weed out those by hand.

The great benefit of this approach is to be able to read the thoughts of the originator of the idea (eg Pribaz's prefabrication, Snodgrass' TIP, Rigotti's fat grafting) or an expert in the field (eg Julia Tertzis, John Thompson) describing just one topic. Finding and reading these articles does take a while, even with good Athens access (or equivalent) but is well worth it in my opinion. Remember, pain goes away but success stays.

OTHERS

Books by Adrian Richards. Read only once as a junior trainee
Books by Hank Giele & Chris Stone. Never read

COPYRIGHTS & TRADEMARKS

Bactigras® and Jelonet® are trademarks of Smith & Nephew. Biobrane® temporary synthetic wound dressing is a registered trademark of Bertek Pharmaceuticals Inc. and sold in UK by Smith & Nephew, UK. Flowtron® intermittent pneumatic compression system is a registered trade mark of ArjoHuntleigh (Malmo, Sweden). Integra® dermal regeneration template and Integra® Bilayer matrix wound dressing, are registered trademarks of Integra Lifesciences corporation. Kerlix™ AMD antimicrobial bandage roll is a trademark of Covidien (now Medtronic Minimally Invasive Therapies, Minneapolis, MN, USA). Mitek GII® anchor and Mini Quickanchor® anchors are registered trademarks of DePuy Synthes Companies. Natrelle® Style 410 is a registered trademark of Allergan Inc. (NJ, USA) now Actavis. Onyx® liquid embolic system is a registered trademark of Micro Therapeutics Inc. (Irvine, CA, USA). Strattice™ is a registered trade mark of Lifecell™ (Bridgewater, NJ, USA). Synthes Compact Hand is a product and copyright of DePuy Synthes companies of Johnson and Johnson. Zimmer® Electric Dermatome is a registered trademark of Zimmer Biomet Inc.

Trauma

Trauma - Burns

CORE KNOWLEDGE
Burns classification
Jackson's model. Douglas Jackson 1953.
Sterling equation/equilibrium
Burn shock
Inhalation injury
Burn size estimation
What types of burns to refer
Burn centre, unit, facility (National burn care review)

APPROACH TO PATIENT - HISTORY
(For diagnosis of inhalation injury, see p.45)
Mechanism of burn
Time of burn
Agent, esp. any accelerant
Environment (closed or open)
Duration of contact, entrapment or unconsciousness
Any other injury sustained? e.g. by a fall or head injury
In children, always consider NAI and whether the stated mechanism is consistent with developmental age

First aid. What? and for how long? Whether any delay?
Management so far, including analgesia and fluids
AMPLE history = PMHx, Meds, Allergies
Tetanus status

APPROACH TO PATIENT - EXAMINATION
Combined ATLS & EMSB protocol (see below)

APPROACH TO PATIENT - TREATMENT
(Depends on the extent of the burn but the following will be common)
Analgesia, Tetanus cover
Cling film
Debride bliters (see below)

EXPECTED CLINICAL QUESTIONS
- Assessment of burn size (65-75% surgeon agreement. Jaskille, J Burn Care Res 2010)

- Assessment of burn depth
- Parkland (is a place)
- Monitoring by urinary output, BE, lactate
- Why Hartman
- What other fluids. [Crystalloids / Colloids. N/Saline, Hartman's, Hypertonic, Human Albumin, FFP, Dextran/Starches (discontinued in EU)]
- What other formula. [Mount Vernon]
- Fluid creep

- When would you take the patient to theatre
- Why early excision and grafting
- How to minimise blood loss (tourniquet on limbs, infiltration & its composition)
- Alexander technique (Cuono technique). [Alexander, J Trauma 1981]
- Meek technique
- Escharotomies. Definition, incisions, when and where to do them
- Priority areas for grafting

- Scar contracture and methods to address this
- Metabolic response
- Sepsis
- Baux score / ABSA
- Mechanism of electrical burn (compartment syndrome, myoglobinuria)
- Chemical antidotes (more relevant in MCQs)
- NAI
- TSS

RECOMMENDED PAPERS

1. EMSB manual
2. Cartotto R. Fluid resuscitation of the thermally injured patient. *Clin Plast Surg.* 2009 Oct;36(4):569–81.
3. Williams FN, Herndon DN, Jeschke MG. The hypermetabolic response to burn injury and interventions to modify this response. *Clin Plast Surg.* 2009 Oct;36(4):583–96.
4. Greenhalgh DG. Topical Antimicrobial Agents for Burn Wounds. *Clin Plast Surg.* 2009 Oct;36(4):597–606.
5. Greenhalgh DG et al. American burn association consensus conference to define sepsis and infection in burns. *J Burn Care Res.* 2007;28(6):776-90
6. Singer M et al. The third international consensus definitions for sepsis and septic shock (Sepsis-3) *JAMA* 2016;315(8):801-10

7. Gibran NS, Wiechman S, Meyer W, Edelman L, Fauerbach J, Gibbons L, et al. American Burn Association Consensus Statements *J Burn Care Res.* 2013;34(4):361–85.
8. Serghiou M, Cowan A, Whitehead C. Rehabilitation After a Burn Injury. *Clin Plast Surg.* 2009 Oct;36(4):675–86.
9. Wainwright DJ. Burn Reconstruction: the Problems, the Techniques, and the Applications. *Clin Plast Surg.* 2009 Oct;36(4):687–700.
10. Orgill DP, Ogawa R. Current Methods of Burn Reconstruction. *Plast Reconstr Surg.* 2013 May;131(5):827e – 836e.

Burns referral system in UK

In UK, wards which care for burn injuries are classified (in the National Burn Care Review) as a:

1. Burn facility (any plastic surgery unit),
2. Burns unit (a plastic surgery unit with at least one burns consultant and a weekly burns theatre list, or
3. Burns centre (dedicated burns beds, with on call burns consultant and access to dedicated theatre and ITU beds).

A burn maybe *complex* because of the patient's age, size of burn, size, presence of inhalation or by its mechanism.

A burn may be *complicated by*
- existing conditions e.g. cardiorespiratory disease, pregnancy, or
- associated injuries like head injury fractures or crush.

A *complex non-burn* is any inhalation without cutaneous burn, or presence of the vesicobullous disorders (e.g. EB, SJS, SSS)

Based on the above definitions, a burn referral may take one of many forms (Ref: Types of burns referrals)

Table: Types of burns referrals

	a complex burn
Acute	a non-complex burn
	a complex non-burn
Non-acute	non-acute burn referral

Management

At the outset consider what worries you about the patient. This could be inhalation injury, major burn, non-accidental injury or high-voltage electrical injury.

Major burns management has the following (somewhat overlapping) stages:
1) resuscitate
2) stabilise
3) early excision and grafting in stages
4) aggressive rehabilitation and long-term follow-up

Initial management

Initial management is a combination of advanced trauma life-support(ATLS) and emergency management of severe burns(EMSB) frameworks. You should have a formal system by which the patient is systematically assessed for

A- Airway with cervical spine control, by a senior anaesthetist.

B- Breathing with ventilation and application of high flow oxygen.

C- Circulatory assessment (with haemorrhage control if needed) with routine bloods and ABGs

D- Disability with neurological status.

E- Exposure of front and back to assess size of the burn (and need for escharotomies) as well as looking for other injuries.

F- Assess the need for fluid resuscitation and if it is the case, the patient will need urinary catheterisation an starting Parklands formula [I'll use 4ml/kg/% TBSA in most patients, unless there is a concern about fluid overload].

G- If more than 30% TBSA burn, then NGT for early feeding.

BEFORE LEAVING THE EMERGENCY DEPARTMENT MAKE SURE THAT:

1. The patient's burns are covered with cling film,
2. iv analgesia has been given,
3. Tetanus status has been checked and
4. You've spoken to all the relevant individuals (Ref: Table)

Table: Important communications to,

Patient, if able to understand
Patient's family esp. the significant other
Senior colleague on call with you (e.g. burns registrar or consultant)
Theatre anaesthetist, if headed to theatre
Theatre sister in charge
ITU anaesthetist
ITU sister in charge
Burns centre nursing staff

IN AN ELECTRICAL BURN, ALWAYS CONSIDER:

1. Arrythmias (Ref: Aside),
2. Compartment syndrome,
3. Myoglobinuria
4. Associated injuries e.g. from a fall, fracture, eye injury.

Hence the following are important in managing electrical burns

- ECG monitoring if appropriate (Ref: Aside)
- Compartment observations,
- Forced diuresis (with Hartman's to keep urine output 1-2 ml/kg/hr) as well as
- Serial CK & K^+ levels

Aside: ECG monitoring

Always do a 12-lead ECG on arrival

If voltage <1000V AND no abnormality on initial ECG AND no h/o LOC, then further ECG monitoring is not needed(Bailey 2007)

Otherwise 24 hour ECG monitoring is important

Surgical management

Patient may be taken to theatre overnight (if more than 30% TBSA burn) or next day (if less than 20% is involved) with a grey area in between. My reasons for taking a major burn to theatre overnight are:

- To secure ETT, by wiring it to the maxillary incisor tooth
- Bronchoscopy (for a broncho-alveolar lavage, or to identify subglottic inhalation injury by the anaesthetist)
- Inserting long lines (venous & arterial) in a clean environment
- Escharotomies (see below)
- Clean & redress in a sterile environment
- To identify the size and depth of burns
- Identify donor sites
- Make a plan for next (& further) theatre trips (for debridement, donor selection as well as personnel requirement)

The long-term care of the burn patient involves multimodality management. It includes the burn surgeon for early excision and grafting, good daily nursing care, dietician for adequate caloric intake, intensivist if in intensive care, physiotherapists for a range of exercises to keep muscle bulk, as well as the clinical psychologist. All of them need to be involved early to achieve best care.

Burns can be classified according to their:
- Mechanism (flames school contact chemical electrical burns),
- Surface area (non-resus, or resus burn if >15% in adult, <u>OR</u> >10% in a child) (Ref: Table)
- Depth (partial or full thickness burn) (Ref: Table)

Table: Methods of determining burn size

Methos	Application	Explanation
Palm size	The palm and adducted fingers of patient's hand = 1% TBSA	Good method for small size burns
Wallace's rule of nines	H&N = 9% TBSA Each upper limb = 9% Anterior torso = 18% Posterior torso = 18% Each lower limb = 18% Perineum = 1%	Quick rule of thumb but not accurate in children (who have different body proportions)
Lund-Browder chart	Detailed description of each limb. Age specific for children	If available, this is the most accurate method

Methos	Application	Explanation
Serial halving	Whether more or less-than-half of any body area is burnt. Count as all-or-none e.g. if more than half of lower limb is involved, count it as 18% otherwise count as zero percent.	Gives a good estimate esp. in the rapid assessment of a major burn

Table: Partial vs Full thickness burns

	Superficial PT	**Mid dermal**	**Deep dermal**	**Full thickness**
Color	Pink	Dark pink	Cherry red / crimson	Black/ white / leathery
Capillary refill	Brisk	1-2 sec	2+ sec	None
Sensations	Yes	Yes	+/-	No

Resuscitation fluids

The reason of using resuscitation fluids is to prevent burn shock. Burn shock is a form of hypovolaemic shock due to translocation of protein rich fluid from intravascular compartment to interstitial compartment, causing edema as well as decreased circulating volume.

PATHOPHYSIOLOGY OF BURN SHOCK

Burn → injury → inflammation → release of histamine and prostaglandins → increase capillary permeability → protein translocation and movement of fluid from intra-vascular to interstitial compartments → ↑tissue edema + ↓circulating volume.

This fluid movement in the microcirculation is governed by the Starling equation (Ref: Figure). The aim of resus fluids is to restore the intravascular volume (and hence the arteriolar hydrostatic pressure) to maintain end organ perfusion and prevent burn shock.

Figure: Starling's equilibrium in normal skin. Thick arrows represent hydrostatic pressure (P) & thin arrows represent colloid osmotic pressure(π), numbers are in mmHg (Ref: Herndon's Total Burn Care, Chapter 8)

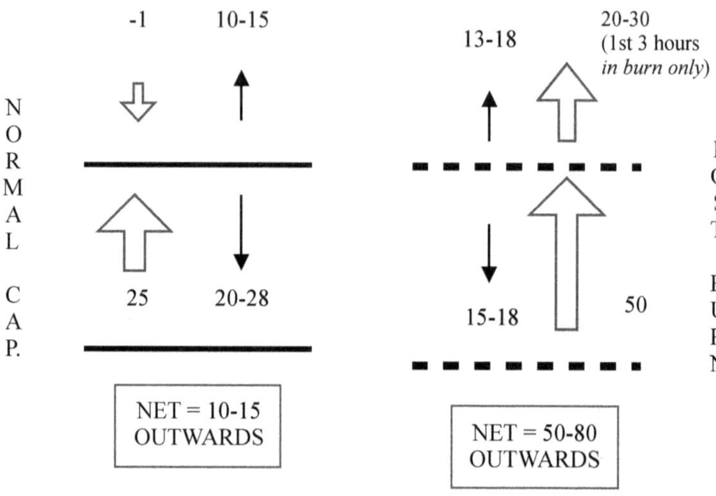

Figure: Fluid changes in a major burn, simplified a) Body fluid compartments in a 70kg adult b) Post burn.

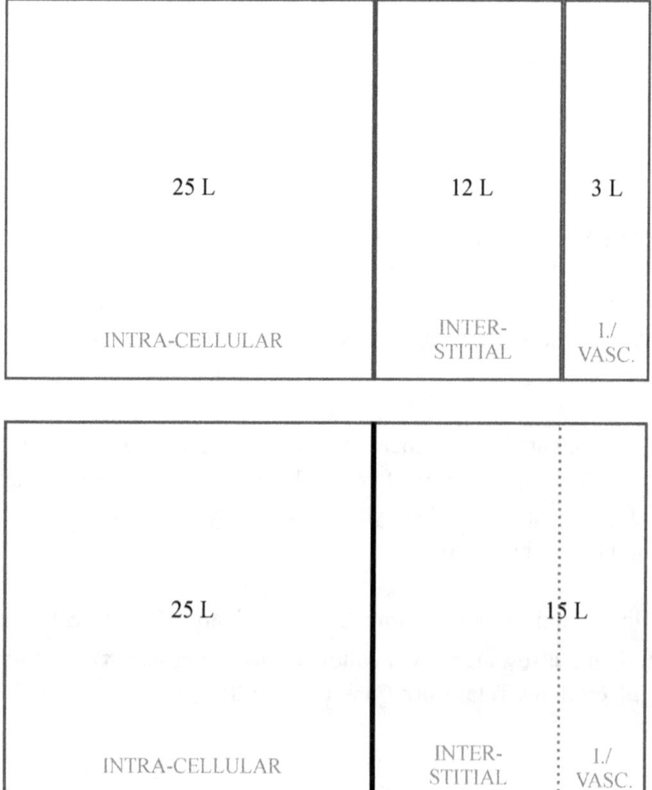

Aside: Fluid changes in first 24hrs in major burns.

Due to high capillary permeability the intravascular proteins leak in to interstitium, causing the intravascular and interstitial compartments to behave almost as one. The migration of proteins takes away water with it ("3rd spacing") → ↓intra-vascular volume → ↓capillary pressure → ↓tissue perfusion ("burn shock").

Note that the iv fluids administered also redistribute in these compartments which means that

i.   ECF behaves as a single 15litre compartment (in which you are pouring fluids)

ii. only the fluid that stays in the intravascular part (of this new 15L compartment) contributes to the tissue perfusion

iii. a large amount of fluids are needed to keep the intravascular compartment topped-up (until capillary permeability returns to baseline)

iv. these fluids contribute to edema formation, hence the age old controversy between crystalloids and colloids. In brief, crystalloids stay in circulation for less time and cause more edema. In contrast, colloids stay in circulation for somewhat longer before redistributing across interstitial and intra-vascular compartments. The capillary permeability returns to baseline level after 24 hours trapping colloid in interstitial space. (This is the reasoning for some regimens starting colloids only 24 hours post burn).

The choice of resuscitation fluid may be a
- Crystalloid (as either N/Saline, Hartman's, or hypertonic saline), or
- Colloid (albumin, fresh-frozen plasma) i.e. Evans / Brooke's formula

The commonest fluid regimen is the use of Hartmann's formula:
First 24 hr total fluid requirement *since the time of burn* = 4ml / kg / %TBSA burn, of which half is given in the first 8 hours *from the time of burn*, and rest is given over the next 16 hours.

Another choice of fluid resus regimen is the Mount Vernon formula:
1 aliquot = (%TBSA burn x weight) / 2
3 aliquots in first 12 hours,
2 aliquots in next 12 hours, and
1 aliquot in next 12 hours (i.e. fluid resus over 36 hours).

Opinion:

You will find that people dwell on whether Parkland is 2, 3 or 4 ml/kg/%TBSA. You have to remember that irrespective of everything else, this number is a *starting point* only. The reason you *start* resus fluids is to restore intravascular volume which you should do asap to help restore tissue perfusion. Assuming the patient has no comorbidities (e.g. CCF), 4ml/kg/%TBSA is the fastest way to do it.

Once you have started the fluid regimen, the 2, 3 or 4 becomes rather meaningless. That is because you are *monitoring* your response with urinary output(UO) and need to *actively adjust* the resus fluids to keep a steady hourly urine output. This urine output (which is a surrogate for GFR & hence tissue perfusion in the kidneys) is a more accurate indicator of tissue perfusion that any formula devised. The only time UO may be inaccurate is if there is a physical blockage in the renal tract. (Also, be more conservative if patient has a history of cardiovascular disease).

So resist the temptation of loading your patient with a volume of fluid simply because a formula says so. The formulas do not take in to account if your patient has been eating and drinking all day, or has been working in the sun all day with little fluid intake - identifying and responding to UO is a lot more physiologic.

If you keep pouring fluids in the circulation even when the UO is adequate, being crystalloids they 3rd space very quickly and make the patient very edematous. Even in presence of good renal function, this edema may take many days to settle. And in case of a major burn, this may contribute to abdominal compartment syndrome.

FLUID CREEP

Fluid creep (coined by Pruitt) is the trend towards giving higher and higher resuscitation fluid volumes to burn patients. Its possible cause includes presence of inhalation injury (i.e. a large surface area burnt, which is not represented on conventional burn charts).

PATHOPHYSIOLOGICAL CHANGES IN MAJOR BURNS
(Ref: EMSB manual)

1) Local response = Jackson's burn wound model (Douglas Jackson, 1953 Br J Surg)
   - Zone of coagulative necrosis = rapid cell death. Irreversible
   - Zone of stasis = impairment of microcirculation. At risk
   - Zone of hyperaemia = area where inflammatory mediators released from damages tissues produce dilation of blood vessels (covers the whole body if burn > 25%). Not at risk of necrosis

> **Aside:**
>
> Note the main aim of burn wound's first aid and early management is to prevent the zone of stasis changing in to zone of necrosis.

2) General response
   - Burn edema
   - $\downarrow$volemia & $\downarrow$myocardial contractility → $\downarrow$cardiac output
   - Stress response = $\uparrow$cortisol,catecholamines & glucagon → $\uparrow$gluconeogenesis & proteolysis → $\uparrow$catabolism & insulin resistance
   - Loss of gut barrier
   - Lung changes → ARDS without inhalation injury
   - Immunosuppression
   - Long term changes = $\uparrow$central fat deposition, $\downarrow$muscle growth/bone mineralization/longitudinal growth of body

Inhalation injury:

MECHANISM OF INHALATION INJURY
A. Airway injury above the larynx → edema and possible obstruction (esp. in children)
B. Airway injury below the larynx from inhalation of products of combustion,
   - direct chemical injury
   - inhaled chemicals + water in respiratory mucosa → acids/alkalis →chemical injury
   - from soot causing irritation pneumonitis
C. Systemic toxicity

PROBLEMS CAUSED BY INHALATION INJURY

1. It increases the risk of mortality by three times (Shirani & Pruitt, Ann Surg 1987, n=1058, inhalation alone=20% increase in mortality, pneumonia alone=40% increase, both=60% increase),
2. Fluid resus volume increases by up to 50% (due to large surface area involved)
3. Associated with haemodynamic instability
4. Parenchymal injury causes poor gas exchange, pneumonia and ARDS

MECHANISM OF CARBON MONOXIDE (CO)

A. Competitive binding to haemoglobin. CO has (200-250x) higher affinity than O_2, to bind to Hb
B. Left shift of O_2-Hb dissociation curve (Ref Figure). Hb saturates with lesser amount of O_2
C. Binds to intracellular enzymes & represents 10-15% of body's CO stores

PROBLEMS CAUSED BY CO

1. CO binds to Hb a lot more easily than O_2
2. Once bound to Hb, it does not let O_2 bind any more
3. It is very difficult to remove this bound CO

Table: CO levels (see also table for toxicities of local anaesthetics as well, & don't confuse between them)

CO%	Symptoms*
<15%	None (smokers, lorry drivers)
15 - 20%	Headache, confusion
20 - 40%	Nausea, fatigue
40 - 60%	Hallucinations, ataxia, syncope, convulsions, coma
>60%	Death

* You're expected to know these symptoms, but you should not wait of any of the symptoms to develop. Have a high index of suspicion based on history. The patient should have ABGs done as soon as possible in ED, and if carbon monoxide is raised, 100% O_2 is started and thereafter ABGs are repeated at regular intervals.

Note that other reasons for similar symptoms are:
- Hypoxia
- Hypoglycaemia
- Head injury

Aside: Clinical significance of CO half life

The half life of CO is 240min (=4hours) without supplemental O_2, and 40min with 100% O_2. It means:

1. If the inhalation injury is identified early and supplemental oxygen given (via non-rebreathing mask or ETT), the effects of CO can be counteracted 6x faster.
2. The first set of ABGs need to be taken early, otherwise the CO level may be falsely low.

Figure: a) O_2-Hb dissociation curve b) CO-Hb dissociation curve. The curves are not to scale.

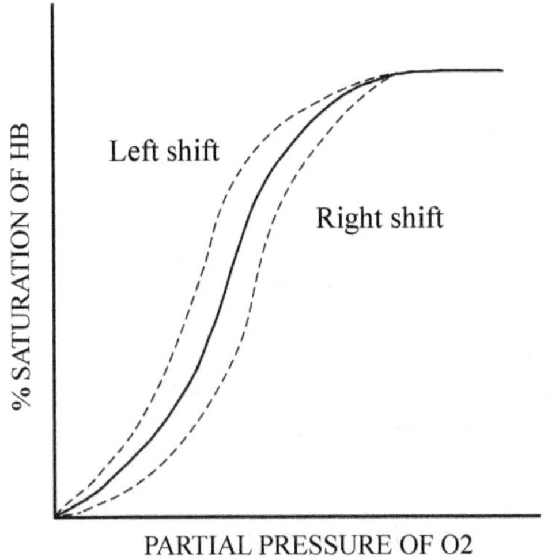

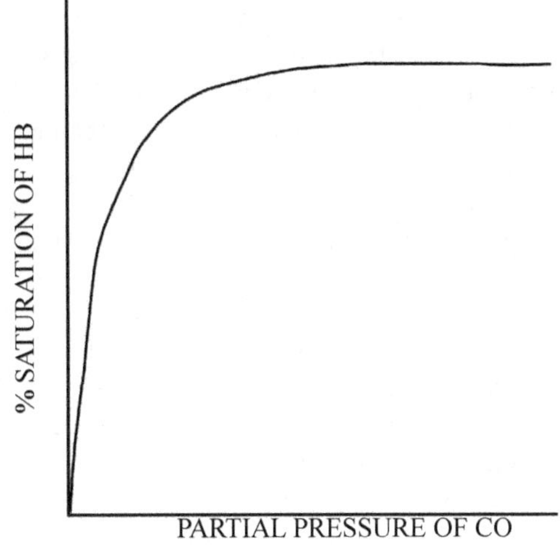

Aside: Hb dissociation curves

The O_2 dissociation curve is sigmoid shape due to the cooperative binding of oxygen to the haem moiety. Starting at the origin of the curve, it is relatively difficult to get the first oxygen molecule to attach i.e. it takes a certain amount of oxygen presence to saturate the haemoglobin molecule, which means that the initial part of the curve has a shallow slope.

Once the first oxygen molecule has attached, it induces a conformational change in the haemoglobin molecule which makes it easier for the next oxygen molecule to attach i.e. oxygen molecules attach quickly (and saturate the Hb molecule) with only a slight increase in oxygen partial pressure. This gives the near vertical shape of the sigmoid curve.

When the haemoglobin molecule is nearly saturated, it takes more effort for the final oxygen molecule to attach i.e. a large increase in partial pressure is needed to increase the Hb saturation. This gives the upper flat part of the curve.

To imagine what happens when the O_2 is released at the tissues, it is easier to consider the four oxygen molecules as a square of four postage stamps. You need to tear off two sides to release the first stamp (aka the oxygen molecule) hence a flat curve at the top. The next stamp needs one side to be torn off so a steep curve. And the last two molecules only need one tear to separate them.

In oxygen rich environments you want haemoglobin to be saturated as quickly as possible. So at the lungs, the curve is left-shifted i.e. has a steeper curve. The Hb saturates more for any given amount of oxygen in the vicinity. Conversely, in oxygen deprived areas e.g. when delivering oxygen into the tissues, you want the haemoglobin molecule to shed its oxygen load as quickly as possible and not hang onto it. This is why the O_2 dissociation curve is right shifted i.e. as the molecule is fully saturated only a small fall in oxygen pressure causes it to release its oxygen. The factors which shift O_2 curve right or left are specific for the oxygen rich or relatively hypoxic environments.

On the other hand carbon monoxide has very high affinity with haemoglobin. It does not need the help of the first molecule to help the other ones. Even a tiny amount of carbon monoxide will find any available haemoglobin and attach very strongly to it i.e. a large increase in saturation (of Hb with CO) with even a tiny amount of carbon monoxide available. This gives the near-vertical shape of the haemoglobin carbon monoxide dissociation curve.

There is no formal guideline about when to stop the supplemental oxygen but most centres would keep it on for at least 24 hours.

DIAGNOSIS OF INHALATION INJURY:

Always have a high index of suspicion to allow for rapid diagnosis and management.

1. History
   - Agent. Flame/ other burning material
   - Environment. Confined space
   - Contact. Prolonged exposure, due to pt unconscious, intoxicated, physically frail or associated injury (eg fracture)
2. Examination
   - Singed facial hair, eyebrows, nasal hair
   - Erythema / swelling / soot in oral cavity
   - Productive cough +/- soot
   - Altered voice

A definitive diagnosis is only made by:
   - Inspection of swelling/erythema in upper airways
   - Finding soot in lower respiratory tract on bronchoalveolar lavage (BAL)

TREATMENT OF INHALATION INJURY:

1. Treatment of inhalation above larynx,
   - Humidified high flow O_2 (Note that EMSB says 8 liters/min while ATLS says 15liter/min ;)
   - Anesthetic review +/- ETT
   - Protect C-spine

Remember: if in doubt, intubate

2. Treatment of inhalation below larynx
   - Humidified high flow O_2
   - Anesthetic review +/- ETT
   - Bronchial lavage
   - Consider IPPV, if not responding otherwise
3. Treatment of systemic toxicity
   - Respiratory support, high flow O_2
   - C-spine protection ,esp if unconscious, or intubated
   - Await natural washout of CO
   - Cyanide takes much longer to washout

CYANIDE INHALATION

If the patient's lactate and base excess levels have not returned to normal levels within a few hours of adequate resuscitation, this may represent cyanide poisoning.

Mechanism

Rapid lung absorption $\rightarrow$ binds to cytochrome $\rightarrow$ uncouples oxidative phophorylation $\rightarrow$ inhibition of cell function $\rightarrow$ LOC, neurotoxicity & convulsions

There is no readily available test for cyanide inhalation. Clinically pt's COHb is normal, ventilation is ok, but lactate is raised & BE may be negative. At the time of this writing, the antidote for cyanide poisoning is not widely available in burns units in UK (which is cyanocobalamin).

The management is still supportive with high flow oxygen and monitored with regular ABGs until they return to normal.

In case you get asked in an MCQ, normal level = 0.1mg/L in smokers, lethal level=1.0mg/L

CAUSES OF UNCONSCIOUSNESS AFTER BURN
- Related to burn e.g. CO poisoning
- Not related to burn e.g. hypoxia, hypoglycaemia, head injury

Escharotomies

see EMSB manual for incisions

Escharotomies should only be done in theatre. Why? Because they bleed enormously, even after infiltration in theatre. [You have been warned]. That is also the reason you should ***never*** be in a position where you have to consider escharotomies in ED. If the circumferential burn is around the chest, your anaesthetist should be telling you sooner that the patient is getting difficult to ventilate. [Talk to your anaesthetists - they are good people. Ask them how the patient is bagging]. If the circumferential burn is around a limb, elevating it temporarily will buy you enough time to arrange for theatre.

In theatre, you will need cross matched blood (anything up to 4 units, or more), infiltration solution, monopolar and bipolar diathermy, diluted adrenaline solution, (large!) burn mops and several pairs of hands to help.

Burns wound excision:

INDICATIONS
- Deep burns (DD/FT) burns which are not expected to heal by themselves within three weeks,
- Mixed depth burns which have failed to progress.

EVIDENCE

1. Dietch 1983, J Trauma. 80% risk of HT scar if healing takes >21 days
2. Tompkins, Burke 1986, Ann Surg. In adult pts (without inhalation injury) ↓in mortality from 24% to 7% after early excision and grafting
3. Burke 1974, J Trauma .Total excision of FT burn and allograft in children → ↑survival,↓hospital stay & ↓metabolic complications

Techniques: I - Tangential excision

Janzekovic 1970 (initial description) & 1975 (follow up study)

ADVANTAGES

Removes burnt skin while preserving underlying viable tissue, and body contours are better preserved.

INSTRUMENTS

1. Watson knife, standard technique
2. Weck knife, for smaller areas
3. Versajet, has been used recently as well for smaller areas or those of indeterminate depth [but its not a "standard" answer. One possible indication is in children whose thin skin can be more accurately debrided with Versajet]

END POINT

- PT burn: white shiny dermal surface with punctate bleeding (assuming there is no tourniquet;)
- FT burn: viable subcutaneous tissue with a yellow glistening fat, without thrombosed veins

Dullness, purple discoloration or thromboses vessels imply non viable tissue

Techniques: II - Fascial excision

"Skin and subcutaneous tissue is removed en bloc, down to investing fascia"

INDICATIONS

1. To decrease blood loss in an massive burn
2. Life-threatening / invasive wound infection
3. Large areas of failed graft take in a major burn

DISADVANTAGES

- Contour & cosmetic deformity, Lymphedema

Methods of controlling blood loss

1. Operate within 24 hours (high levels of thromboxanes decrease the blood loss).
2. Use tumescent techniques
3. Use tourniquets for limbs
4. Rapid excision
5. Immediate coverage with adrenaline soaks & compressive bandages

Aside: Evidence of decreased blood loss with early surgery

Ref: Desai, Herndon 1990, Ann Surg

Operate @ <24hr	→ 0.4ml/cm² burn, blood loss
Operate @ 2-16 day	→ 0.75ml/cm² burn, blood loss
Operate @ >16 days	→ 0.5ml/cm² burn, blood loss

Grafting techniques, Sheet / Meshed grafts

Sheet graft

- Advantage = better cosmetic and functional outcome
- Disadvantage = risk of haematoma with loss of graft and can only cover small areas
- Indications = small & cosmetically sensitive areas e.g. on face (respecting the aesthetic subunits)

Meshed graft

Allows the graft to be expanded to cover a wider area then its original size.

Common meshes = 2:1 or 3:1 esp. in major burns (although 1.5:1 is used in smaller TBSA burns, 1:1 mesh for anterior neck & fenestrated sheet grafts for face are also used). 2:1 mesh allows for easy handling (than 3:1 mesh)

(After meshing, the deeper surface of the graft is more shiny than superficial surface & is has a tendency to be concave as a result of meshing process).

Common meshers

1. Those that need a board which determines the size of mesh. Width is limited by the size of the board
2. The mesher itself determines the size of the mesh. Allows wider grafts to be taken

TECHNIQUES OF APPLICATION OF MESHED GRAFT
1. Alexander technique
It is an overlay coverage of a widely meshed graft using allograft to decrease the risk of graft loss. The allograft is applied at 90° orientation to the autograft in a sandwich pattern (so it is easier to tell them apart when removing the allograft later).

2. Meek technique.
Originally Meek (1958 Ann J Surg) and modified by Kreis (1993 Burns, who added allograft sandwich). It uses autographed cut into small squares with a special dermatome and cork board. The squares are passed on to pre-folded pleated gauze that is expanded/opened up in four directions giving islands of autograft which are then applied to the wound bed. Expansion up to 9:1 can be achieved (but the intervening area heals by second intent). With the availability of skin substitutes, this technique is very rarely used.

HOW TO COVER A LARGE BURN AREA
The exact choice and sequence depends on amount of donor site available as well as the availability of skin substitutes, theatre time, surgical, anaesthetic & intensivist expertise. This is a suggested sequence (Ref: next page)

1. Neck & groin
2. Back
3. Large confluent areas
4. Fingers

SKIN SUBSTITUTES
- Integra™ it is a bilaminar dermal regeneration template with protective silicone layer and a dermal scaffold made of bovine collagen and shark chondroitin sulphate.
- Biobrane™ is a temporary synthetic skin substitute composed of nylon mesh impregnated with porcine collagen, bonded onto a thin silicone membrane.

Many more are available now with varying handling properties.

Opinion: Grafting priorities for major burns

Neck and groins are very important to place long lines and trachy for the major burn patient. You want these to heal fast and have a robust cover, hence put your best graft here and do it early. Groin may be spared in many large burns but neck is very often involved. This means that the first long lines are often placed in femoral vein in the ED. This location needs to be rotated on a regular basis, partly because ED is not an ideally sterile environment. Neck is a better place for a long line but it may have been burnt. A 1:1 meshed SSG allows for both egress of fluid and heals to a robust coverage in a week's time.

Major burns patients have to spend a considerable amount of time lying on their back. Warmth & moisture (baseline sweating + warm room + layers of dressing and gamgee!) make it prone to colonisation by skin flora. Plus the immunosuppression from the burn makes it ideal for opportunistic infections as well. Excision & grafting removes up to 18% of necrotic tissue, modifies the burn response considerably and decreases chances of graft loss from infection.

From there on, it is a balance between form and function. You want to excise (and cover) large areas so that patient's inflammatory response and metabolic rate decreases. At the same time you want to cover joints so that range of motion exercises can begin early to prevent joint contractures and keep the muscle mass. The exact order is determined by the location of burn and the size and quality of donor sites.

Hands and fingers tend to use a lot of anaesthetic time and graft which may not always work. So you don't want to spend too much time here, too early in the course of events.

Electrical burn

MECHANISM

Heat generation due to tissue resistance + direct denaturing of proteins + electroporation.

RESULT

1. Arrythmias, from interference with the cardiac pacemaker at the sinoatrial node

2. Compartment syndrome. It is a surgical emergency where limb viability is at risk due to increased tissue pressure in a closed myofascial compartment over a prolonged period of time.

3. Myoglobinuria, which is the presence of myoglobin in the urine from rhabdomolysis. As myoglobin is a protein, once it is filtered through the glomerulus, there is no mechanism for its reabsorption. Moreover, it is not a readily soluble substance, hence there is risk of myoglobin precipitating in the renal tubules and causing renal failure. The urinary levels are usually not monitored, but aim for urine output of 1-2ml/kg/hr and do serial serum CK levels to guide the adequacy & duration of diuresis.

Aside: Mechanism of electrical burn injury

↑bone resistance to passage of electrical current

→ ↑heat generation by Joule heating ("$Q \sim I^2R$")

→ coagulation of adjacent muscle

→ inflammation & edema

→ ↑tissue pressure in a tight space → ↓perfusion

→ hypoxia → ↑tissue damage (& r/o compartment syndrome), eventually

→ muscle cell death and rupture (rhabdomyolysis) → myoglobinuria & raised CK

+ electroporation (formation of ionic leak channels in the cell membrane from the passage of high voltage electric current)

Burn infection:

Ref: Greenhalgh et al. ABA consensus paper. J Burn Care & Research. 2007

Burn erythema is redness around the burn injury that is not a partial thickness burn and is not an infection. It is characteristically non-tender and is present from day 2-3, up to day 5-6.

Folliculitis, esp. on the scalp is from S. aureus and can cause graft loss ("melting", or "ghosting"). Manage by daily washes, deroofing any abscesses, trim hair and consider topical mupirocin/flammazine shave

Burn wound colonisation, bacteria present at surface concentration @ $<10^5/$ gm. There is no invasive infection.

Burn wound infection, bacteria present in wound or eschar @ $>10^5/$gm. There is cellulitis with warmth, erythema and tenderness, usually from S aureus.

Treatment is by thorough cleaning, topical antimicrobials and systemic antibiotics.

Toxic shock syndrome (TSS)

TSS is a severe soft tissue infection classically in a child with a small burn (<10% TBSA) that was expected to heal by itself. Incidence = 2-3% @mean age 2yr.

- Cause = toxin producing Staph aureus (TSST-1, or enterotoxin), or Strep pyogenes.
- Clinically a prodrome of 1-2 days, with fever, D&V, malaise, usually (but not always) with a rash.
- Treatment is with supportive (admit, iv fluids) & empiric Abx (iv fluclox).
- Untreated, it will rapidly lead to shock, with a nearly 50% mortality [so WARN *every* parent of *every* child with even the smallest unhealed burn that if their child is unwell, they need to return to nearest ED asap].

Burn sepsis

"It is a change in the burn patient that triggers a concern for infection". It is a presumptive diagnosis and the triggers include any three of

1. ↑temperature (remember that major burn pts., usually run a core temp of 38°C as "normal")
2. progressive tachycardia,
3. progressive tachypnea,
4. thrombocytopenia,
5. hypoglycaemia,
6. inability to continue enteral feeding

PLUS, a documented infection, which may be

- a +ve culture
- id of pathologic source
- clinical response to Abx

The source of this infection can be pneumonia (from tracheobronchial tree, or hematogenous), blood stream infection (BSI), catheter-related BSI, abdominal sepsis (may be specific to burns, but don't forget abdominal emergencies), ophthalmic infection, chondrites of ears, urospesis etc.

Sepsis 3.0

Ref: Singer et al. 3rd international consensus definitions for Sepsis & septic shock. JAMA 2016

SOFA = Sequential (Sepsis-related) Organ Failure Assessment
(PaO2:FiO2 ratio, GCS, MAP, need for vasopressors, platelet count, serum creatinine & bilirubin)
qSOFA = quick SOFA (altered mentation, RR$\geq$22/min, Systolic BP$\geq$100mmHg)

If qSOFA is positive, then look for evidence of organ dysfunction using SOFA scoring system. An acute increase in SOFA $\geq$2 points implies **sepsis**.

Septic shock = Sepsis + serum lactate >2mmol/L + need for vasopressors to keep MAP$\geq$65mmHg *in a normo-volemic patient.*

Burn outcome

PREDICTION OF MORTALITY
1. Baux score. Age + TBSA > 100 is high risk
2. Modified Baux score. Baux score + add 17 for inhalation injury
3. Abbreviated burn severity index (ABSI). Includes age, gender, inhalation, total TBSA & %FT burn.

Long term complications

This is not an exhaustive list. Ref: Wainwright 2009

1. Form - Scar related
   - Contracted
   - Hypertrophic
   - Itchy
   - Unstable
2. Form - Joint related
   - Contractures
   - Loss of function
3. Function - Limb
   - Inability to feed them-self
   - Loss of mobility
   - Loss of independence
4. Function - Orifices
   - Eyes
   - Nose
   - Mouth
   - Genitals
5. Neurological
6. Psychological. [In exam, mention it last but in your clinical practice, think of it as Number One!]

Trauma - Lower limb

CORE KNOWLEDGE
BOA-BAPRAS standards of care. [These are not guidelines any more]
Initial asesment & management
Gustilo Anderson classification
Operating sequence in theatre
Coverage options - upper, middle and lower third
Degloving injury

APPROACH TO PATIENT - HISTORY
Knowing the mechanism of injury is crucial. Speaking to the ambulance crew is the ideal for that. You need to know, in addition to when it happened and how,

1. Suspected injuries to this patient, based on
    * whether found at scene of accident / details of extraction,
    * blood loss at scene,
    * vitals and GCS at scene and during transfer,
    * any procedures needed en route
2. Injuries to any other person
3. Damage to vehicle(s) involved

PMHx, Medication, Allergies, Last meal
Has the next of kin been informed

APPROACH TO PATIENT - EXAMINATION
Full ATLS

APPROACH TO PATIENT - MANAGEMENT
Read BOA-BAPRAS standard of care consensus document & follow it to the letter.

EXPECTED CLINICAL QUESTIONS
[Expect to see a picture with a lower limb injury. Describe what you see. What can you see in the *whole* picture. Classify the defect e.g. Gustilo Andreson & what tissues are missing. *Remember* the information trickled in by the examiner.]

"You are the on call consultant & get called to ED and this is what you see"
* What can you see
* What will you do

- How will you classify it [Know Gustilo Anderson in detail and the principle of at least one more]
- Stepwise management [These are some of the commonest injuries seen so expect a detailed questioning on what you will do and why]
- Compartment syndrome
- Fasciotomies
- Topical negative pressure therapy

RECOMMENDED PAPERS

1. Nanchahal J. et al. Standards for the management of open fractures of the lower limb. London: Royal Society of Medicine Press Ltd.; 2009.
2. Hallock. EBM: Lower extremity trauma. *Plast Reconstr Surg.* 2013; 132(6): 1733-41
3. Gustilo RB, Anderson JT. Prevention of infection in the treatment of one thousand and twenty-five open fractures of long bones: retrospective and prospective analyses. *J Bone Joint Surg Am.* 1976 Jun;58(4):453-8.
4. Anderson JT, Gustilo RB. Immediate internal fixation in open fractures. *Orthop Clin North Am.* 1980 Jul;11(3):569-78.

5. Godina M, Arnez ZM, Lister GD. Preferential use of the posterior approach to blood vessels of the lower leg in microvascular surgery. *Plast Reconstr Surg.* 1991 Aug;88(2):287-91
6. Godina M. Early microsurgical reconstruction of complex trauma of the extremities. *Plast Reconstr Surg.* 1986 Sep;78(3):285-92
7. Godina M. Arterial autografts in microvascular surgery. *Plast Reconstr Surg.* 1986 Sep;78(3):293-4
8. Godina M, Bajec J, Baraga A. Salvage of the mutilated upper extremity with temporary ectopic implantation of the undamaged part. *Plast Reconstr Surg.* 1986 Sep;78(3):295-9.

9. Byrd HS, Cierny G 3rd, Tebbetts JB. The management of open tibial fractures with associated soft-tissue loss: external pin fixation with early flap coverage. *Plast Reconstr Surg.* 1981 Jul;68(1):73-82
10. Gopal S, Majumder S, Batchelor AG, Knight SL, De Boer P, Smith RM. Fix and flap: the radical orthopaedic and plastic treatment of severe open fractures of the tibia. *J Bone Joint Surg Br.* 2000 Sep;82(7):959-66

11. Cavadas PC. Arteriovenous vascular loops in free flap reconstruction of the extremities. *Plast Reconstr Surg.* 2008 Feb;121(2):514-20
12. Arnez ZM, Khan U, Tyler MP. Classification of soft-tissue degloving in limb trauma. *J Plast Reconstr Aesthet Surg.* 2010 Nov;63(11):1865-9

13. Khan U, Smitham P, Pearse M, Nanchahal J. Management of severe open ankle injuries. *Plast Reconstr Surg*. 2007 Feb;119(2):578-89

LEAP Study: (this is a selection and many papers are available for free from PubMed)
14. Webb LX, Bosse MJ, Castillo RC, MacKenzie EJ; LEAP Study Group. Analysis of surgeon-controlled variables in the treatment of limb-threatening type-III open tibial diaphyseal fractures. *J Bone Joint Surg Am*. 2007 May; 89(5):923-8
15. Cannada LK, Jones AL. Demographic, social and economic variables that affect lower extremity injury outcomes. *Injury*. 2006 Dec;37(12):1109-16.
16. Archer KR, Castillo RC, Mackenzie EJ, Bosse MJ; LEAP Study Group. Physical disability after severe lower-extremity injury. *Arch Phys Med Rehabil*. 2006 Aug;87(8):1153-5
17. Smith JJ, Agel J, Swiontkowski MF, Castillo R, et al.; LEAP Study Group. Functional outcome of bilateral limb threatening: lower extremity injuries at two years postinjury. *J Orthop Trauma*. 2005 Apr;19(4):249-53
18. MacKenzie EJ, Bosse MJ, Kellam JF, et al.; LEAP Study Group. Factors influencing the decision to amputate or reconstruct after high-energy lower extremity trauma. *J Trauma*. 2002 Apr;52(4):641-9. Erratum in: *J Trauma* 2002 Jul;53(1):48
19. Pollak AN, McCarthy ML, Burgess AR. Short-term wound complications after application of flaps for coverage of traumatic soft-tissue defects about the tibia. The Lower Extremity Assessment Project (LEAP) Study Group. *J Bone Joint Surg Am*. 2000 Dec;82-A(12):1681-91

Opinion:

A lower limb injury in isolation is unlikely to kill the patient. However a mechanism that had the energy to cause significant bony & soft tissue injury to the lower limb, can certainly cause other injuries which may be rapidly life threatening. Hence the need, in acute situation, to expedite a complete ATLS assessment & management.

You need to be confident to systematically assess the patient for life threatening injuries using the ATLS methodology - it is ideal to have acted as the trauma team leader. For the purpose of the exam, avoid getting in to the details of the ATLS assessment - it is not an A&E exam. You'll score marks once you are *safely* past this point and discussing plastic surgery.

Gustilo Anderson classification

JBJS 1976. It is based on the state of soft tissues associated with an open fracture.

[An open fracture is one where the fracture haematoma communicates with the exterior].

Type		Description
1		< 1cm wound, clean, no significant soft tissue damage
2		> 1cm wound, clean, no significant soft tissue damage
3		Significant soft tissue injury, with soft tissue stripping off the bone
	3A	bone can be covered
	3B	bone *cannot* be covered
	3C	Arterial injury

Gustilo 3B is where plastic surgery team is typically involved. Gustilo-Anderson classification may not incorporate every injury pattern but it is simple to remember & is widely understood.

The classification can only be truly applied *after* surgical debridement in theatre. What started out as a 3A in ED can very easily become a 3B after e trip to theatre.

Antibiotic regimen

This is from the BOA-BAPRAS standards - hopefully made a little simpler to read & recall.

	1st line*	AND	Until
In ED (within 3hrs of injury)	co-amoxiclav 1.2gm 8hrly, OR cefuroxime 1.2gm 8hrly		first debridement
At first debridement	co-amoxiclav 1.2gm 8hrly OR cefuroxime 1.2gm 8hrly	gentamicin (1.5mg/kg) once only	Earlier of, soft tissue closure OR 72 hr
At skeletal stabilisation	vancomycin 1gm OR teicoplanin 800mg	gentamicin (1.5mg/kg) once only	

* If penicillin allergic: give clindamycin 600mg iv 6 hours *preoperatively.*

Opinion:

There are a few things that the standards are moot on e.g.
- if patient is given a dose in ED and then taken to theatre soon afterwards do you give another dose of co-amoxiclav (and how long a gap is acceptable),
- most times you will stabilise the fracture with an exfix (& at times it is not possible to do a definitive fixation any time soon e.g. due to associated injuries) should you give co-amox. or vanc./teic. with gent. on induction at first debridement,
- giving clinda. 6 hours pre-op assumes that you know exactly when the patient will go to theatre - something which is not easy to forecast for inpatients. Acute admissions tend to go to theatre within 6 hours of injury so clinda may not be given on time either.

Compartment syndrome

It is a condition where limb viability is threatened by increased tissue pressure in a fixed fascial compartment in the body, over a prolonged period of time.

Causes

[This is not an exhaustive list]

1. Pressure from outside
   - Prolonged crush
   - Severe crush for short duration
2. Pressure from inside
   - Extravasation deep to deep fascia
3. Both

Pathophysiology

Pressure (from outside/inside)

→ increased tissue pressure

→ tissue damage (directly related to amount and duration of applied pressure)

→ inflammation

→ swelling

→ increased tissue pressure → disruption of Starling equilibrium* → tissue hypoxia → more inflammation (& a +ve feedback loop that causes tissue hypoxia. Muscle is most sensitive to hypoxia due to increased metabolic requirements)

→ eventual venous compression → rapid stasis → further increase in tissue pressure.

Diagnosis

AWAKE & COOPERATIVE PATIENT

- Pain on passive movement (esp. stretch) of affected muscle compartment, which is out of proportion to the injury and not relieved with adequate analgesia. [The term "adequate" analgesia is not well defined]. Pain on toe extension suggests involvement of deep posterior compartment, while pain on toe flexion suggests anterior compartment involvement.
- Paraestheia in the distribution of nerves running in the involved compartments.

* Ref: Pathophysiology of Burn shock

UNCOOPERATIVE / UNCONSCIOUS PATIENT

- Index of suspicion based on mechanism
- Compartment pressure (serial) monitoring. The typical procedure involves turning on the manometer and "zeroing" its reading. Attach a 21G (green) needle on one side of the manometer and a 10ml syringe filled with normal saline on the other end. Insert the needle in the given compartment and measure the pressure.
- Commercially available manometers differ in exact details of the procedure e.g. whether to inject any saline in the compartment and whether to read the compartment pressure immediately or let it equilibrate (for a few seconds) before taking the reading.
- A compartment pressure reading *within* 30mmHg of diastolic pressure should prompt fasciotomy. If the clinical picture is evolving, it my be appropriate to repeat this measurement. Note that elevation of limb may reduce tissue edema by gravity, but be careful as in arteriopaths this manoeuvre may decrease the perfusion pressure and be counterproductive.

Opinion:

Compartment pressures are ideally measured using a commercially available manometer for this purpose (or marketed for CSF pressure monitoring). Although some colleagues have reported using a green needle with a giving set and a CV/arterial line transducer and associated monitor, it is prone to errors and is not recommended.

Be sure that you are familiar with using the particular manometer available in your unit because you will base your decision to do fasciotomies on this method.

Management

1. High index of suspicion
2. Early detection
3. Expedite investigation and managment of concurrent injuries
4. Prompt adequate fasciotomies (see BOA-BAPRAS guidelines for details of incision placement etc.).

Draw a cross section of lower leg

This is a cross section of the middle 1/3rd of right lower leg

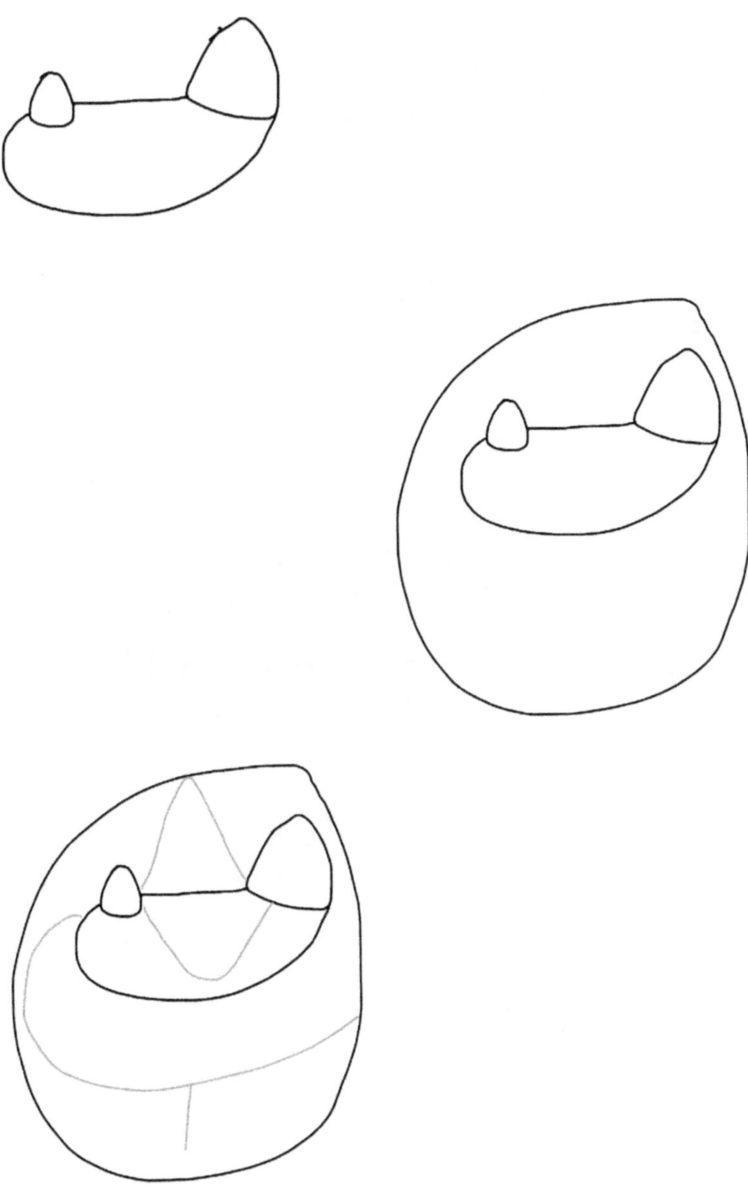

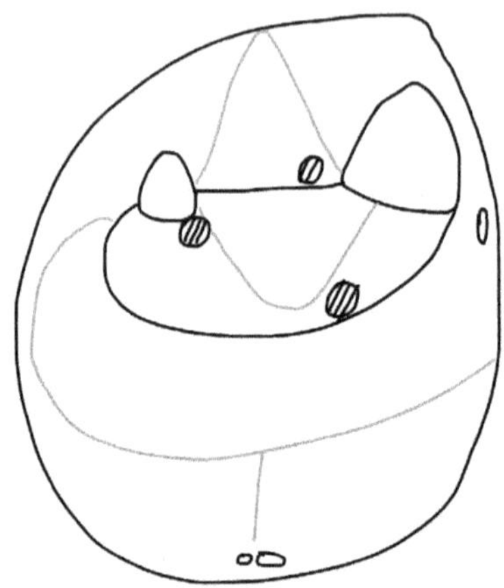

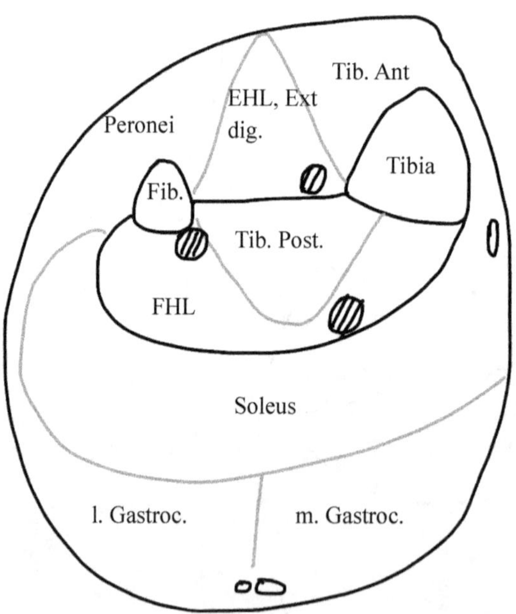

Tib. Ant
EHL, Ext dig.
Peronei
Tibia
Fib.
Tib. Post.
FHL
Soleus
l. Gastroc.
m. Gastroc.

Degloving injury

MECHANISM

Degloving injuries occur due to a tangential force that shears the skin from subcutaneous tissue. Depending on the energy involved, the degloving may also occur in deeper planes e.g. between subcutaneous fat & deep fascia, or multiple planes within the subcutaneous fat. This differential shearing disrupts the perforators coming from deep vessels (anterior, posterior tibial & peroneal) to supply the angiosomes. Since there isn't another axial source of blood supply for the skin, large areas may necrose.

CLASSIFICATION

Table: Degloving classification (Arnez, Khan & Taylor. JPRAS 2010)

Type	Pattern	Implication
1	Limited degloving with abrasion/ avulsion	• Usu. over bony prominences causing exposure of e.g. malleoli. • Minimal debridement but need free flap cover
2	Non-circumferential	Skin graft / flap reconstruction result in good healing
3	Circumferential single plane	Do not close primarily & await demarcation
4	Circumferential multiple plane	Plan staged reconstruction

MANAGEMENT

1. **Management of patient** - ATLS approach
2. **Management of limb** - orthoplastic approach and decision making
3. **Management of degloving** - by serial debridements & evaluation of tissue viability at each layer. Consider CT angio if free tissue transfer is anticipated. If large areas of skin appear nonviable at first operation, consider harvesting SSG from them and either storing [Ref: Human Tissue Act, UK] or primary grafting.

Opinion:

In practice there are very few degloving injuries that you'll close at the first operation. The mechanisms of injury severe enough to cause a limb degloving are mostly RTAs or industrial accidents, both of which are associated with risk of foreign body contamination so a second (or third or more) look & washout +/- debridement is important.

The use of negative pressure therapy has revolutionised the management of lower limb injuries considerably. It is worth remembering that in acute lower limb injuries TNP is primarily a wound *management* system and not a magical wound healing device.

The TNP keeps the wound a closed system so the patient does not have to undergo bedside dressing changes for strike through. It does encourage granulation but only on well vascularised beds. There is no substitute for decontamination by good washout of wound and adequate surgical debridement while allowing tissues to declare, followed by a sound surgical plan for wound coverage.

That surgical plan should take in to account the expected zone of injury, to decide between delayed primary closure, local flap options or free tissue transfer. (SSG on the primary lower limb defect, in most cases, does not provide a stable, reliable long term wound cover). Do stay away from people who like to TNP to infinity and beyond!

Trauma - Hands trauma

In hand surgery, more than anywhere else, think of "function, function, and function". Note that the basic pattern of history is broadly similar.

CORE KNOWLEDGE

Fractures
Flexor & extensor tendon injuries
Tendon rehab regimens
Finger tip injuries
Flexor sheath infection
Replants - single/multiple digits, thumb, different levels

APPROACH TO PATIENT - HISTORY

Age, occupation, hand dominance, hobbies, smoking, who is at home
PMHx, Tetanus status, Allergies, (last meal)

Mechanism of injury
Time since injury
Are any other injuries likely (Higher the energy involved in the accident, more likely to have associated injuries e.g. Ask specifically if the "isolated" nail bed injury happened as a result of a car roll over?)
First aid - at the scene
Any other management since then - ?been to a walk-in centre / another hospital before arriving at the hand surgery unit

APPROACH TO PATIENT - EXAMINATION

- Finger cascade & whether it is maintained on active flexion & extension of digits (with wrist supinated)
- Note any missing parts, lacerations, bruising/swelling or cellulitis (+/- ascending lymphangitis) - [In exam, only comment on what is there]
- In acute scenario - Have a systematic approach e.g. sensory before motor, distal to proximal.
- Never forget potential injuries proximal to what u can see e.g. Can there be a brachial plexus injury. The mechanism of injury is a very strong indicator for it, hence the need for accurate history.

APPROACH TO PATIENT - MANAGEMENT

ATLS approach (depending on the history & mechanism)

The definitive management of an isolated hand injury takes into account, patient factors:
1. Occupation
2. Hand dominance
3. Functional status
4. Expected compliance

as well as the injury:
a) Site of the defect
b) Size of defect
c) Which digit is involved
d) Exposed bone

Presuming it is an isolated injury and patient does not qualify for a full ATLS resuscitation, you need to think of initial management as well as definitive management.

Initial management (after taking detailed history and examination) includes analgesia, antibiotics, tetanus cover, x-ray, washout under a ring block, backslab. Definitive management involves providing adequate soft tissue cover to allow early primary healing and early return to pre-morbid function.

[Note brachial plexus injuries are dealt with in the section on cold hands].

EXPECTED CLINICAL QUESTIONS
- Fingertip injuries, and coverage of soft tissue defects of various size and at different locations
- Thumb recon
- Flexor & extensor tendon zones
- Flexor & extensor tendon rehab protocol
- Principles of fracture management
- Fracture management, of different configuration fractures on phalanx and MC
- Transportation of an amputated digit, warm and cold ischeimia times
- Evaluation of an amputated digit [ideally a 2 surgeon approach]
- Sequence of replant in theatre
- Compartment syndrome, pressure monitoring indications, methods & fasciotomy incisions
- Hand replant

RECOMMENDED PAPERS

1. Boyer MI, Strickland JW, Engles DR, Sachar K, Leversedge FJ. Flexor tendon repair and rehabilitation. J Bone Joint Surg Am. 2002;84(9):1684–706.
2. Chao JD, Huang JM, Wiedrich TA. Local hand flaps. Journal of the American Society for Surgery of the Hand. 2001 Feb;1(1):25–44.
3. Chin SH, Vedder NB. MOC-PSSM CME Article: Metacarpal Fractures. Plast Reconstr Surg. 2008 Jan;121(MOC-PS CME Coll):1–13.
4. Chung KC, Alderman AK. Replantation of the upper extremity: Indications and outcomes. Journal of the American Society for Surgery of the Hand. 2002 May;2(2):78–94.
5. Friedrich JB, Vedder NB. An Evidence-Based Approach to Metacarpal Fractures. Plast Reconstr Surg. 2010 Dec;126(6):2205–9.
6. Giuffre JL, Kakar S, Bishop AT, Spinner RJ, Shin AY. Current Concepts of the Treatment of Adult Brachial Plexus Injuries. The Journal of Hand Surgery. 2010 Apr;35(4):678–88.
7. Isaacs J. Treatment of Acute Peripheral Nerve Injuries: Current Concepts. The Journal of Hand Surgery. 2010 Mar;35(3):491–7.
8. Kang R, Stern PJ. Fracture dislocations of the proximal interphalangeal joint. Journal of the American Society for Surgery of the Hand. 2002 May; 2(2):47–59.
9. Lehfeldt M, Ray E, Sherman R. MOC-PS(SM) CME Article: Treatment of Flexor Tendon Laceration. Plast Reconstr Surg. 2008 Apr;121(Supplement): 1–12.
10. Lemmon JA, Janis JE, Rohrich RJ. Soft-Tissue Injuries of the Fingertip: Methods of Evaluation and Treatment. An Algorithmic Approach. Plast Reconstr Surg. 2008 Sep;122(3):105e – 117e.
11. Moran SL, Steinmann SP, Shin AY. Adult brachial plexus injuries: mechanism, patterns of injury, and physical diagnosis. Hand Clinics. 2005 Feb;21(1):13–24.
12. Muzaffar et al. CME: post traumatic thumb reconstruction. PRS 2005
13. Ratner JA, Peljovich A, Kozin SH. Update on Tendon Transfers for Peripheral Nerve Injuries. The Journal of Hand Surgery. 2010 Aug;35(8): 1371–81.
14. Rhee PC, Jones DB, Kakar S. Management of Thumb Metacarpophalangeal Ulnar Collateral Ligament Injuries. The Journal of Bone and Joint Surgery (American). 2012 Nov 7;94(21):2005.
15. IFSSH flexor tendon committee report 2007. Journal of Hand Surgery: European Volume. 2007 Jun;32(3):346–56.

Fingertip injury / defect

Consider describing it as dorsal/volar side of right/left hand of a patient showing transverse / dorsal oblique/ volar oblique amputation at the level of (e.g.) DIPj or middle phalanx (or similar).

Relevant questions

Age, Occupation
Hand dominance, Hobbies / functional status
Smoking
Who is at home

PMHx, Medications, Allergies

Mechanism of injury - detailed
Time since injuring
Whether it is isolated
First aid & any management since

Principles of management

The goals of management are to provide
- Sensate,
- Well padded,
- Durable cover to the finger tip

Options of management

Options depend upon the
- level of injury,
- direction of amputation and
- the state of soft tissues and underlying bone.

These options are:
1. Bone shortening and primary closure of skin
2. local random pattern flaps
3. local axial pattern flaps
4. homodigital neurovascular flaps

Opinion:

The following is not a complete list. It is biased towards my preference for closure of these defects. At the end of the day, you have to consider the amount of bone stock available and cover it with available soft tissue. And this needs to be done with minimal loss of function.

For all of the types of injuries given below:
1. If bone is not exposed and <1.5cm^2 pulp defect - allow to heal by 2nd intent
2. Trim bone and primary closure. However, this strategy runs into problem
   A. when there is relatively more soft tissue loss than bony, or
   B. when shortening the bone will demand sacrifice of a tendon insertion or need to go proximal to a joint. You can't leave an articular condylar surface under a terminalised finger tip. That articular surface needs to to be removed and bone shortened to a tip, which means sacrificing a lot of bone stock. This is especially a problem in,
      - amputations at proximal P3 level, or
      - at mid P2 where bone shortening may mean loss of FDS insertion (consider if you should be replanting this digit instead)

DORSAL OBLIQUE INJURIES
i.e. volar skin is preserved
Atasoy V-Y advancement flap (Ref: Figure)
Tranquili-Leali flap (Ref: Figure)

LATERAL OBLIQUE
At distal P3: Lateral pulp flap to cover bone (effectively a unilateral Kutler flap) and allow the rest to heal by 2nd intent

TRANSVERSE
1. Trim bone and direct closure, e.g. at distal P3
2. Homodigital island flap (Ref: Figure), esp if terminalisation will endanger FDS/FDP insertion or require the terminalisation level to be moved proximal to a joint (resulting in significant loss of length).

Opinion:

Personally I don't use Kutler bilateral advancement as they move little and need more sutures than there is tissue. I either shorten to cover the bone, or use a homodigital advancement flap.

Figure: A) Tranquili-Leali flaps, and B) Atasoy

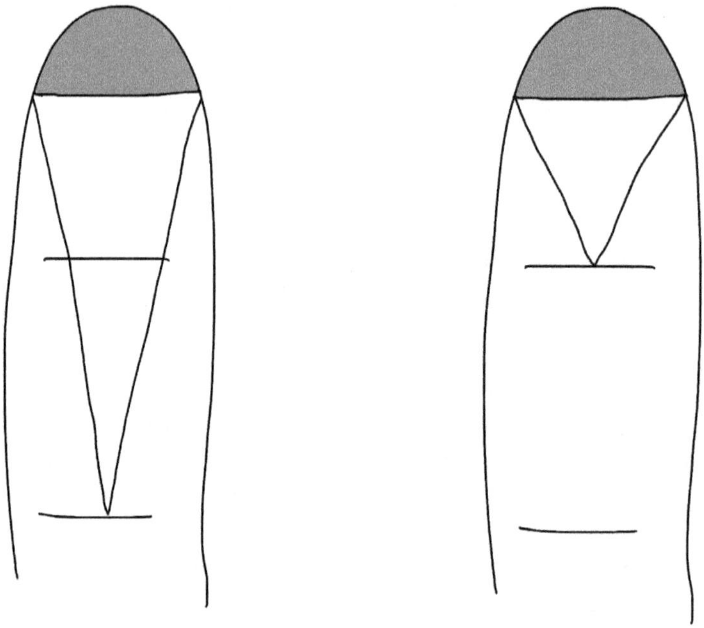

Figure: Kutler bilateral V-Y advancement

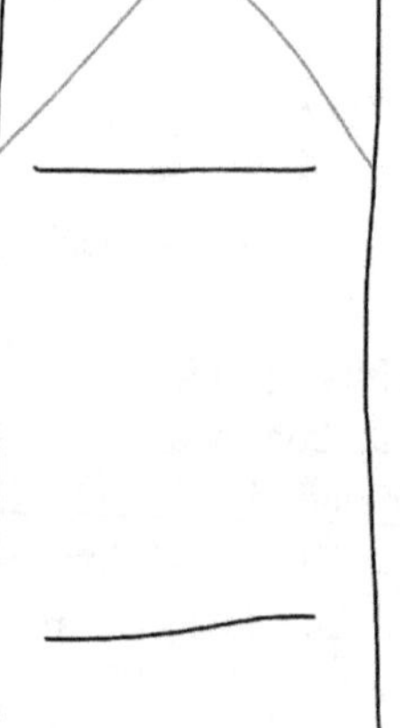

VOLAR OBLIQUE

Homodigital island flap

1. Segmuller (1976). Soft tissue is raised based on neurovascular bundle that can be dissected proximally as needed to allow adequate flap movement (up to interdigital crease or up to the bifurcation of the common digital artery, or as far proximally as its origin at the superficial arch. Skin apex (of the classic description) is at the DIPj crease. The flap takes tissue up to digit's volar midline only & hence can be designed as bilateral flaps (Ref: Figure)
2. Extended Segmuller (Elliott 2000) has apex at P2 close to PIPj crease.
3. Venkatswami. Original description of the technique was for lateral oblique injuries, using the contralateral pedicle

Figure: Homo-digital island flaps a) Extended Segmuller b) Venkatswami

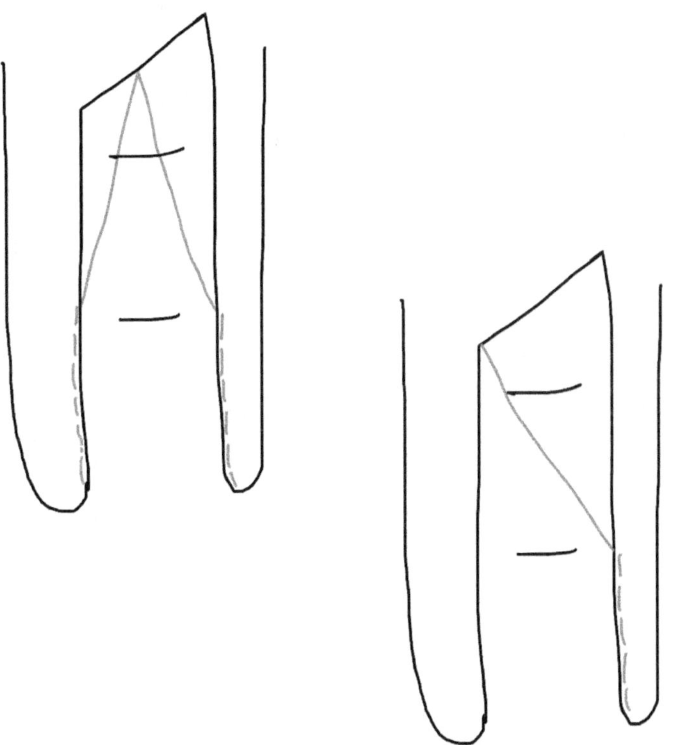

Opinion:

There *are* a few confirmed methods of starting a riot in a room full of plastic surgeons - ask them about the best dressing for skin grafts, favourite pinnaplasty technique and ideal management of fingertip injuries.

In my opinion, the random pattern flaps for fingertips are over-rated. Although the pictures in the books look great, once you have incised the skin on an Atasoy flap and then slide the tenotomy scissors to release the septae from P3, pause and think where is the blood supply coming from. At best, it can come from the remaining horizontal attachment of the septae between flap and the adjacent pulp. These very septae limit the movement of the Atasoy flap to only a few millimeters. Similarly Kutler bilateral advancement flaps, I feel, are more like small composite grafts as the blood supply becomes very tenuous if you release the flap from its deeper surface. But if you don't release it from the deeper surface, it moves very little. On the other hand, homodigital islanded flaps provide a reliable sensate padded tissue whose pedicle can be dissected (if needed) as far as the bifurcation of common digital artery to provide 1cm or more of advancement.

Replantation of digits

Replantation is the restoration of an amputated part of the body. Most commonly it is from the upper limb, but may be lower limb, pinna or nose.

Clinical scenario

You may come across a hand/forearm with one or many digits missing.

Before you can plan any management, you need to know about
1. The patient
2. The injury
3. The management so far

Relevant questions

Age, Occupation
Handedness, Hobbies / functional status
Smoking
Who is at home

PMHx, Medications, Allergies

Mechanism of injury - clean cut/ crush / avulsion / combination
Time since injury
Whether it is an isolated injury

First aid to patient (immediately)
Management so far (in ambulance or in A&E)
Fate of the amputated part and method of its storage and transport
Warm and cold ischiemia times

Principles of management

Remember your immediate goal is to save life, and in long term to return the patient to premorbid level of function and appearance within a reasonable length of time.

Rule out life threatening injuries
Stabilise the patient
Consider an operation to:
   • Explore

- Washout
- Debride
- Attempt replant, in a timely fashion

The decision on whether to replant (or not) takes into account:

A. Mechanism of injury - sharp guillotine with minimal tissue injury & contamination, vs avulsion vs (prolonged) crush
B. The level of amputation - muscle has less ischiemia time
C. Time since injury & ischiemia time - proximal injuries should have an indicative warm ischiemia time of <6hrs or cold ischiemia time <12hr (limited by muscle damage). Distal injuries i.e. digits, can tolerate warm ischiemia of up to 12hr or cold ischiemia of 24 hours. Of course your priority should be to keep any ischiemia time to a minimum to minimise reperfusion injury.
D. Which digits are involved, & how many
E. Condition of amputated part(s)

In addition to patient characteristics (occupation, co-morbidities, functional status & expected compliance).

> **Opinion:**
>
> I'll argue that even a decision *not* to replant should only be taken in theatre (with some exceptions). A theatre is a much better place to examine the limb and the amputated part in a clean environment, under good lighting, magnification and with appropriate instruments. A second surgeon is invaluable who can take the amputated part to theatre (after it has been x-rayed) to identify damage and tag structures. The patient, in the mean time, can be investigated and stabilised prior to transfer to theatre suite. The exceptions to this routine are if the amputated part is too small, too damaged or has a clearly adverse ischiemia time.

How to store an amputated digit

"In moist gauze *inside* a plastic bag *on* ice"

Transport the amputated part in mildly moist gauze (i.e. damp, but not wet). The gauze should go in a clear plastic bag (duly labelled with patient details, identifying multiple digits if possible). This plastic bag needs to be sitting on a container containing ice cubes.

The idea is to keep the amputated part cold without letting it dry out and without freezing it. Drying will desiccate tissues while freezing forms microscopic ice crystals which mechanically damage tissues.

> **Opinion:**
>
> Suggest to the referring hospital that they write down your instructions and follow them closely. In at least one incidence, an amputated digit was sent over in a hastily washed formalin jar!

Options of management

1. Attempt replant
2. Attempt multiple replants
3. Amputate

Strong indicators for replantation

- Thumb amputation
- Multiple digits
- Amputation in a child
- Amputation at the level of palm/wrist/forearm

Note, that all of these relate to preservation of function.

ATTEMPT REPLANT

One sequence may be

1. Hand pronated, fix bone (plate or double ended cross K-wires in retrograde fashion), repair extensor tendon.
2. Supinate hand and fix flexor tendon and then both digital arteries and nerves. (Otherwise the arterial anastomosis may be at risk from movement during flexor tendon repair).
3. Pronate hand again. Identify and repair veins.

For proximal replants, consider skeletal stabilisation followed immediately by vascular repair to avoid further muscle damage.

ATTEMPT MULTIPLE REPLANTS

Have a priority order to replant different digits with. Your options are either to start with the most functionally important ones (Thumb > IF > LF > MF >RF), or the least damaged ones first (depending on the mechanism and findings of exploration), or a combination.

AMPUTATE
See contra-indications to replantation (below)

Contra-indications to replantation of digit

[Some of these are set in stone, some are not. If in doubt, seek a second opinion]
- Concurrent life threatening injuries
- Severe co-morbidities
- Excessive ischiemia time
- Crush- avulsion injury
- Multiple level injury

Challenging situations

REPAIR UNDER TENSION

This is probably the most common situation to encounter. You can predict it from the mechanism of injury (e.g. circular saw or other cut-avulsion type injuries) and counsel the patient appropriately. Importantly, resist the temptation to stretch neurovascular pedicles in an attempt to avoid grafting - you will likely struggle with the repair and either tear the vessel wall or give traction injury to the nerve.

The possible solutions are:
- Bone shortening, which may allow primary repair of neurovascular defect, in some cases.
- Vein graft, e.g. from volar forearm
- Nerve graft, e.g. lateral cutaneous of forearm, terminal branch of PIN, sural nerve

The following situations have been described in literature as well.
1. Heterodigital replants. When all digits can't be replanted, the one in best condition is replanted at the most functionally important place
2. AV fistulas. When venous outflow in a distal amputation in not possible
3. Peri-arterial sympathectomy, for atherosclerotic arteries
4. E2S anastomosis to radial artery in anatomical snuff box

Postoperative care

Splint, and position it across the chest
Analgesia
iv fluids and urinary catheter
Monitor colour, capillary refill, temperature and turgor

Rehabilitation

- Start at 7-10 days postop
- PROM in un-involved joints
- Active ROM after removal of any K-wires (usually 4-6/52)

Salient complications

Failed replant
Primary amputation
Delayed amputation
Joint stiffness
Tendon adhesions
Malunion
Cold intolerance

Secondary procedures that may be needed

Bone	Bone graft
Joint	Capsulotomy, arthrodesis
Tendon	Tenolysis
Nerve	Nerve grafting / neurolysis
Skin	Secondary coverage / revision
Delayed amputation	

Ring avulsion injuries

Urbaniak Classification

I	Circulation adequate
II	Circulation inadequate
II A	Circulation inadequate, only arterial damage
III	Complete degloving

Kay Classification
(JHS 1989)

I	Circulation adequate	
II	Circulation inadequate	IIA = Artery only problem
		IIB = Venous only problem
III	Circulation inadequate + fracture	IIA = Artery only problem
		IIB = Venous only problem
IV	Complete degloving	

Principles of management are the same as replantation. Save life before digit!

Emergent operation is indicated if circulation is inadequate, to identify the cause and mitigate it.

> **Opinion:**
>
> Despite the popularity of these (and other) classifications, you have to think what is wrong and then address that problem. Any classification exists to help plan your management. If it takes you away from management planning (e.g. MESS scoring system) return to basics and restore form and function - very rarely will you go wrong.

Post-traumatic thumb reconstruction

Goals

Sensation
Stability
Length
Mobility
Pain free function

Options

Ref: Muzaffar et al. PRS 2005

IPJ and beyond

Aim: Provide good soft tissue cover.

Principle: Since the length (and attachment of EPL & FPL) is preserved, a reasonable amount of function is expected.

Options:
1. Homodigital flap. Moberg (gives 1-1.5cm advancement) +/- V-Y on thenar eminence
2. Heterodigital flap. Cross finger, or Foucher

Opinion:

Although described as such by Moberg, I would not flex the IPj to "increase the reach" of the flap. It leaves the patient with a very thin pulp once IPj is extended which in turn compromises pinch.

Most of P1 intact

Aim: Deepen the first web (to improve the span and hence the grasp).

Principle: Long flexor and extensor are missing, so the power comes from small muscles of the hand (thenar and 1st dorsal interosseous).

Options:

Option	Example	Comments
Local flap	4 flap Z-plasty 5-flap Z-plasty Transposition flap from dorsum	Mainstay. Other options are only considered if local skin is not suitable, eg extensive injury / burn to dorsum
Regional flap	Reverse RFF PIA flap	
Free flap	Lateral arm flap (or any other)	

Most of P1 missing

Aim: To provide length as well as soft tissue.

Options:

In acute situation consider microvascular transfer of another digit, or pollicisation of e.g. IF stump (if it is injured already)

Otherwise or for late presentation, distraction osteogenesis of 1st MC (which needs compliant patient, a good length of MC and good soft tissue cover) or toe to thumb transfer (see below) may be considered.

Proximal 1/3rd of 1st ray

Aim: Stable sensate post for pinch and opposition.

Principle: Anything better than a "post" is a bonus, but anything less is not acceptable as patient will lose opposition and the ability to grasp any object.

Options:
1. Pollicisation (see below)
2. Toe to thumb transfer (see below)

Pollicisation

Principles

1. Transposition of a digit on its neurovascular pedicle
2. Skeletal realignment
3. Muscle stabilisation
4. Appropriate incision design

Choice of digit

1st choice: Injured, but sensate finger
2nd choice: IF
Next choice: RF then MF

Some of the issues with the particular choice of digit

	Pros	Cons
IF	• No cross-over of structures • MF compensates automatically as the "new IF" • Removal of 2nd MC deepens 1st webspace • Origin of adductor longus is preserved	
MF		Causes rotation and overriding of IF and RF
RF	• Shorter than MF • Adductor pollicis origin is preserved on 3rd MC	

Operative steps

Ref: Green's operative hand surgery. Note that these steps are for a congenital case

1. Skin incision
2. Isolate n/vasc bundle
3. Microdissection of CDN
4. Ligate RDA to MF
5. Release A2 of IF
6. Elevate dorsal skin while preserving veins
7. Free extensors
8. Elevate and release, thenar muscles, 1st DIO

9. Identify and tag lateral bands at PIPj of IF
10. Incise inter-metacarpal ligament
11. MC epiphysiodesis to shorten IF
12. Reposition IF in hyper-extension (as IF MCPj can hyper-extend but thumb CMCj can't. If this is not done, then the new thumb will hyperextend every time the patient tries to grasp an object causing functional problems).

For toe-to-thumb transfer, see congenital section

Principles of fracture fixation

> 1. (Atraumatic) Anatomical reduction
> 2. (Appropriately) Stable fixation
> 3. Respect for fracture biology
> 4. Early mobilisation

Function w.r.t. hand injuries

The primary aim of fixation of any hand fracture is to restore function in as short a time as possible. The function of the hand can be described as

- three pinches,
- three grips,
- a grasp and
- open hand.

The pinches consist of:

PINCHES	Formation	Notes
Fine pinch	Between the very distal ends of IF & thumb	e.g. picking a pin
Pulp to pulp	Between finger and thumb pulp	e.g. turning pages of a book / newspaper, fastening a zipper
Key pinch	Between radial side of (usually the) IF & thumb pulp	e.g. holding & turning a key in a door lock

The three grips include the

GRIPS	Formation	Notes
Chuck/tripod	Using IF, MF & Thumb to twist an object	e.g. turning door knobs, twisting open/close water taps
Power grip	Rolling the fingers around a cylindrical object for a firm hold	e.g. lift a kettle, turn door handles, using a hammer
Hook	Lifting objects with MCPjs extended and IPJs flexed	e.g. lifting shopping bags

As well as

	Formation	Notes
Grasp / Span	Holding a large (cylindrical) object	e.g. glass of water
Open palm	Palm is fully flat with thumb either in neutral or adducted	e.g. when pushing open a door

After a complex condition or injury, it is very useful to know which functions of the hand have been affected so that the management can be tailored according to patient's activities of daily living.

Principles of fracture fixation

The principles of fracture fixation are:

- anatomical reduction,
- appropriate stable fixation,
- respect for fracture biology and
- early mobilisation.

Management of a fracture primarily depends upon its position and stability (Ref: Figure). If the fracture fragments are aligned anatomically and stable no further management may be needed (except a short period of resting splint for comfort).

If the fragments are not in an anatomical position, closed reduction may be attempted and if the fracture is then deemed to be stable, it can be managed in a plaster cast.

Fractures which are not anatomical and/or unstable need operative management.

Anatomical Reduction

In order to reduce a fracture to its anatomical position one needs to restore its full length, alignment and rotation (i.e. all three dimensions). Presence of any intra-articular fragments necessitate accurate reduction of articular surface. This may involve elevation of depressed fragments (and may need bone graft e.g. in die punch fracture of the distal radius by the lunate).

Figure: General decision tree about fracture position and stability

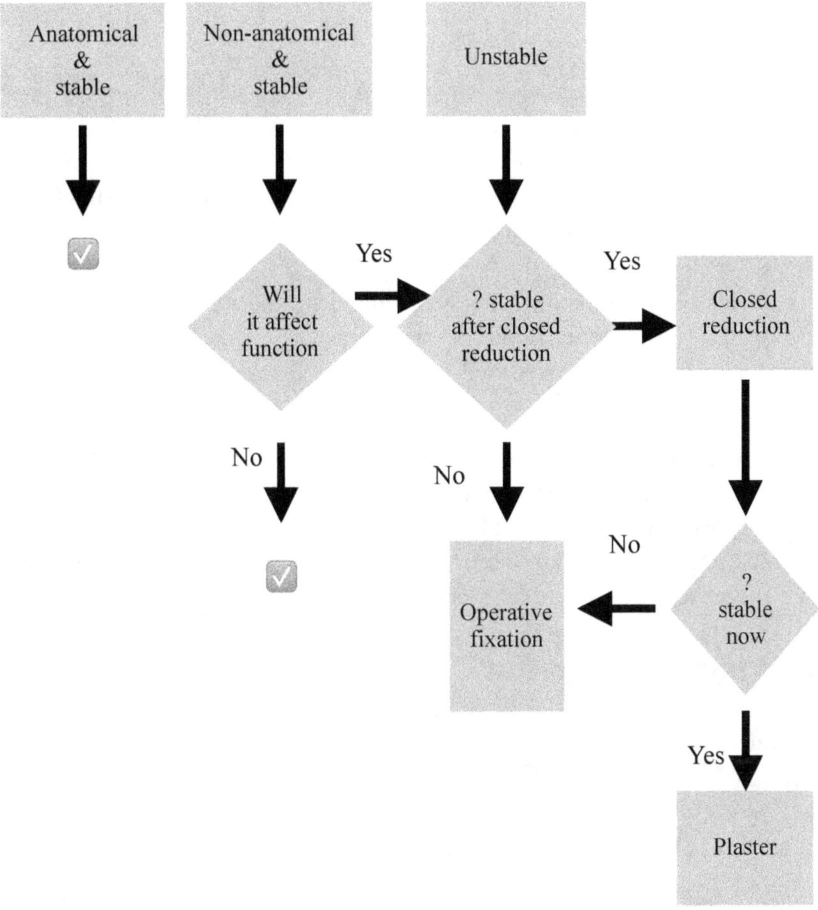

Stable Fixation

A fracture may be fixed in a position of relative stability or of absolute stability.

Absolute stability is achieved by a construct that does not allow any discernible macro movement at the fracture site, and in turn, allows primary bone healing. This is only possible if there are large fracture fragments which can be compressed together without destabilising the bone. In contrast, a fracture in a position of relative stability heals by callus formation. This process tends to be faster than primary bone healing.

Absolute stability can be achieved by the use of compression plates or lag screws. Relative stability may be achieved by the use of K wires or bridging plate. Although described in terms of all-or-none categories, the conditions of stability occupy a spectrum.

K wires are made of medical grade stainless steel. In the hand surgery their commonly used sizes vary from 0.9-1.5 mm. These can hold a fracture in position but do not offer any compression at the fracture site. Out of the different methods of using K wires, using crossed K wires is a more stable construct then using them in parallel or individually.

The implants used for fixation are standardised by the AO-ASIF group from Switzerland. The generic implants are known by the AO prefix while commercial manufacturers have their proprietary systems.

AO-Screws

A screw is a mechanical device that converts torsion to linear motion by virtue of helically wound threads around a (usually) solid core. (The exception being cannulated screws e.g. used in hip fixation). Screws may be used by themselves or in combination with a plate for fixation of fractures.

ANATOMY OF A SCREW

Anatomically a screw is divided into head, core, thread, pitch. The diameter of a screw refers to the diameter of the core *and* that of the adjacent thread. (Ref: Figure)

Figure: Parts of a screw a) fully threaded screw, b) partially threaded screw

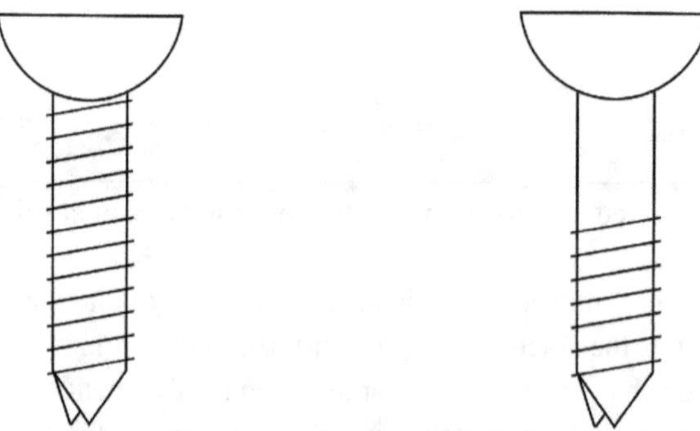

Then there are special anatomical types of screws such as the headless (Herbert screw and its modifications) and the variable pitch screw.

Tapping vs non-tapping

By design, the screws can be described as a tapping or non-tapping. Most of the screws used in hand surgery are self-tapping screws which means that the inclination of the spiral is such that the screw cores out a thread for itself in the distal cortex.

Locking vs non-locking

According to design the screws may be locking or non-locking (also called "conventional") screws. Locking screws have a threaded *head* (Ref: Figure) which engages in a reciprocally threaded slot in the specially designed plate (called the "locking plate"). In addition to being threaded, the two surfaces (the one on the screw and the other on the plate) are trapezoidal in sagittal section so the screw cannot be tightened beyond a certain amount, which contribute to its locking.

Figure: Head of a locking screw. Note the trapezoidal shape which prevents it from over-tightening. The threads of the screw fit in with reciprocal grooves in the associated plate (called a "locking plate").

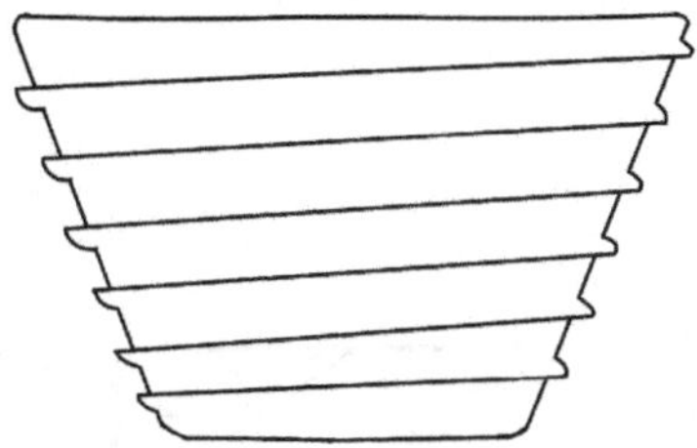

FUNCTIONAL CLASSIFICATION

According to function the screws may be classified as a lag screw or a reduction screw.

Lagging is a principle which allows compression at the fracture site by one or more screws inserted at right angles to the fracture plane.

The proximal cortex (also called "near" or "cis" cortex, Ref Figure) is made with a drill-bit whose diameter is equal to the diameter of the screw to be inserted ("over drilling"). After over-drilling the screw threads cannot engage the proximal cortex and instead the screw is free to slide up and down the glide hole now created. The screw head limits how deep that screw can go in that glide hole.

Figure: Naming the near & far cortices

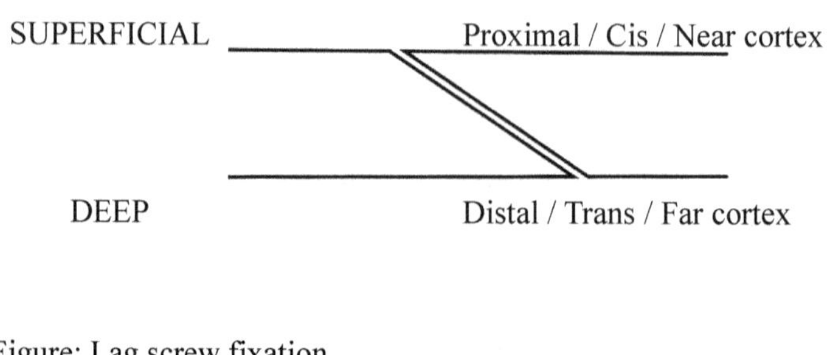

Figure: Lag screw fixation

Overdrill the *proximal* cortex

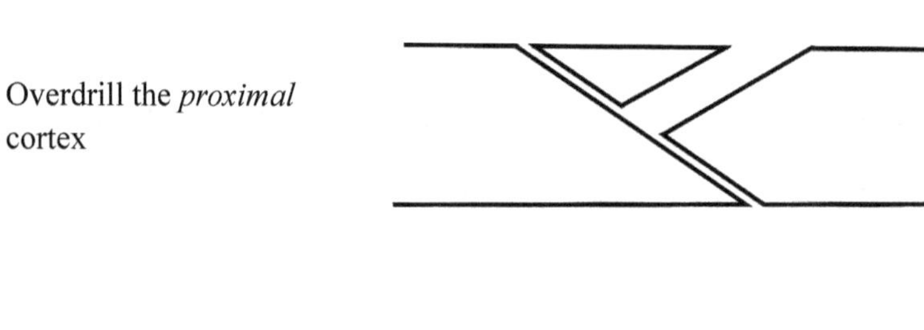

The screw will now slide in and out without resistance

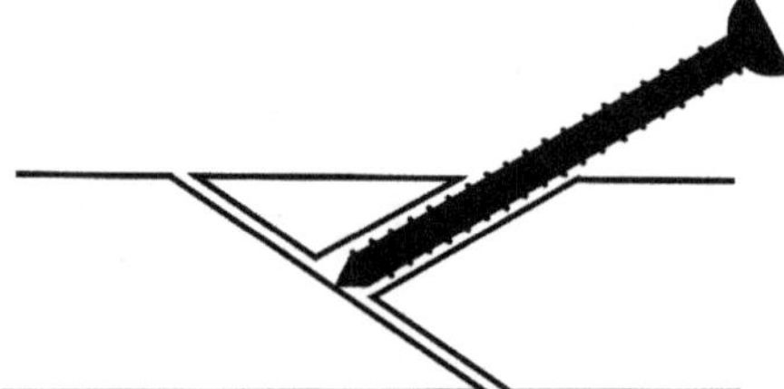

Drill the *distal* cortex with same drill size as the core diameter of the screw

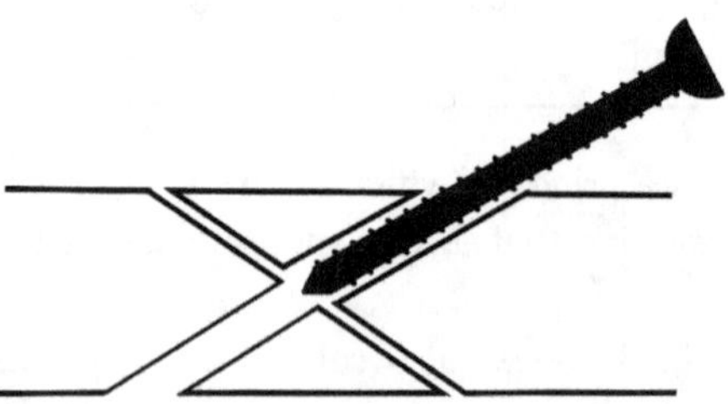

Figure: Lag screw fixation (contd.)

As the screw is advanced, its threads take purchase on the distal cortex only

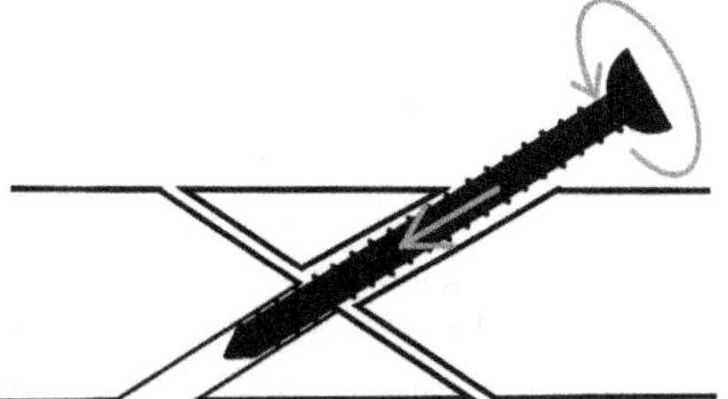

As the screw is tightened, its head engages the proximal cortex and hence compresses the two bone fragments

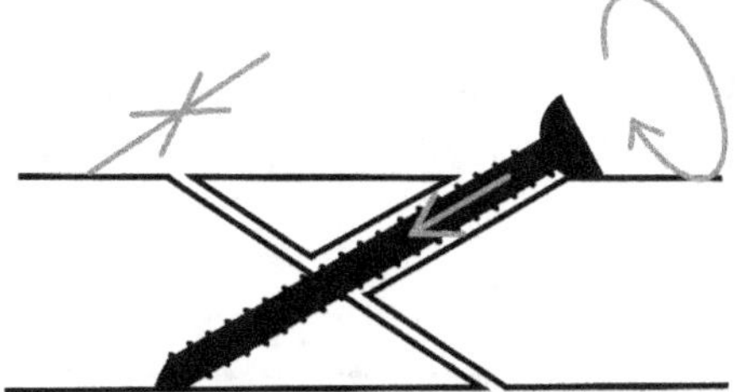

The distal cortex is drilled the same size as the diameter of the core of the screw. This means that the screw threads can take purchase in the distal (also called 'trans') cortex to make the screw advance in a linear direction. After both cortices have been drilled appropriately and the screw is advanced, it takes purchase in the distal cortex only while gliding in the proximal cortex. As the screw advances, the screw head pulls the proximal cortex with it and compresses it against the distal cortex.

Care needs to be taken to **position** the screw at least one screw-diameter away from any fracture, otherwise the intervening bone may split, compromising fracture stability &/or position. The **direction** of the placed screw needs to be perpendicular to the fracture plane through which it is passing, otherwise you will introduce a shear force that will distract the fracture again.

If a single lag screw is placed across a fracture (as in a short oblique fracture) it can act as a pivot and allow rotation around it. This rotational tendency can be counteracted by another lag screw in a different plane to the first (ideally perpendicular). This rotational tendency can also be neutralised by fixation of a length of bone with a plate (called a "neutralisation plate").

Aside: Countersinking

Sometimes you will find that the side of a screw lies proud of the surface (of the bone). It may be palpable or rub against a tendon. This situation is more likely if the screw is placed more obliquely. To prevent these functional issues, you can "countersink" the cis-cortex to create a niche that accommodates the deeper side of the screw head, which prevents the head from sitting proud.

Figure: Countersinking. a) No countersinking, note the prominence of the screw head. This may be palpable through the skin, or abrade overlying tendons or soft tissue. b) Countersunk screw, note that the screw head sits less proud and hence less likely to be palpable or abrade an overlying tendon. Also note that with countersinking you need a smaller length screw, than otherwise.

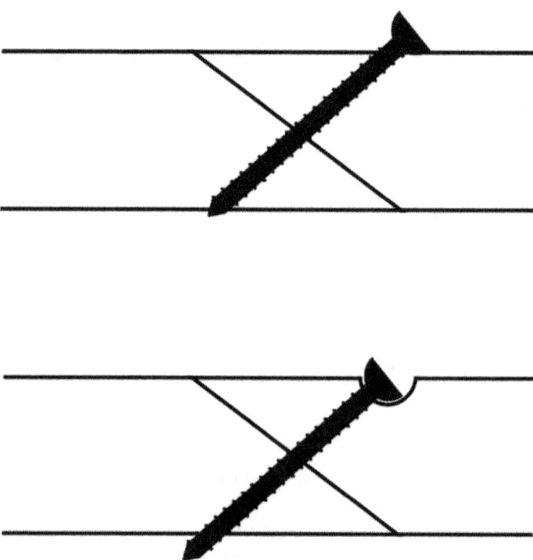

AO-Plates

The plates used for internal fixation can be classified by their size (1.1, 1.5, 2 mm), shape (e.g. dynamic compression plate DCP, low contact DCP LC-DCP) or according to their function (e.g. bridging or buttressing plates). Ref: Table and Figure

Tables 1 & 2: Classification of plates. Note that a particular shape plate may be used for different functions

Functional classification
Compression
Neutralisation
Bridging
Buttress

Anatomical classification
DCP (dynamic compression plate)
LC-DCP (Low contact DCP)
Locking plate
LCP (Locking compression plate)

Figure: Any given shape of plate may be used for different functional purpose depending on the fracture type (except e.g. that locking plate can't compress)

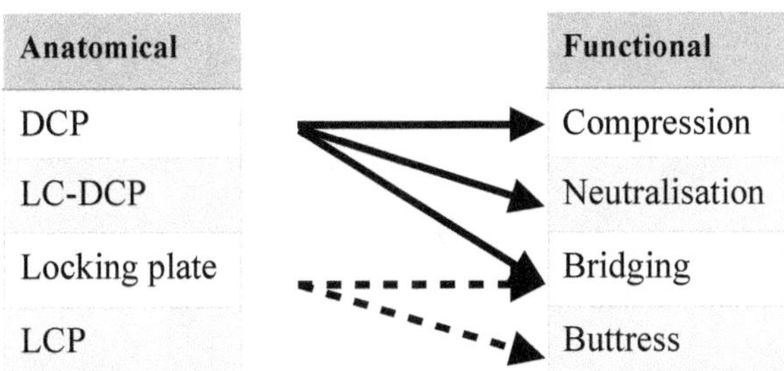

ANATOMICAL CLASSIFICATION OF PLATES

1. DCP
2. LC-DCP
3. Locking plate
4. LCP

DCP (Dynamic compression plate)

Dynamic compression plates are not used anymore (the current AO standard being the LC-DCP, see below) but they are the historical standard against which everything else is compared. The DCP consists of a flat under surface and has oval shaped screw holes with bevelled edges. Note that because of the oval shape of the screw holes, the screws/screw heads cannot prevent the plate from sliding longitudinally along the bone. The major factor preventing this slide is the friction at the plate-bone interface (except when screws are inserted off-centre, see below).

Figure: Dynamic compression plate (not to scale)

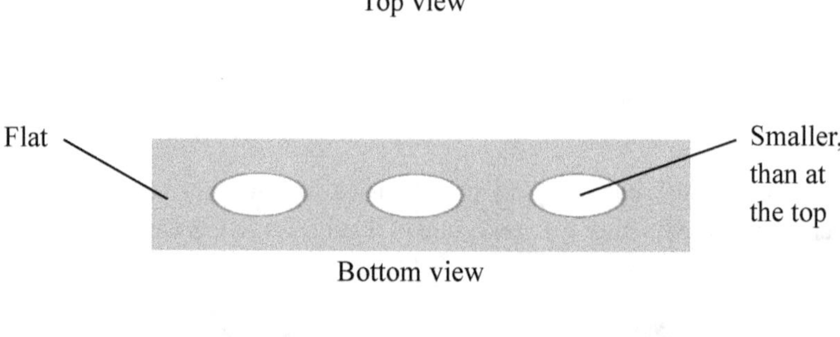

Off centre insertion of screws (away from the fracture site) lets the screw head engage the bevelled edge of the screw hole in the final stage of tightening. As the ellipsoidal screw head is tightened it tries to slide down the bevel of the screw hole (Ref: Figure).

The first screw inserted in the plate (e.g. in the proximal fracture fragment) effectively creates a fragment-plate construct. When the second screw is inserted (off centre) in the distal bone fragment, the distal bone fragment moves relative to the 'proximal fragment-plate' construct. This is because the threads of the screw are firmly fixed in the bone so the bone moves as the screw head slides down the edge of the glide hole. This advances the bone towards the fracture site, causing compression at the fracture site. The amount of compression can be controlled with the degree of tightening of the screw head.

The problem with these plates tuned out to be that the pressure of the plate on the bone interfered with the periosteal blood supply and caused resorption of underlying bone followed by implant fatigue and failure. So AO replaced DCPs with a low-contact plate (see below) as their standard.

Figure: Role of screw position in dynamic compression (also see Figure on page 97)

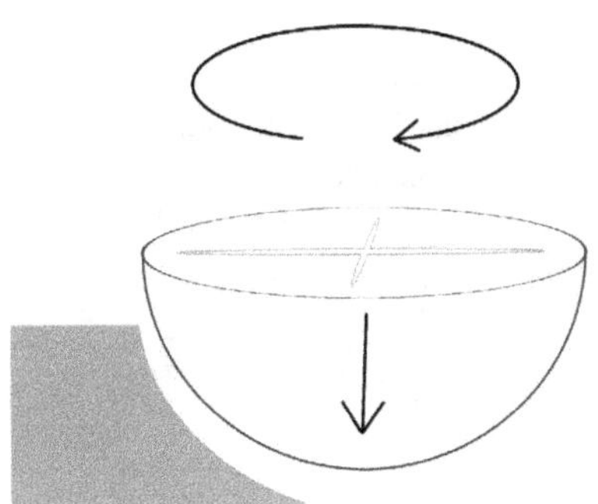

The head of the screw is hemispherical which matches the sagittal profile of the screw hole in the DCP. This allows both to slide smoothly in relation to each other.

The point of insertion of the screw fixes it in relation to the bone (and the fracture site). The first screw that is inserted off-centre (in its screw hole) in a fracture fragment- its head will contact the sidewalls of the screw hole and try to push it *away* from the fracture site.

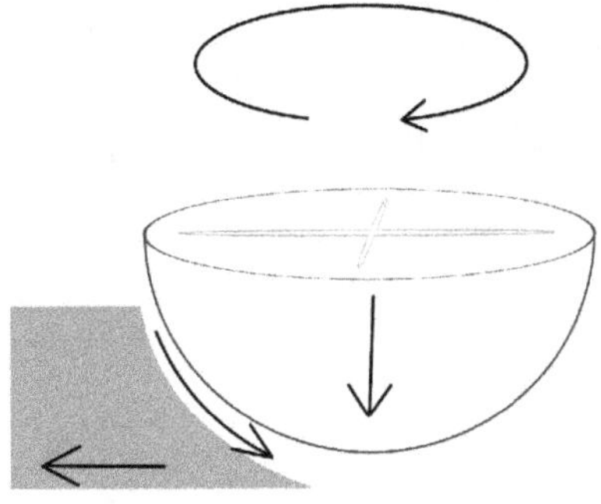

Figure: Role of screw position in dynamic compression (contd.)

> If the plate has been fixed in another fracture fragment already, the plate will carry that fragment *towards* the fracture site, causing compression.
>
> The degree of compression achieved can be adjusted by how off-centre the screw is and how tight it is.

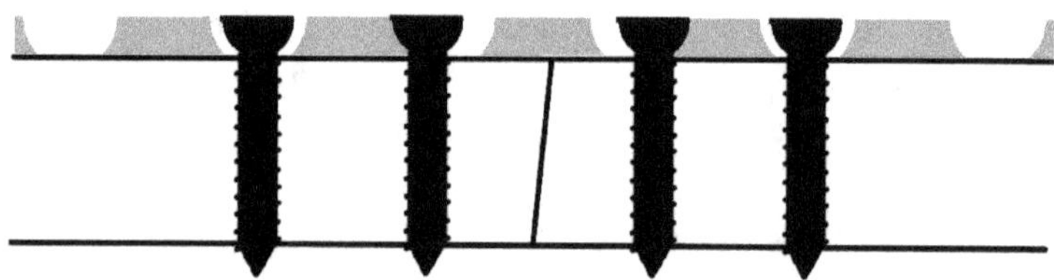

> Whether you do off centre screw holing on only one, or both fracture fragments *does* depend on the accuracy of your reduction. Well reduced fractures may only need one dynamic compression screw.

LC-DCP (Low contact DCP)

Low contact DCP (Ref: Figure) is the current standard AO plate. It has undulations on its deeper surface so that the amount of contact with the bone is limited. This helps in preservation of the sub-periosteal blood supply and decreases bone resorption.

Figure: LC-DCP (not to scale, next page)

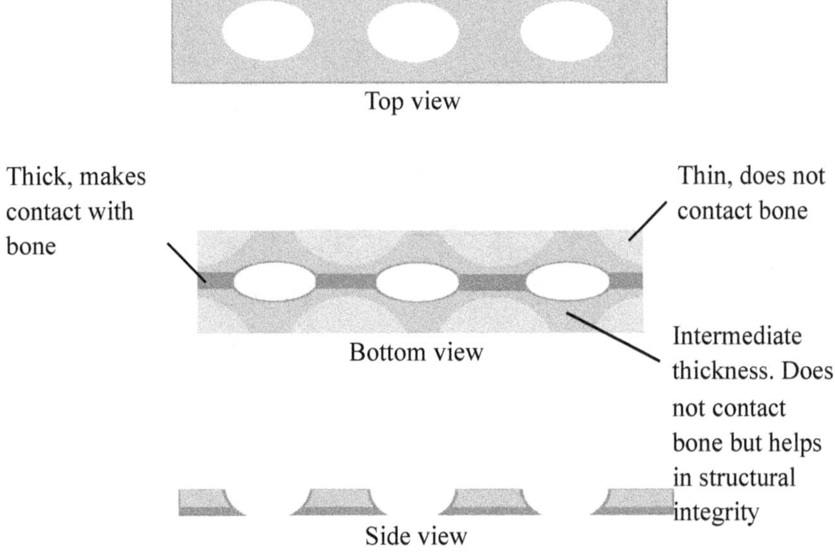

Locking plate

Locking plates do not have oval bevelled screw holes. Their screw holes have threads which only allow a specific screw type (a 'locking screw', with a threaded head). The walls of the screw holes are narrower at the deep surface matching the screw head design, which prevents the screw from advancing beyond a predetermined amount.

Stability is achieved by rigid contact between screw head and the plate, as well as by rigidity at the screw thread-bone interface. Therefore, the plate does not need to rely on friction at the bone-plate interface. In fact when seen from the side, the locking plates are elevated a fraction of a millimetre above the bone surface (hence the name 'internal ex-fix'). This prevents interference with the bone's blood supply.

Its worth noting that the stability at the bone-screw interface depends on the screw thread engaging a certain thickness of cortical bone. In lower limb and proximal upper limb, the cortical bone is considerably thick so the locking screws only need to engage one cortex ('uni-cortical screws'). This is of course, not the case in hand and the locking screws in metacarpals are designed to engage two cortices.

Figure: Locking plate (not to scale). Note that the plate does not make contact with the bone

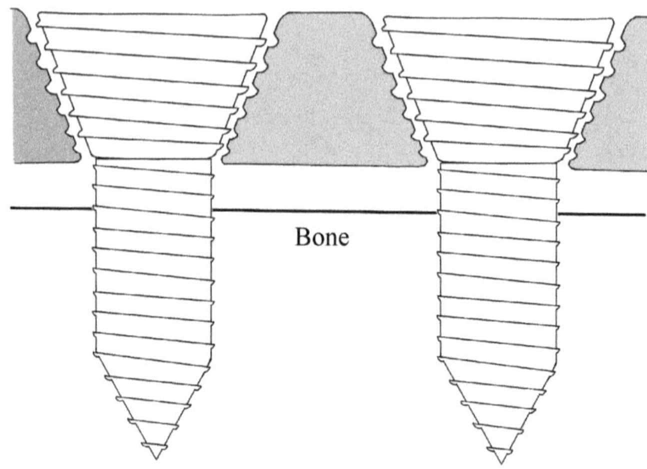

LCP (Locking compression plate)

A locking compression plate (LCP) is a hybrid between a low-contact DCP and a locking plate. It offers the opportunity to apply compression as well as use locking screws. This is because each screw is in fact a combination hole - one half of the oval screw hole is for compression and the other half for locking. In order to achieve compression, conventional screws are applied through compression holes before inserting the locking screws.

FUNCTIONAL CLASSIFICATION OF PLATES

1. Compression plate
2. Neutralisation plate
3. Bridging plate
4. Buttress plate

The plates can serve to compress (compression plate), neutralise the tendency of rotation around a single lag screw (neutralisation plate), bridge over a comminuted segment (bridging plate) or counteract the tendency for a peri-articular fracture to collapse (buttress plate). (Ref: Figure).

Figure: Functional configuration of plates a) compression plate*,
b) neutralisation plate, c) bridging plate

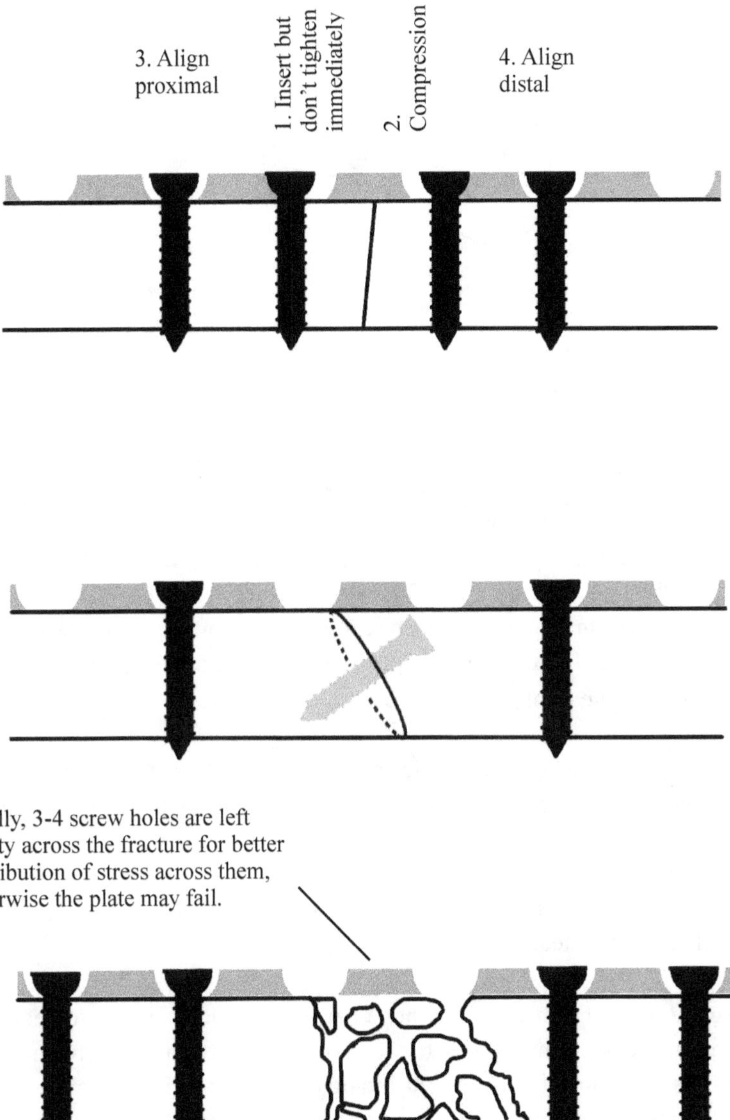

* The sequence described is the standard AO technique. The alternative sequence is proximal alignment → proximal compression → distal compression → distal alignment. I **strongly** recommend reading the online AO surgery reference for details.

Figure (contd.): Functional classification of plates. d) Buttress plate

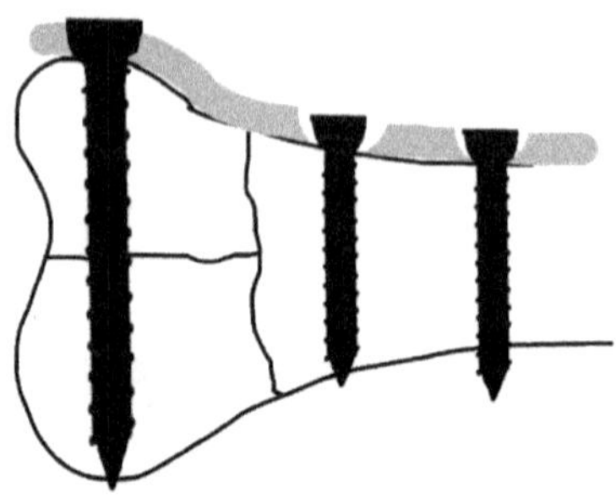

DCP, LC-DCP or LCP can be used for any of these functions. The exception is the locking plate, which due to its design, can only be used to stabilise the fracture ('internal ex-fix').

Respect for fracture biology

Bone heals in one of two ways. Well approximated and rigidly fixed simple fractures heal by primary bone healing, whereby osteons grow directly from one end of the fracture into the other. There is no intervening haematoma and no discernible macro-motion at the fracture site. This allows bone to heal without forming any callus. In fact, there is not much to see on a radiograph as the bone heals and the diagnosis of healing is purely a clinical one.

Alternatively, bone heals by callus formation ('secondary bone healing ') which is the faster of the two mechanisms. Secondary bone healing occurs in fractures that are
• comminuted,
• not rigidly fixed (see conditions of relative stability above) or are
• not well approximated.

Irrespective of the mechanism, the bone needs good blood supply to heal. This comes from the surrounding soft tissues and the periosteum. Interference with the blood supply and the associated biological processes increases the risk of complications (bone resorption, fatigue failure of implant, malunion or non-union).

The most important consideration for surgical technique, in relation to fracture biology, is preservation of blood supply by
• limiting soft tissue dissection and peri-osteal stripping, as well as
• gentle tissue handling.

Denuding the bone of surrounding soft tissues and stripping of periosteum interrupts the respective sources of blood supply. This is especially damaging for small bone fragments which may be completely devitalised. In larger bone fragments, the endosteal flow is already limited (in at least one direction) due to the pre-existing fracture so excessive dissection and mobilisation will increase the chances of delayed union or non-union.

The current generation of implants take advantage of this principle in plate design. While soft tissue dissection is dependant on the surgical technique, periosteal blood supply can be preserved by avoiding pressure on it.

The LC-DCPs have a limited contact with bone. They only contact the bone at the perimeter of the screw holes and even less in-between the screw holes. This reduces the bone demineralisation induced by prolonged direct pressure. The locking plates take the concept even further and do not contact the bone at all, relying instead on the stiffness of design at the plate-screw and screw-bone interface.

Early mobilisation

The benefits of early mobilisation include:
1. Keeps joints through their range of motion
2. Reduced edema
3. Prevents stiffness
4. Reduces muscle loss
5. Improved outcome
6. Better motivation
7. Earlier return to work/job, which is especially important for manual workers, which represent a high percentage of hand injury patients

Draw the extensor mechanism

Figure: Extensor mechanism (dorsal view)

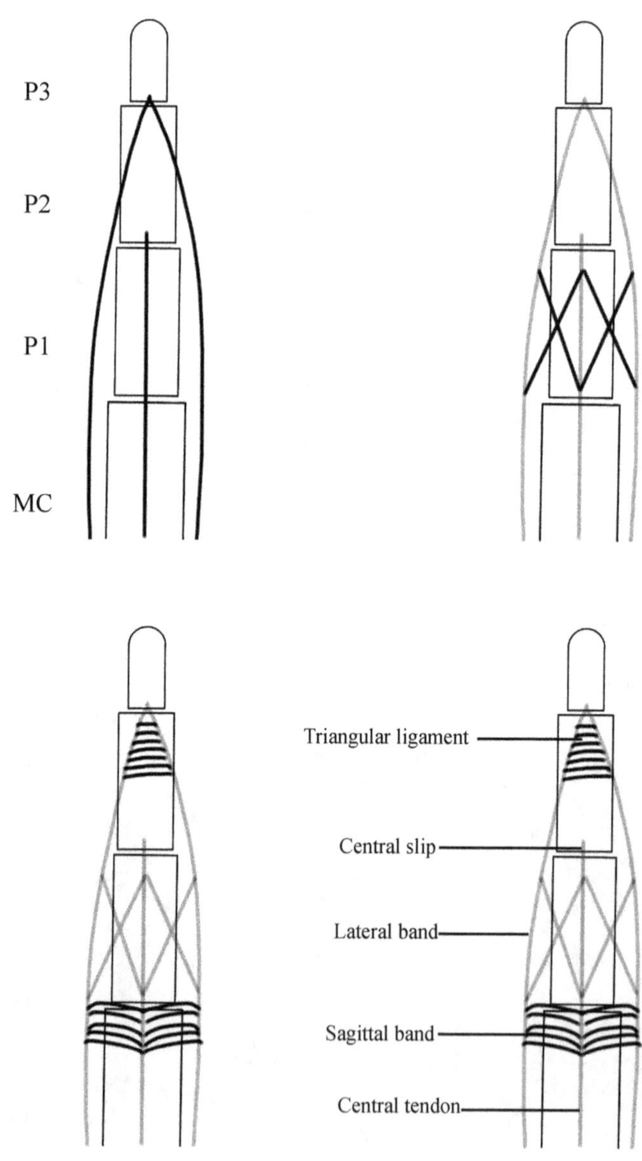

Figure: Extensor mechanism (lateral view)

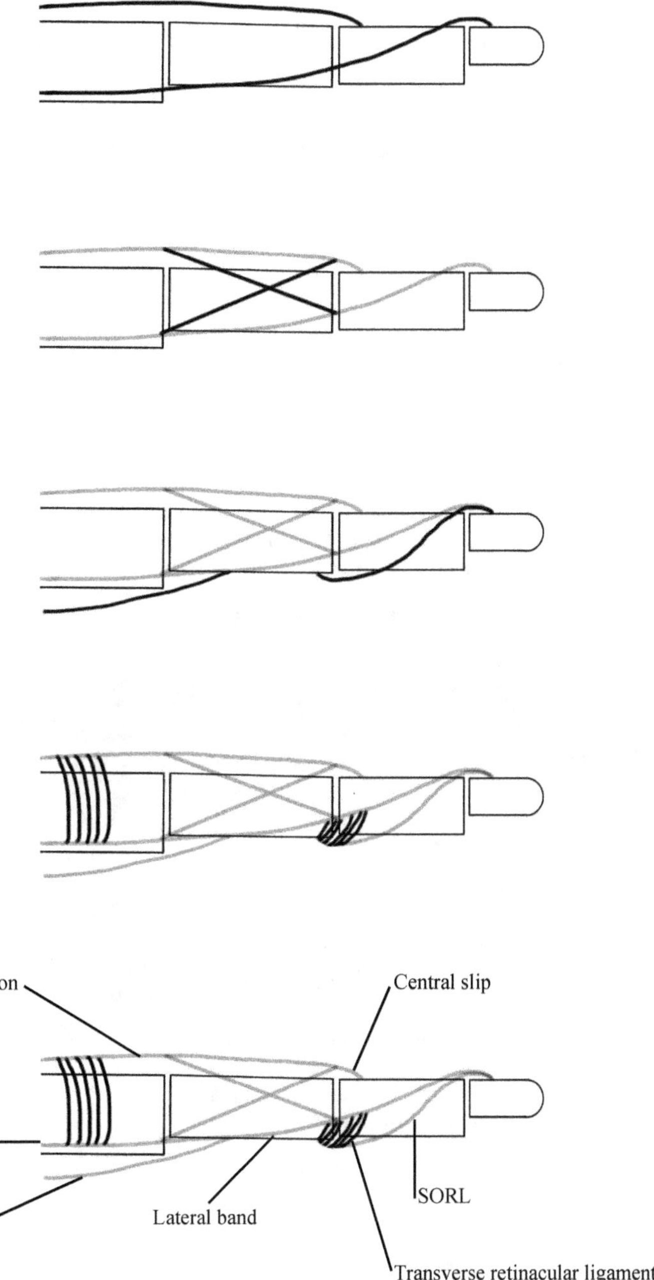

Extensor tendon rehab.

The following protocols assume a compliant motivated patient without any other injury and no postop complications.

Norwich regimen

Ref: Logan et al. 1997, described for extensor zone 4-7 injuries. n=24

Splinting position	W-45, MP+50, IP=0
Start	@ day 2
Excercise	Active combined MP & IP extension Active MP flexion & IP extension
Frequency	x4/session, 4 sessions/day for 4 weeks
@ 5/52	Gentle flexion of MP & IPj (slow if ext lag >30) Night splint only Slowly progress to full power and grip

Birmingham Hand Centre regimen

Goals of management are, 1) scar & edema management, 2) patient education & 3) therapy

Splinting position	W-30, MP+30, IP=0
Start	within 5 days
Excercise	Passive extension all digits Active MP flexion/extension (with IP=0) Active IP flexion/extension (with MP supported in extension)
Frequency	10x hourly during waking hours
@ 4/52	Splint at night & in crowded places Composite flexion & tendon glide*
@ 6/52	Gentle resistance exercise. No splint
@ 10/52	Driving and light ADLs
@ 12/52	unrestricted

* Composite flexion is to curl in the fingers by IPj flexion only. Tendon glide is movement at either PIPj-only or DIPj-only, to favour excursion of the respective long flexor.

Mallet injury:

Splinting position	Static finger based removable TP splint DIP=0, PIP free.
Excercise	MP & PIP active flexion & extension
Frequency	10x / hour
@ 6/52	Remove splint hourly for 10x active extension of DIPj Stop if any extensor lag
@ 7/52	Start flexion at DIPj
@ 8/52	Light ADLs & night splint
@ 10/52	Driving and light ADL
@ 12/52	Unrestricted use

Central slip injury:

Splinting position	Static finger based, PIP=0, DIP=0 Full time for 3/52, except hygiene
Start	within 5 days
Excercise	Active MP flexion Active DIPj flexion while supporting PIPj (lateral band exercise)
Frequency	10x / hour
@ 3/52	• Capener splint at day (hourly active PIPj flexion & lateral band exercises) • Static splint at night
@ 6/52	Remove Capener & active flexion/extension of PIPj, 10x / hour
@ 8/52	Wean off Capener Static night splint Light ADLs
@ 10/52	Driving and light ADLs
@ 12/52	Unrestricted use

Flexor tendon rehab.

Eponymous names

Duran	Controlled passive mobilisation
Kleinert	Passive flexion, active extension
modified Kleinert	as above+ bar at wrist to increase DIPj excursion
Strickland	Place & active hold + tenodesis splint
Belfast regimen	Early active mobilisation*

* Most current tendon rehab regimens are active mobilisations regimens. Exceptions exist for tendon repairs in children, combined flexor/extensor repairs, associated hand fractures

Belfast regimen

Ref: Small et al. 1989, 9% rupture rate

Splinting position	W+30, MP+90, IP=0
Start	@ day 2 postop
Excercise	2 active & 2 passive movements
Frequency	every 2 hours
@ 6/52	movement against resistance
@ 12/52	full power

Manchester regimen

Splinting position	W-20, MP+30, IP=0
Start	@ day 2 postop
Excercise	Passive flexion Active flexion/extension Place & hold
Frequency	hourly
@ 6/52	passive extension and blocking

Birmingham Hand Centre regimen

Splinting position	W=0, MP+70, IP=0
Start	within 3 days postop
Excercise	Full passive flexion Full active flexion/extension Active IPj extension, with MPj held in flexion
Frequency	10x hourly
@ 6/52	Splint at night & in crowded places Active extension & tendon glide Light ADLs only
@ 8/52	Blocking excercises
@12/52	Unrestricted use

Outcome measurements:

- Goniometer at 6 & 12 weeks
- Grip strength at 12 weeks

TAM

The ASSH recommended outcome measurement is TAM (Total Active Motion)

TAM =	sum of active flexion of MP, PIP & DIP MINUS sum of extensor lag at each joint
Normal TAM =	TAM of contralateral side (if uninjured) OR 260 degrees (if other side is injured)
Reported as:	TAM/Normal x 100%

Almost all contemporary flexor tendon rehab regimens are early active mobilisation regimens, which aim to keep the joint range of motion & prevent adhesions using active movement of _un_injured tendons. The repaired tendon is gradually loaded over a period of weeks, in line with its physiologic strength.

Rupture of flexor tendon repair

A typical scenario may be that the physiotherapist calls to say that there is no movement at the joint.

HISTORY
How long ago
How well was patient moving before that
Any trauma
Sudden loss or gradual

EXAMINATION
Whether there is a flicker of movement, or nothing at all
Any passive ROM
State of soft tissues

DIFFERENTIAL
1. Adhesions. Likely to happen over time with a gradual decrease in range of motion
2. Tendon rupture. Likely to be acute with sudden loss of movement after a specific incident

INVESTIGATION
If unsure, consider urgent USS to determine continuity of tendon

MANAGEMENT OF RUPTURE
Re-explore (consent patient for both 1 and 2 stage repairs)
Intra-operative decision is to,
- immediate re-repair (if no tendon-muscle unit shortening), or
- insert a silicone spacer (a "Hunter rod") as a 1st stage procedure

Insertion of Hunter's rod (First stage)
2 incisions. At FDP insertion and at wrist
Size 3 or 4 silicone rod
Insert distally and retrieve at wrist
Fix distally only
Leave in place for 3/12

2nd stage

The ideal time for 2nd stage is when,

- Joints are _s_upple, ideally with full PROM
- Good _s_oft tissue cover
- _S_ensations intact
- _S_table injury e.g. all fractures have healed
- _S_ingle digit problem only (relative indication)

Sources of graft are,

- Palmaris longus tendon (absent in 15%)*
- Plantaris tendon (absent in 8%)

Fixation technique:
Distally, with a button, or using a Mitek™ bone anchor
Proximally, with a Pulvertaft weave and 3/0 prolene

*Given an approximate chance of 15% that one palmaris longus is absent, the chance of both tendons being absent is 0.15 x 0.15 = 0.225 or 2% approx. The risk of absence of a plantaris tendon *and* both plamaris longus tendons is 0.225 x 0.08 = 0.001 = 0.1% or 1 in 1000 patients. This should be mentioned in a consent process.

Trauma - Maxillofacial

The commonest causes are road traffic accidents (RTA) or inter-personal violence.

CORE KNOWLEDGE
ATLS - rapid evaluation!, X-match, max fax input
Systematic history and assessment

APPROACH TO PATIENT - HISTORY
What happened? When?
What other injuries in this patient. Be guided by the mechanism and speed involved [This has to be *very* detailed]
Any injuries to any one else. esp for RTAs know if any fatalities

Any 1st aid
Events and management so far

PMHx, Medications, Allergies, Tetanus status

APPROACH TO PATIENT - EXAMINATION
(see below)

APPROACH TO PATIENT - MANAGEMENT
1. Patient survival. Initial management is according to ATLS
2. Preservation of function
    - Vision
    - Breathing & olfaction
    - Mastication
3. Restoration of form
    - Bony stability
    - Soft tissue redraping

Detailed management as per injury (see below)

EXPECTED CLINICAL QUESTIONS
How to evaluate - be systematic & know your ATLS ["C-ABC"]
Principles of fixation
Mandible fractures

RECOMMENDED PAPERS

1. Evans BGA, Evans GRD. MOC-PSSM CME Article: Zygomatic Fractures: *Plast Reconstr Surg.* 2008 Jan;121(MOC-PS CME Coll):1–11.
2. Guyuron B. MOC-PSSM CME Article: Genioplasty: *Plast Reconstr Surg.* 2008 Apr;121(Supplement):1–7.
3. Kaufman Y, Stal D, Cole P, Hollier L. Orbitozygomatic Fracture Management *Plast Reconstr Surg.* 2008 Apr;121(4):1370–4.
4. Morcos SS, Patel PK. The Vocabulary of Dentofacial Deformities. *Clinics in Plastic Surgery.* 2007 Jul;34(3):589–99.

History

What happened? Exact mechanism*

When

Details of extrication, if any

What other injuries**

PMHx, Meds, Allergies, Tetanus status

* Handover from any para-medical or ambulance crew is invaluable about the scene of the injury especially in RTAs.
** Certain injury patterns occur in combination e.g. falls over six feet (calcaneal fracture, pelvic fracture, spinal burst fractures, head injury, wrist fracture), seatbelt or deceleration injuries (facial injury, chest or intra-abdominal injuries).

Primary Survery

Strict ATLS assessment

A. AIRWAY WITH C-SPINE CONTROL.

Expedite this step in a safe manner - use the expertise of the anaesthetist in your trauma team. Inline immobilisation must be maintained before c-spine is cleared.

Beware of:
- facial fractures bleeding in to the airway
- dental injuries introducing foreign bodies
- associated C-spine fractures.

B. BREATHING

Blunt trauma can cause contusions while sharp objects can result in penetrating injuries to lungs.

C. CIRCULATION

Bleeding from facial lacerations or maxillary fractures can be very dramatic and can compromise the airway, or cause hypovolemia.

Significant nasal bleeding can be controlled by anterior or posterior nasal packing, or both. Uncontrolled bleeding from the maxilla needs urgent maxillofacial input (e.g. for a reduction and inter-maxillary fixation).

D. DISABILITY/HEAD INJURY

Especially in,
- elderly and
- un-cooperative patients.

E. EXPOSURE

Look every where else, including hair bearing scalp and patient's back.
Note patient's temperature
Cover the patient with warming blankets / bear hugger, as appropriate

Opinion:

1. In any significant trauma, consider doing a trauma CT (head, C-spine, chest, abdo and pelvis)
2. If the patient is going to need a CT for any reason, strongly consider extending the study for a CT head & C-spine
3. Involve anaesthetist at the outset and maxfax colleagues early

Secondary Survey:

Much of the head and neck examination is part of secondary survey. Be systematic! e.g. top to bottom and lateral to medial (so scalp, forehead, ears, orbital margins, eyes, maxilla, nose etc)

Inspection:
Swelling, bruising, abrasions, lacerations, traumatic tattooing

Test:
- Test for light touch sensation over face, scalp, ear and compare with the opposite side. (The sensations over the angle of mandible are supplied by the cervical plexus and should not be altered in a facial injury).
- Check for facial nerve function in all its branches. (Frontal branch of facial nerve courses from 0.5cm below the tragus of ear to 1.5cm lateral and above the lateral end of the eyebrow).

For each of the following sites, inspect and then gently palpate if there is a suspicion of a fracture. [In any significant trauma, you will likely have done a trauma CT before this stage and already know if there is a fracture].

Eyebrows

- Palpate for frontal sinus or orbital rim fracture.
- Foreign body, loss of substance

Eye exam

- Inspect for peri-orbital swelling or bruising, conjunctival haemorrhage, epiphora.
- Palpate for the integrity of orbital margin and zygoma.
- Test the extra-ocular muscles by asking the patient to follow your finger in a H-shaped pattern. Inability to look upwards and outwards is classically due to entrapment of the inferior oblique muscle in an orbital floor fracture.
- Check pupil shape, size, direct and consensual response to light and visual acuity.

TESTING FOR RAPD

A swinging pen light test can detect afferent pathway defects ("relative afferent pupillary defect", or RAPD) i.e. in the optic nerve which may be missed with a direct pupillary reflex.

Normally a pupil constricts to both direct light and consensually (when the light is shone in the other pupil). If one pupil appears to dilate as the light is swung away to the opposite pupil, the *defect is the the eye where the light is shining* (i.e. the afferent limb of the pupillary reflex).

VISUAL FIELDS

You can use confrontation method for a quick assessment, if you have a high index of suspicion, refer to the ophthalmologist for a more detailed review. Of course, this requires an awake and co-operative patient.

FLORESCEINE STAINING

Use floresceine stain to look for any corneal abrasion and any foreign body in the conjunctival sac.

Retrobulbar haemorrhage presents with a variable combination of pain, proptosis, ophthalmoplegia and deteriorating visual acuity (assuming an awake and alert patient).

Treat any deterioration of visual acuity, diplopia or ophthalmoplegia with suspicion that it may require emergent surgery.

Eyelids
- Ptosis
- Epiphora
- Levator function
- Canthal integrity - gentle tug

Cheek examination
Figure: Structures at risk in a cheek laceration

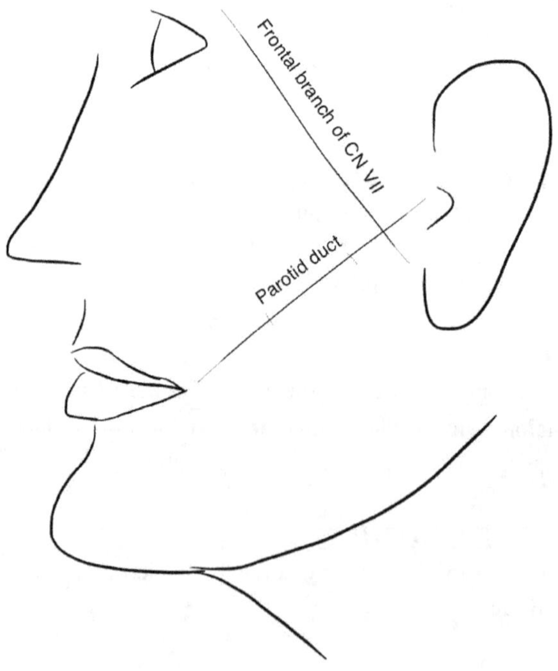

- Facial nerve
- Parotid duct. Is it likely to be injured? Is there any bleeding at the opening of the duct opposite the 2nd upper molar
- Zygoma tenderness

Nose exam

Inspect for shape, symmetry [get a mirror for the patient]

Palpate for,
- tenderness, crepitus or step-off over the nasal bones
- subluxation of septum &/or ULCs

Check for septal haematoma and any rhinorrhea. In high energy trauma, any clear nasal discharge should be considered CSF leak and prompt a CT head.

Examination of lips

Inspect the lips, teeth, mucosa and palate. Identify the landmarks involved in lip laceration (Ref: Figure). What is commonly referred to as a "full thickness laceration" of the lips is more precisely a "through and through" laceration.

Simple small lacerations of the oral mucosa can be managed non-operatively and, rather counter-intuitively, do not require antibiotic cover.

Figure: Landmarks on lip

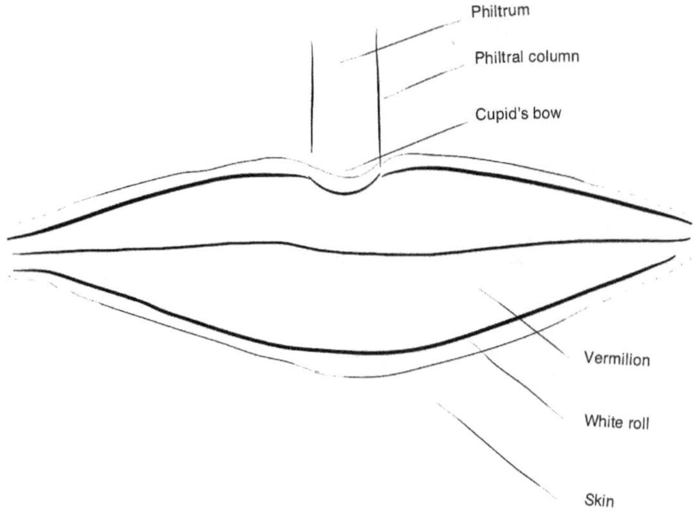

Intra-oral examination

- Is the patient able to open their mouth fully and without discomfort. Note any trismus.
- Look for any foreign bodies, damage to dentition, bleeding in the oral cavity including the palate.
- Specifically ask if the teeth fit normally when the patient closes his mouth and if it hurts to bite.

Any broken tooth is best stored in a (clearly labelled) cup of milk. Imaging may reveal missing dentition in parts of the aero-digestive tract (Casap *et al.*, 2011).

Ear exam

Look for,
- haematoma at the pinna(which requires urgent drainage), or
- retroauricular haemorrhage (Battle sign, suggesting base of skull fracture).

Use an otoscope to examine for,
- bleeding (or CSF) in the external auditory canal,
- integrity of the tympanic membrane and evidence of bleeding behind it.

Investigations

Be guided by the mechanism of injury!

- Facial view Xrays can rule out many (but not all) facial fractures. These may only be used in low energy trauma situation
- CT head with specific sections for the facial fractures provide a lot more information
- Orthopantomogram (OPG) is good to visualize dental injuries and most of the mandible (except undisplaced parasymphyseal fractures).

Amputations

Amputations in this area usually result from inter-personal violence, including human bites. These will normally be repaired by a specialist service, hence the need for optimal preservation of the amputated part.

See the section about digital amputations, for storage and transfer details.

Tessier's principles

Wide exposure

Rigid internal fixation

Bone grafting of any substantial defects

Buttresses

The word buttress is a civil engineering/mechanical term to describe reinforced sections of a structure (usually a building) for the purpose of structural strength and stability.

In facial skeleton, a similar purpose is served by sections of thickened bone arranged in a vertical or a horizontal direction. These are called the vertical or horizontal buttresses of the facial skeleton.

Horizontal. Superior orbital rim, inferior orbital rim, palate
Vertical. Zygomatic (lateral orbital rim), naso-frontal (medial orbital rim), pterygo-maxillary

Word of caution

The following pages divide the maxillofacial trauma in separate entities, which is only strictly true in low velocity injuries. High speed RTAs can result in complex patterns that may follow the Le Fort scheme. However it still is useful as a widely understood classification system.

Similarly, CT scan has replaced Xray as the diagnostic modality of choice. The only exception being low energy trauma where you want to rule out zygomatic arch injury. OPGs are still useful to assess mandibular fractures.

Frontal sinus fracture

Signs & symptoms

GENERAL
Laceration, bruising, swelling, haematoma

SPECIFIC
Localised tenderness
CSF rhinorrhea
Epistaxis
Supra-orbital nerve anaesthesia

Important anatomical relations

Anteriorly	Supra-orbital nerve
Posteriorly	Meninges over frontal lobe, anterior cranial fossa
Inferiorly	Frontal sinus duct (into middle meatus), ethmoid air cells, orbital cavity

Complications

IMMEDIATE
Epistaxis
Intra-cranial haematoma
CSF leak
Meningitis

DAYS TO WEEKS
Sinusitis
Mucocele
Meningitis

MONTHS TO YEARS
Mucocele
Osteomyelitis
Intra-cranial / orbital abscesses

Management principles

Anterior wall minimally displaced fracture	Conservative
Anterior wall depressed fracture	Open reduction (via a coronal incision, to lift the bone fragments while keeping their periosteal blood supply intact)
Posterior wall undisplaced fracture	Conservative
Posterior wall comminuted fracture +/- CSF leak	Cranialisation (by neurosurgery team). It removes the whole posterior wall and the frontal lobe moves in to obliterate the space. A galeal flap is needed to obliterate the frontonasal duct and to keep the intracranical contents separate.

Naso-orbito-ethmoid (NOE) fractures

Signs & symptoms

GENERAL

Laceration, bruising

SPECIFIC

Signs of injury to the globe:
- Blood in anterior chamber (hyphaema)
- Subconjuctival hemorrhage
- Direct and consensual pupillary responses
- Change in visual acuity

Signs of injury to structures around the globe:
- Globe malposition (are they both at the same horizontal level and the relation between medial and lateral canthi is same bilaterally? Ref: Figure)
- Diplopia
- Ophthalmoplegia
- Bony tenderness +/- step-off

Signs of injury to the nose/ethmoid:
- Flattening of dorsum
- Nasal deviation
- Telecanthus (=increased distance between medial canthi, as opposed to "hypertelorism" which is true displacement of the bony orbit)
- Septal haematoma

An orbital fracture may involve the floor, medial wall (ethmoid air cells), lateral wall (with or without a zygomatic fracture) or apex.

Figure: Globe mal-position, with inferior dystopia of left globe [easily missed if you are not looking for it]

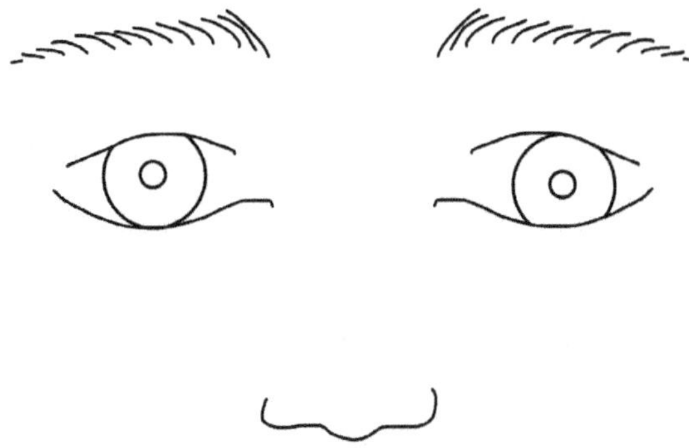

ORBITAL BLOWOUT FRACTURE

It is a pattern of injury of orbital floor where a localised sudden force applied to the inferior orbital rim (e.g. baseball or a fist) sets up a wave that transmits that force posteriorly. The initial force may be absorbed well by the thick buttress of bone provided by the inferior orbital rim and transmitted posteriorly. The posterior bone (i.e. the floor of the orbit) is very thin and readily fractures.

If the fracture is large enough, inferior orbital fat +/- inferior rectus can herniate through and become trapped. Clinically, the patient will have inferior orbital dystopia and inability to gaze upwards. Classically, the herniated fat looked liked a tear drop hanging from the roof of maxillary sinus ("tear drop sign"). In 2015, you should have a CT of the facial bones (helps you rule out intra-cranial, facial and c-spine injuries).

Pure blow out fractures only involve the orbital floor, while "impure blowout fractures" involve the adjacent bones too.

RELATIVE AFFERENT PUPILLARY DEFECT (RAPD)

= Marcus Gunn pupil

Injured pupil constricts when light is shone in *opposite* pupil, but not when directly into it. It implies a problem with retina / optic nerve (the afferent pathway) while the efferent pathway of pupillary reflex(oculomotor nerve) is intact.

Management of retrobulbar haemorrhage

It is a vision threatening condition due to bleeding behind the globe which compresses the optic nerve.

Signs include bruising around the eye, proptosis, increasing pain and ophthalmoplegia. Decrease in vision is relatively late and implies active compression of the optic nerve and immediate need for decompression. Hence check for extra-ocular muscle ROM and formal vision assessment *regularly* and document.

Management includes, good analgesia, head up positioning. If the surgeon is not immediately available acetazolamide and mannitol may buy some time (see section on Blephroplasty as well). Definitive treatment is lateral canthotomy. Make a subciliary incision at the lateral extent of lower lid. Carry it laterally over the lateral orbital rim. Use the lower lid tarsus to find the lateral canthal tendon. Protect globe and release the lateral canthal tendon near its attachment at the rim.

Important anatomical relations of orbit

Superior	Anterior cranial fossa
Medially	Ethmoid cells (separated by the very thin lamina papyracea)
Inferiorly	Infra-orbital nerve and vessels, maxillary sinus
Infero-lateral	Zygoma
Lateral	Lesser wing of sphenoid
Superior orbital fissure structures	CN 3,4,6 & V_1
Inferior orbital fissure structures	V_2 and branches, branches from pterygopalatine ganglion, infra-orbital vessels, emissary veins

Principles of management

Assuming ATLS assessment and that any other injuries have been appropriately addressed/prioritised, the principles are restoration of form and function.

FUNCTION

Maintenance of
- binocular vision,
- ocular mobility &
- patent bilateral nasal airway

FORM
- Stabilisation and reconstruction of buttresses

- Reconstruction of orbital walls
- Restoration of mid-face width
- Re-draping of soft tissues in normal anatomical relationship

Approaches to orbital floor

(see also, the approaches to facial fractures)

1. Transcutaneous
   - Subciliary. Incision at grey line down to the tarsus. Lift OO with skin. Stay on top of tarsus until its inferior edge to find the septum. Stay superficial to the septum until the inferior orbital rim. Then change plane by incising the septum to access the orbital floor. Gives an aesthetic scar.
   - (Converse's) Sub-tarsal. Incision at grey line but stay superficial to OO (i.e. skin only flap). Lift the skin-only flap to the level of lower border of tarsus. At the level of lower border of tarsus, go through OO to reach the superficial surface of the septum. Stay superficial to the septum until the inferior orbital rim, and then incise it to reach the orbital floor.
   - Skin only flap, up to the infra-orbital margin has been described but is very prone to ectropion.
2. Transconjunctival. Protect globe with malleable retractor. Incise conjunctiva at level of lower border of the tarsus. Go through capsulopalpebral fascia *and the septum* to reach the plane between OO and the septum. Dissect inferiorly until the inferior orbital rim, then incise the septum again to reach the orbital floor

Figure: Approaches to orbital floor

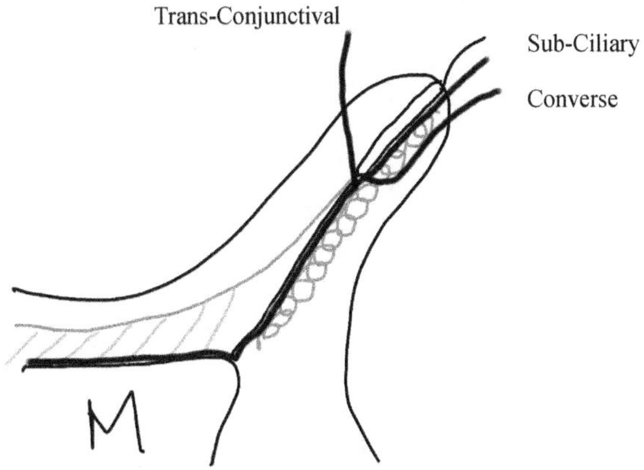

IMPLANT MATERIAL

Potentially, these can be autologous (e.g. split calvarium, iliac crest) or alloplastic (Titanium, Medpor etc.). Most places in UK use titanium mesh plates.

Complications

SUPERIOR ORBITAL FISSURE SYNDROME

1. Ptosis
2. Proptosis
3. Ophthalmoplegia
4. Forehead anaesthesia (from CN 3,4,6, V1 and swelling behind globe)

ORBITAL APEX SYNDROME

= Sup. orbital fissure syndrome + blindness (from Optic nerve compression)

NOSE

- Deviation
- Saddle nose deformity
- Septal perforation

Zygomatic fractures

Signs & symptoms

GENERAL
Laceration, bruising

SPECIFIC
Numbness of the cheek (Infra-orbital nerve or its branches)
Altered width of the mid face

Principles of management

(Assuming ATLS assessment and that any other injuries have been appropriately addressed/prioritised)

INDICATIONS FOR NON-OP. MANAGEMENT
Undisplaced fractures that are not comminuted

OPERATIVE INDICATIONS
Displaced, comminuted

OPERATIVE APPROACHES
1. Trans-oral approach using a buccal sulcus incision, insert a flat tipped elevator and lift the fracture fragment in place. Works well for isolated zygomatic arch fractures.
2. Temporal / indirect approach (Gillies' lift), which involves passing a flat ended instrument in Layer 4 (Ref: Neligan's Plastic surgery, volume 2*) to elevate the fracture fragments.
3. Bicoronal approach, for ORIF. Despite the large scar, exposure of zygoma is not very good.
4. (Direct approach), with an incision directly over the zygoma. Uncommonly used.

* Richard J. Warren, Peter C. Neligan MB. Plastic Surgery: Volume 2: Aesthetic Surgery (Expert Consult - Online and Print), 3e. 3 edition. London ; New York: Saunders; 2012. 924 p. Also see the discussion on anatomical basis of facelift.

Complications
Decreased width of face, asymmetry

Maxillary fractures

Signs & symptoms

GENERAL
Laceration, bruising
Crepitus

SPECIFIC
(see below)

LEFORT TYPES
Patterns of fractures described originally from cadaveric experiments, and before modern mechanism of injury were available [road traffic accidents]. Most modern fractures are comminuted and may not strictly adhere to this classification, but it is easy to remember and communicate.

	Fracture pattern	Clinical finding
Le Fort I	Transverse fracture of the maxilla. Pyramid not involved.	Maxillary teeth separated from rest of the facial skeleton. Occlusion altered. Crepitus
Le Fort II	Fracture line passes through the pyramid, but no higher	as above
Le Fort III	Fracture line passes through orbit. Craniofacial disjunction= if all 3 vertical buttresses are disrupted	The entire facial skeleton may slide inferior and posteriorly (in relation to the cranium). High risk to Airway!

Principles of management
(Assuming ATLS assessment and that any other injuries have been appropriately addressed/prioritised)
Restoration of form and function by
- Re-establishing buttresses, to restore mid facial height and projection [note that width is mostly due to zygoma]
- Restoration of occlusion

Complications
Malocclusion
Flattening of face

Mandibular fractures

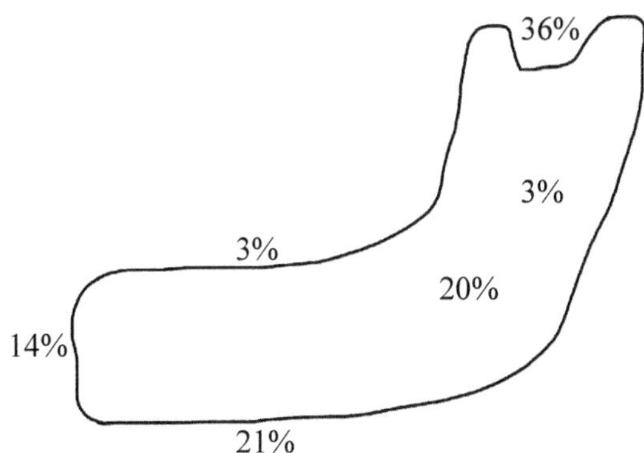

Figure: Incidence of fractures of mandible by location

Signs & symptoms

GENERAL
- Laceration &/or bruising, either on the skin, or intra-orally (FOM, bucco-gingival sulcus)
- Mal-occlusion
- Crepitus

SPECIFIC
- Numbness of chin (mental nerve)
- Trismus

Principles of management

(Assuming ATLS assessment and that any other injuries have been appropriately addressed/prioritised)

Mandible fractures can be described as favourable or unfavourable depending on how the muscles attached to the major fracture fragments interact with the fracture configuration. A favourable fracture is where the fracture configuration prevents displacement, while an unfavourable fracture is where it does not.

The tendency for displacement (or its prevention) may be in the vertical plane or horizontal, hence the terms vertically or horizontally favourable/unfavourable. (Ref: Figure)

Figure: Forces acting to displace the mandible

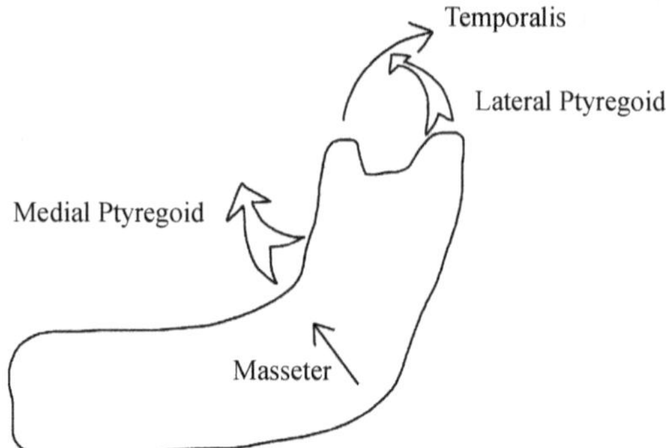

Figure: a) Vertically favourable, b) Vertically *un*favourable fracture

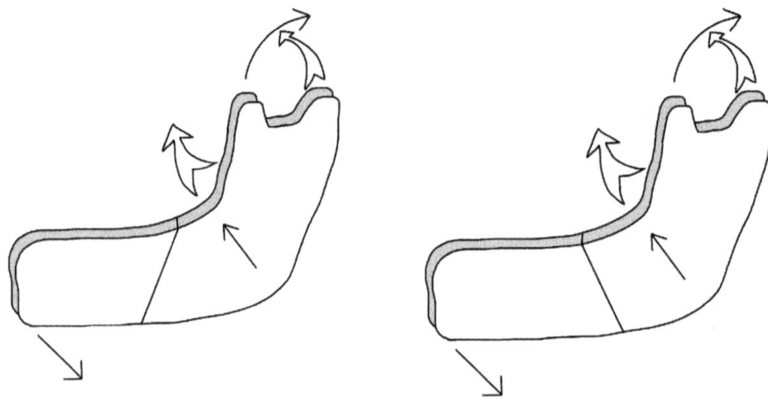

Figure: a) Horizontally favourable, b) Horizontally *un*favourable fracture

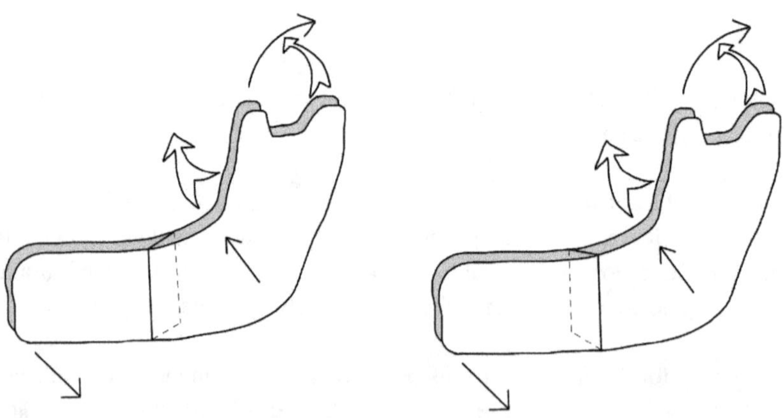

In addition to the muscular forces, mandible is also subject to occlusal forces. In this case, the ramus and body of mandible behave like a cantilever. These forces tend to rotate the free edge of the cantilever down, resulting in a tension force across the top of the cantilever (i.e. the dental/occlusal surface) and a corresponding compression force at its caudal surface (Ref: Figure).

Figure: Principle of fixation of madibular ramus. a) the lateral view resembles a cantilever, b) Tendancy for deformation of the cantilever under an applied force, c) plane of zero net force

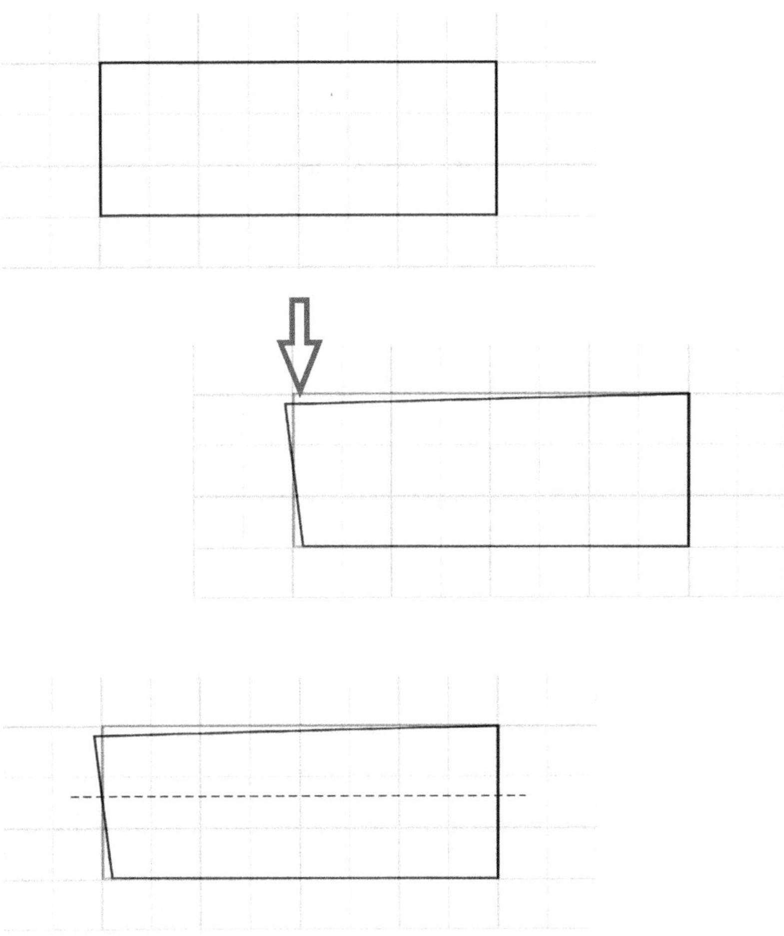

Naturally, there is a plane somewhere in the thickness of the cantilever, where the tension forces (from the top) and the compression forces (at the bottom) cancel out. This is the ideal position for the placement of a mini-plate (to fix an underlying fracture). Anatomically, this corresponds to the line between the mental foramina for fixation of para-symphyseal fractures. (More laterally, you have to take into consideration the location of the roots of the teeth, and presence of mental nerve).

Complications

Skin & soft tissues

- Scars
- Infection

Bone & joint

- Malunion
- Nonunion
- Failure of metal work, from movement at fracture site +/- infection
- TMJ ankylosis, from prolonged immobilisation

Panfacial fractures

GENERAL

Laceration, bruising

(Beware of intra-oral bleeding, that may compromise breathing)

SPECIFIC

Specific to each site involved

(Assuming ATLS assessment and that any other injuries have been appropriately addressed/prioritised)

There are 2 ways to sequence the reconstruction of the facial skeleton. In either sequence, reconstruction of the buttresses takes priority. In any complex injury, 3D reconstruction of CT can guide approach, sequencing and fixation.

1. Establish occlusion and then address the more cranial fractures.
   - If either dental arch is intact (i.e. mandible intact, maxilla intact, or Le Fort I fracture only), it is fairly simple to identify occlusion and establish maxilo-mandibular fixation.
   - If both dental arches are disrupted, the situation is more difficult. Reconstruct one and use it as template to reconstruct the other.
2. Start cranially and proceed caudally. Reconstruct the mid-face and then proceed caudally

FORM

Scars, Edema, Atrophy of tissues, Asymmetry

Mucocele

FUNCTION

Occlusion, Mastication

TMJ dysfunction

Sensory-motor dysfunction

Head and neck

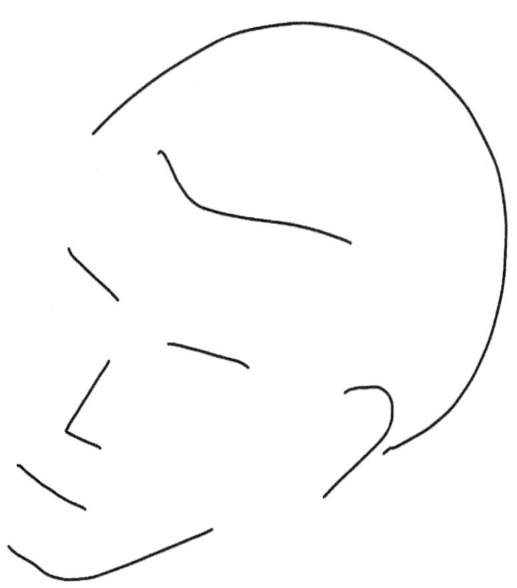

Head & neck cancer

CORE KNOWLEDGE
Principles of management
SCC
Parotid
Neck dissection

APPROACH TO PATIENT - HISTORY
Age, occupation, hobbies, who is at home
PMHx, Meds, Allergies

Risk factors for primary. Alcohol, smoking, ill fitting dentures, Betel nut chewing (esp. south asian population)

Symptomatic synchronous tumour Blocked nose, sore throat, hoarseness, dysphagia

The swelling in question
Duration
Symptoms e.g. pain, sore throat, hoarseness, dysphagia
Any previous malignancies
What management has been done so far?
Is there a current MDT / other management plan? (Of course, in exam you will have to come up with this plan)

APPROACH TO PATIENT - EXAMINATION
Intra-oral examination:
- Swelling. Site, size, shape, fixity etc
- Systematic intra-oral examination. Palate, alveolus, buccal mucosa, BOT, RMT
- Bimanual intra-oral examination

Regional lymph nodes +/- FNA of any accessible node
Direct / indirect laryngoscopy

APPROACH TO PATIENT - MANAGEMENT
See below for an overview. Please refer to the NCCN or SIGN90 guidelines for details.

EXPECTED CLINICAL QUESTIONS

- Management of "lump" in neck
- Neck dissection. Types, Levels & their boundaries
- Parotid swelling

RECOMMENDED PAPERS

1. Chummun S, McLean NR, Ragbir M. Surgical education: neck dissection. *Br J Plast Surg*. 2004 Oct;57(7):610–23.
2. Pfister DG. American Society of Clinical Oncology Clinical Practice Guideline for the Use of Larynx-Preservation Strategies in the Treatment of Laryngeal Cancer. *J Clin Oncology*. 2006 May 25;24(22):3693–704.
3. Shah JP, Gil Z. Current concepts in management of oral cancer – Surgery. *Oral Oncology*. 2009 Apr;45(4-5):394–401.
4. McCammon SD, Shah JP. Radical neck dissection. *Operative Techniques in Otolaryngology-Head and Neck Surgery*. 2004 Sep;15(3):152–9.
5. Mehanna H, McQueen A, Robinson M, Paleri V. Salivary gland swellings. *BMJ* [Internet]. 2012;345. Available from: http://www.bmj.com/content/345/bmj.e6794
6. SIGN 90 guidelines: Diagnosis and management of head and neck cancer.
7. Effective head and neck cancer management: Third consensus document. British Association of Otorhinolaryngologists Head and Neck Surgeon. London, 2002

Principles of management

A. Obtain a tissue diagnosis of the primary
B. Assess local involvement (clinically, radiologically initially with OPG, then later with CT. MRI may be needed in select cases to know the resectability of disease)
C. Clinical Staging to assess regional and distant involvement (Primaries with high risk of mets needs surgical staging procedures as well)
D. Discuss in the MDT, where further management is the dictated primarily by disease factors (site, size, resectability, risk of occult disease) but also by patient factors (e.g. comorbidities)

MDT panel:
- ENT, MaxFax, Plastics Head & neck surgeons
- Radiologist, Pathologist, Specialist nurses

Diagnostic investigations

1. OPG, is a screening tool to rule out mandibular invasion
2. Tissue diagnosis by incision biopsy (under GA) +/- FNA of any suspect lymph node

Staging investigations

1. **Endoscopy by ENT**. SIGN90 guidelines say flexible nasoendoscopy for everyone and symptomatically directed direct laryngoscopy, oesophagoscopy and bronchoscopies. (In practice if the patient is having a general anaesthetic for a biopsy/endoscopy most people would perform panendoscopy in the same procedure. Each endoscopy involves visualising the respective structures, taking tissue samples from any suspicious lesion and taking random samples from high-risk areas like base of tongue).
2. **CT head & neck**, as there is 20% risk of occult mets at diagnosis
3. **CT Chest**, to identify metastases or synchronous tumours.
4. (MRI), in difficult cases to identify tissue planes and determine resectability

Management of primary

Surgery is (theoretically) equivalent to radiotherapy, but (practically speaking) if patient has a recurrence after radiotherapy, doing salvage surgery is a lot more difficult. Therefore most surgeons prefer surgery first and reserve radiotherapy for poor surgical candidates.

Surgery involves wide local excision of the tumour, to achieve histologically clear margins.

MARGINS

- Surgical margins for WLE of primary disease are ideally 1.5 to 2 cm
- Histological clearance of more than 5 mm is considered a "clear" margin
- Histological clearance of less than 5 mm is considered "close" margin

(Of course tumour abutting any histologic plane is an "involved" margin)

MANAGEMENT OF INVOLVED MANDIBLE

- Rim resection, if the mandibular canal is not involved
- Segmental resection, if the mandibular canal is involved. The reason being that extension of tumour in the mandibular canal can result in rapid (& wider) spread.

Management of neck

1. Clinically (=exam + CT) negative necks (N0 neck)

CONSIDERATION

- >20% occult mets in oral primaries
- >50% metastases in oropharyngeal primaries
- Despite regular follow up, some patients with occult disease can progress to in-operable tumors

RX

- Rx options are surgery or radiotherapy (but surgery chosen for same logic as above)
- Surgical staging is done by supra-omohyoid dissection (Levels I-III) on intra-oral cancers

2. Clinically N1 neck

CONSIDERATION

Neck dissection is as effective as radiotherapy

RX

Appropriate selective neck dissection only

(Post neck dissection) If high-risk, then external beam radiotherapy (EBRT) for,

- closed/involved margin,
- any neural/lympho-vascular invasion,
- >3 cm node, extracapsular spread

3. Clinically N2/3 neck

Comprehensive neck dissection,

Followed by EBRT +/- cisplatin ("chemo-radio")

4. Elective dissection of contralateral neck

For

- Advanced tumour
- Midline tumour
- Multiple ipsilateral nodal involvement

5. Chemo-radio

Can be offered as adjuvant treatment, or (rarely) as a primary modality

Indications for radiotherapy + cisplatin chemotherapy

- Tumour cannot be adequately protected
- Patients condition precludes surgery
- Patient does not wish to have surgical resection

PRE-OP ASSESSMENT:

1. Nutritional. To determine postop nutritional requirements and whether those could be met with orally (unusual), via NG (if tolerated and for short periods only) or gastrostomy (more likely)
2. Dental. Esp. if postop. radiotherapy is expected (large tumor, marginal resection, aggressive histology - see below)

Surgical approaches to primary

1. Per-oral, esp. small anteriorly placed tumours
2. Sagittal split osteotomy, for relatively posterior tumours
3. Visor flap, esp. FOM / midline
4. Lower cheek flap
5. (Upper cheek flap) via Weber Ferguson incision if maxilla is involved

The exact choice of approach also depends on whether you are doing a neck dissection at the same time ;)

Post surgical considerations

INDICATIONS FOR POSTOP RADIOTHERAPY

= high risk of recurrence

- >3cm node
- extra capsular spread
- close / +ve surgical margins
- perineural / vascular invasion

Management of recurrence

Re-stage with CT

Assess resectability with MRI

Discuss in MDT

Re-operate if resectable, else radiotherapy +/- chemo

Oral cancer

Sites:

Buccal mucosa, FOM, anterior tongue, alveolar ridge, RMT, hard palate

Table: Summary of management strategies for oral cancer

	Early	Advanced
Rx option	Surgery = RT* Brachy better than EBRT Note, RT gives r/o ORN if bone is involved	Combination surgery & RT Accelerated RT/ hyperfractionation
	20-40% ↑ r/o extracapsular midline have ↑ r/o bilateral involvement	N2 & N3 need surgery + chemo-radio
Commonest levels involved	I, II & III <1% r/o level V involv. wrt locoregional control & survival: RND = MRND supraomohyoid > MRND	

*Surgery = RT but a recurrence after surgery is easier to manage (re-operate +/- RT) than a recurrence after RT (because its a poor surgical plane & you can't redo RT as well).

Parotid tumors

APPROACH TO PATIENT - HISTORY

Age, occupation, fit and well
How long ago, suddenly, slowly
One side or both
Pain or redness, discharge inside mouth
Changes with meals
Weakness of face
Tingling on face

APPROACH TO PATIENT - EXAMINATION

Look:

- Site
- Size
- Skin induration/involvement
- Facial asymmetry

Feel:

- Fixity of skin
- Lymph notes
- CN VII
- Intra oral examination. Bimanual parotid, Stenson's duct

APPROACH TO PATIENT - INVESTIGATIONS

USS guided FNA indicates benign vs malignant (pro= simple, inexpensive. con=inconclusive result does not rule out malignancy). Many centres do USS guided FNA within the MDT clinic setting, allowing rapid access and results.

If USS shows malignancy,
- Staging CT (to identify loco-regional disease) and
- MRI (for better visualisation of tissue planes, esp. deep lobe of parotid)

Tissue diagnosis for an unspecified lump is either FNAC or biopsy. FNAC may miss invasive cancer so for high risk swellings of the parotid tissue, diagnosis is best done by a biopsy. Due to presence of the facial nerve, a trucut biopsy is not a good option. An adequate "biopsy" specimen for the parotid is superficial parotidectomy. For benign lesions it is therapeutic, and for malignant lesions the procedure can be upstaged to total parotidectomy and combined with a neck dissection if needed.

RECOMMENDED PAPER
Mehanna et al. BMJ 2012

Causes of salivary swellings

1. Obstruction
2. Infection
3. Inflammation
4. Systemic conditions
5. Neoplasia
    A. Benign
    B. Malignant

Benign parotid tumors

[Note that most of these are adenomas]
Pleomorphic ademona, 50%
Papillary cyst-adenoma (Warthin's tumor) 5-10%
Other adenomas (basal cell, cancalicular), 5-10%
Oncocytoma, 1%

Malignant parotid tumors

Muco-epidermoid CA, 15% (of all parotid tumours)
AdenoCA, 10%
Adenoid-cystic CA, 5%
Acinic cell CA, 5%
CA ex pleomorphic adenoma

CONCERNING SIGNS
The following should prompt concerns about invasive CA in parotid (which may be primary or secondary)
On history
- Rapid increase in size
- Increasing pain

Patient's PMHx
- Known skin CA (esp scalp)
- RT to H&N
- Autoimmune condition eg Sjogren's

Examination
- Overlying skin ulceration / fixity
- CN VII weakness
- Adjacent cutaneous paraesthesia

Examination is like that of any "surgical lump", but emphasise these:
Look
- Swelling
- Skin
- Induration
- Ipsilateral facial droop

Feel
- Tenderness
- Fixity to skin
- Bimanual examination (with a gloved finger)

Move
- Muscles of facial expression (i.e. branches of CN VII)
- (In the end, check stapedius and ask for tears and taste)

Neck dissection

Types

Although many classifications have been devised, Medina's classification is the most widely known and understood.

A. Selective. According to levels of dissection
B. Comprehensive. Removes Levels I-V
    1. Radical (RND). Also removes IJV, SCM & CN XI
    2. Modified radical (MRND). Preserves one or more of the above structures. *
       • Type 1, preserves CN XI
       • Type 2, preserved CN XI & IJV
       • Type 3, preserves CN XI, IJV & SCM
    3. Extended radical neck dissection. Removes another non-lymphatic structure e.g. parotid

* It is best to document in the op note as to which structures you are preserving, to minimise any confusion later

Indications

FOR SELECTIVE NECK DISSECTION

Clinically negative necks (cN0), as a staging procedure in cancers at high risk of occult metastases

FOR MODIFIED RADICAL NECK DISSECTION

Some clinically +ve necks e.g.
- mobile, <3cm nodes
- removing residual disease after down staging with RT

FOR RADICAL NECK DISSECTION

T3 (>6cm primary)
Gross extra-capsular spread
Involvement of structures wanting to preserve

Procedure

INCISIONS

- Tri-radiate, 3 straight lines meet over the carotid bifurcation
- Hayes-Martin, "wine-glass" shape
- Schobinger / modified Schobinger, commonest
- McFee, for irradiated necks

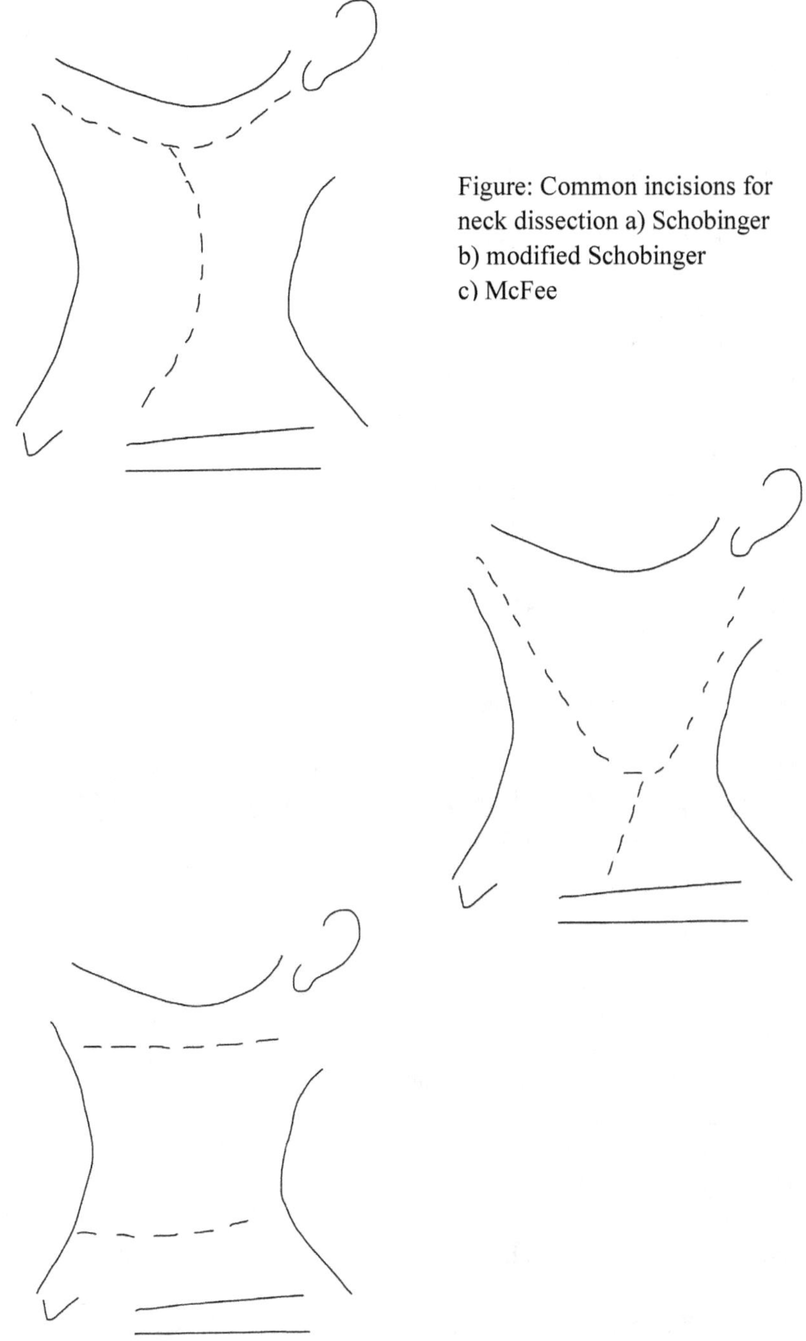

Figure: Common incisions for neck dissection a) Schobinger b) modified Schobinger c) McFee

Each surgeon has a favourite incision for the procedure. Schobinger (and its modifications) are the commonest incisions used for neck dissection. It avoids placing the confluence of two scars over the carotid bifurcation (which was the down side of Hayes-Martin "champagne glass" or tri-radiate incisions). McFee incision is a bipedicle flap used in irradiated necks which though difficult to raise, preserves better blood supply.

POSTERIOR SKIN FLAP
CN XI
Great auricular nerve
Omohyoid
Transverse cervical vessels
Brachial plexus, Phrenic nerve
Lymphatics

ANTERIOR SKIN FLAP
Carotid sheath (IJV, common carotid artery, CN X)
Ansa cervicalis, whch leads to CN XII superiorly

SUPERIOR SKIN FLAP
Marginal mandibular nerve
Facial vessels
Sub-mandibular gland + lingual nerve & Wharton's duct

Surgical complications
[The following is not an exhaustive list]

Scar
Bleeding, needing transfusion
Haematoma, needing urgent return to theatre
Wound infection / breakdown

Loss of sensation over lower half of pinna (great auricular n.)
Paraesthesias (temporary / rarely permanent):
- marginal mandibular nerve → oral incontinence
- CN XI (if preserved) → shoulder drop
- CN XII → weakness of tongue

Arrythmias (mediated by carotid body)

Chyle leak, which may necessitate fat free diet (for several days to a few weeks)

Rare but important:

- Upgrading to bilateral neck dissection intra-operatively.
- Tracheostomy (in bilateral neck dissection, esp. if both IJVs need to be removed)
- Head and neck plethora (in bilateral cases after removal of both IJVs)
- Death

Management of IJV bleed

Avoid, avoid, avoid!
The risk of injury is much higher if the tumour is encasing the IJV

- Inform anaesthetist, scrub nurse and theatre team
- Direct pressure to stop haemorrhage until you get everything ready
- Arm your assistant with a suction cannula
- Assess if you have/can get proximal and distal control
- Ask for partially occluding non-traumatic clamps
- Gentle release and suction to identify bleeding point
- Many a times it is a small side branch requiring careful bipolar cautery
- Any injury to IJV proper needs an appropriate repair while maintaining control of the vessel with a partially occluding non-traumatic clamp.

Levels of neck dissection

	Anterior	Posterior	Superior	Inferior
I **(Anterior triangle)** Ia=submental Ib=sub mandibular	Midline	Clinically: posterior belly of digastric Radiologically: posterior border of submandibular gland	Mandibular border	-
II **(Level of upper 1/3rd of SCM)** IIa = anterior to XI IIb= posterior to XI	Clinically: Lateral borders of sterno- & stylo-hyoid muscles (approx. anterior border of SCM) Radiologically: posterior boundary of level I	Posterior border of SCM	Skull base	Clinically: junction of upper and mid 1/3rds of SCM = Hyoid bone

	Anterior	Posterior	Superior	Inferior
III **(Level of middle 1/3rd of SCM)**	Lateral border of sternohyoid (approx. anterior border of SCM)	Posterior border of SCM	Clinically: (inferior border of) hyoid	Clinically: inferior border of cricoid cartilage
IV **(Level of lower 1/3rd of SCM)**	Lateral border of sternohyoid (approx. anterior border of SCM)	Posterior border of SCM	Clinically: inferior border of cricoid cartilage	Clavicle
V **(Posterior triangle)** Va = above level of cricoid arch Vb= below the level of cricoid arch	Posterior border of SCM	Lateral border of trapezius	-	Clavicle
VI **(Para- tracheal and paraesophge al)**	-	-	Skull base	Thoracic inlet
VII **(superior mediastinm)**				

Note, that Level I sits astride the midline and a "unilateral" neck dissection at Level I involves going across the midline to the contralateral anterior belly of digastric.

Head & Neck - Major recon

CORE KNOWLEDGE
Approach to head and neck cancers
BOT

APPROACH TO PATIENT - HISTORY
Primary diagnosis
Its prognosis
What treatment has been given so far? Excision/re-excision/XRT
What treatment is planned? esp XRT
What is the MDT decision? Named McMillan nurse?

PMHx, Meds, Allergies

Social situation
How is it currently affecting ADL
Consider how will the recon affect ADL

APPROACH TO PATIENT - EXAMINATION
Defect - site, size, sub-units involved, layers involved
Surrounding area - signs of loco-regional spread, laxity of tissues, potential donors
Regional lymph nodes
Distant donor sites - for free tissue transfer

APPROACH TO PATIENT - TREATMENT
Manage underlying condition in a MDT setting
Recon option are based on the missing tissue layers and defect size
Rehab will depend on the ADLs affected and patient's social situation

EXPECTED CLINICAL QUESTIONS
Any number of small, medium and large size defects on various anatomical locations

RECOMMENDED PAPERS
1. Selected Readings in Plastic Surgery
2. Urken, ML, Weinberg, H, Vickery, C, Buchbinder, D, Lawson, W, and Biller, HF. Oromandibular reconstruction using microvascular composite free flaps. Report of 71 cases and a new classification scheme for bony, soft-

tissue, and neurologic defects. *Arch Otolaryngol Head Neck Surg.* 1991; 117: 733–744

Oropharyngeal reconstruction

Depends on the size of the defect and the missing tissues (like any where else in plastic surgery)

Defect	Reconstruction option
Small soft tissue only	SSG
Large soft tissue only eg. FOM, gums, buccal mucosa	Free tissue transfer eg RFFF
Mandible	
Rim resection	Restoration of dentition
Segmental resection Central / Lateral / Hemi-mandibular	Free fibula (usually contralateral)

Figure: a) rim resection, if mandibular canal is not involved, b) segmental resection

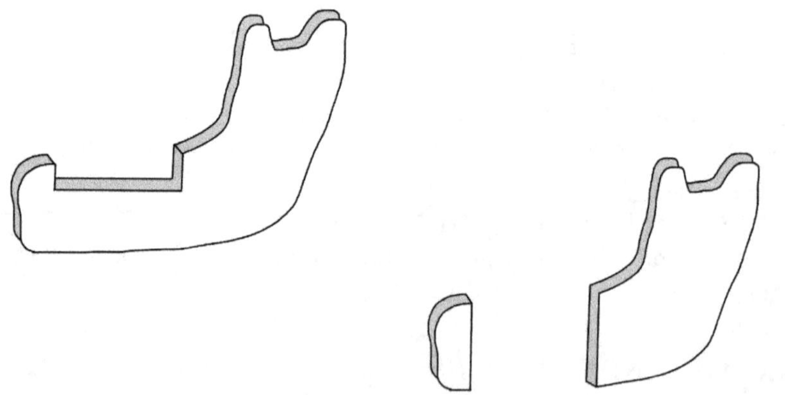

Scalp reconstruction

Assuming it is not amenable to direct closure

Option	Notes
Heal by 2nd intent	Rarely used (e.g. donor site of forehead flap)
FTSG	For small areas, if pericranium is intact. eg. small skin cancer removed
SSG	For large areas, if pericranium intact eg. skin cancers with large area of field change
Skin substitute + SSG	
TE	Can cover up to 50% of scalp. Commonly used in younger patients. CI = infection, irradiation
Random pattern flaps	eg rhomboid, or V-Y advancement from the more lax temporal skin. Pin wheel flap is a modification of several rhomboid flaps for defects on the vertex
Axial pattern flaps	eg. as described by Juri (based on superficial temporal artery), Orticochea (multiple transposition flaps based on superficial temporal and occipital vessels) (Ref: Figure)
Free tissue transfer	most common recipient vessels are the superficial temporal

Figure: Juri flap, is a local transposition flap that hides the scar in the anterior hair line.

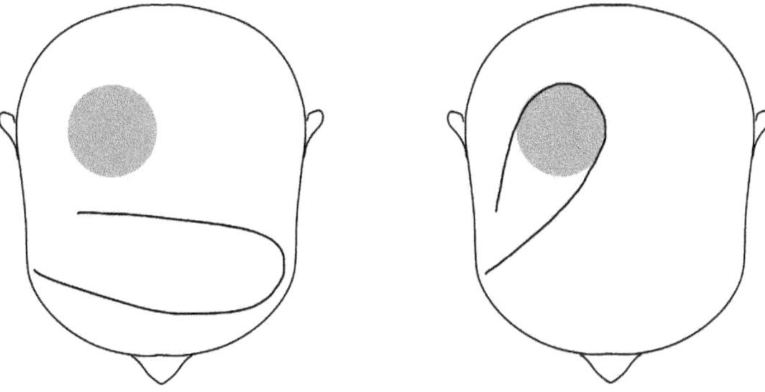

Opinion:

While planning a reconstruction (esp.) with any flap, you have to consider
- the underlying pathology,
- its prognosis,
- risk of field change and,
- a bailout procedure if the disease recurs/extends.

Most commonly encountered skin cancers are related to a field change in the area, the skin in very thin in this patient group and deep clearance is not always guaranteed. Also, the patient is at risk for developing further lesions, hence local flaps are not a good option for that.

Large defects (of scalp alone) are most commonly reconstructed using a 2 stage procedure employing a dermal substitute.

Large composite defects need free tissue transfer (probably over a titanium plate by the neurosurgical colleagues).

So the large local flaps (e.g. Orticochea's 3 flap or 4 flap) , at best, occupy only a small niche of defects e.g. when the outer table has been breached but you want/need to cover the defect with a single stage procedure (may be your patient isn't the fittest), or you are in a part of the world with no skin substitute or microsurgical facility. There is a reason that most books only show line drawings of these flap procedures and reference a book written in 1970s i.e. the pre-free flap era.

Forehead reconstruction

Do consider the sub-unit principle

Option	Notes
(2nd intent)	rare
Direct closure	consider if the best scar will be horizontal or vertical
SSG alone	e.g. sheet graft from supra-clavicular donor site
SSG over a periosteal flap	
(SSG using "Crane principle")	i.e. 2 stage procedure where a donor tissue is brought as a local flap, allowed to gain a vascular bed, then the top layer ("the crane") is moved back to its original site leaving a vascularised graftable bed. Almost by definition it means there is no periosteum for a conventional graft. Leaves scars at 2 places. Rarely used now, considering availability of skin substitutes and free tissue transfer
SSG with dermal substitute	Modern approach to reconstructing any sizeable clean defect
Local flaps	Small defect: e.g. Bilateral uni-pedicle advancement ("H-flap"), "yin-yang" flap, bilateral V-Y advancement, rhomboid (on temporal area). Large defects: shutter flap, Worthen flap (Ref: Figure)
TE	
Free tissue transfer	

Figure: a) Shutter flap

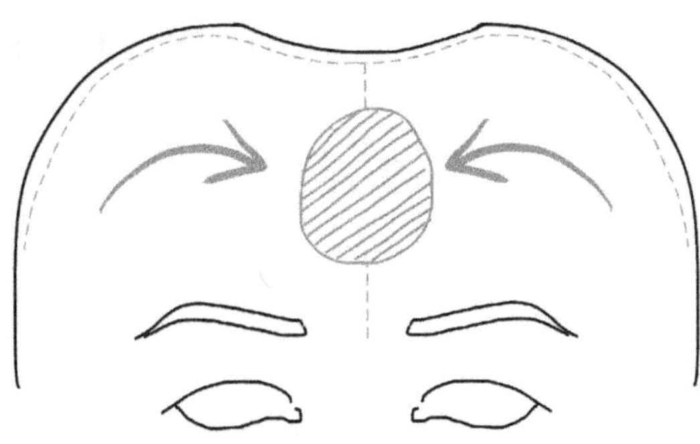

Figure (contd.): b) Worthen flap

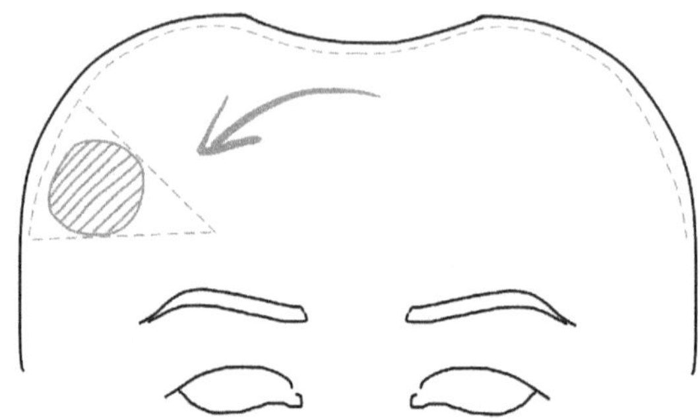

Eyebrow reconstruction

PROBLEMS
Hair are very thin, slow growing, oriented along different directions and come out nearly horizontal

PARTIAL DEFECT
Consider local flaps, as long as they don't move the land marks

LARGE PARTIAL / TOTAL DEFECT
1. Hair transplant. As long as there is a good vascularised (non-scarred) bed, this is a very good option as the hair direction can be addressed.
2. (Hair strip grafts). Need a vascularised bed and the grafted hair will all align in their own direction.
3. (Pedicled scalp flap) have been described but don't add a major benefit.

Eyelid reconstruction

[The best algorithm is in Grabb & Smith, although you will want to modify it according to your practice.]

Key points:
- Correct abnormality of bony orbit
- Provide eyelid opening / closing and lacrimal drainage
- Proper positioning of lateral and medial canthi

Figure: Cross section of upper and lower eyelids

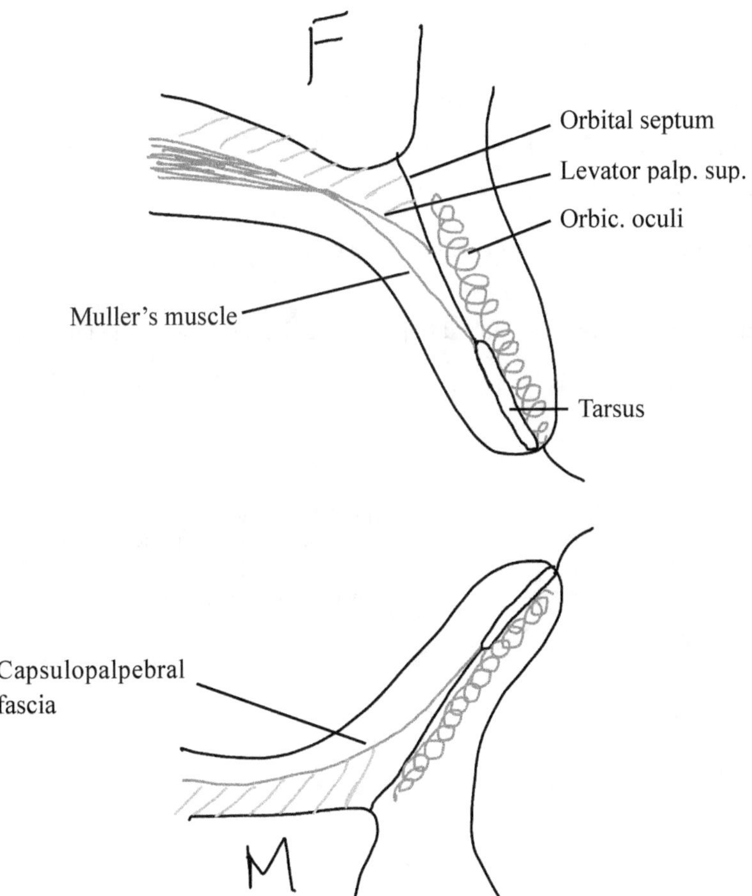

Nose recon

SKIN ONLY

Random pattern flap	Banner flap Bilobed flap ("Zitelli") Glabellar flap
Axial pattern flap	Reiger flap Nasolabial flap Cheek flap
Regional flap	Forehead flap Washio flap

Common options are:

Forehead flap	For large reconstructions
Nasolabial flap	For alar rim
Reiger flap	For dorsum
Bilobed flap	For side wall (see below)

Figure: Construction of a bilobed flap (assume the defect is on the left sidewall of nose)

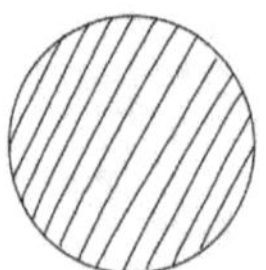

Find the line where you want to hide your scar. This tends to be at the border of lateral nasal wall and cheek aesthetic subunits.

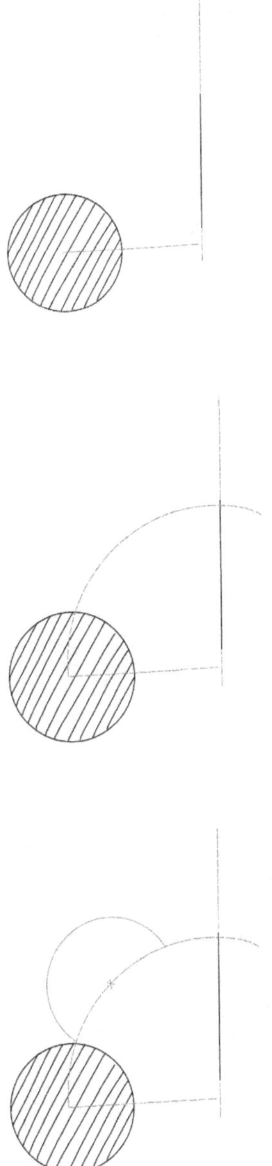

Extend this line in either direction.
Join the centre of your defect with your first line at an angle of 90-100°. This gives you your pivot point.

With this pivot point as the centre and radius equal to the defect centre, draw an arc from your defect to the line of closure.

On this arc, mark a semicircle of diameter exactly same as the defect. This is the first "lobe".

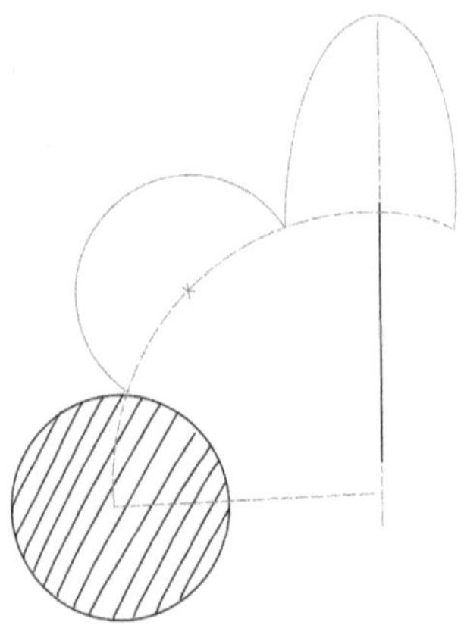

From the distal end of the semicircle, to the previously marked straight line, is *half width* of the 2nd lobe.

First judge the complete width of the 2nd lobe. Your previously marked straight line should bisect it. Then pinch this width (of 2nd lobe) to make sure the defect will close.

The vertical dimension of the flap should preferably keep the tip at/ below the level of medial canthus.

With its width & length determined, draw a curve to join all three, aiming to enclose an area approximately the same that of the 1st lobe.

Undermine up to the pivot point and transpose the flap.

Start closure from the defect left by the 2nd lobe.

Figure: Nasolabial transposition flap

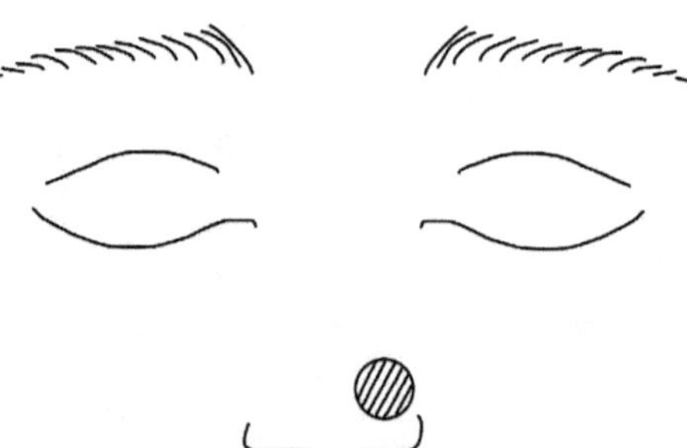

Figure (contd.): Nasolabial transposition flap

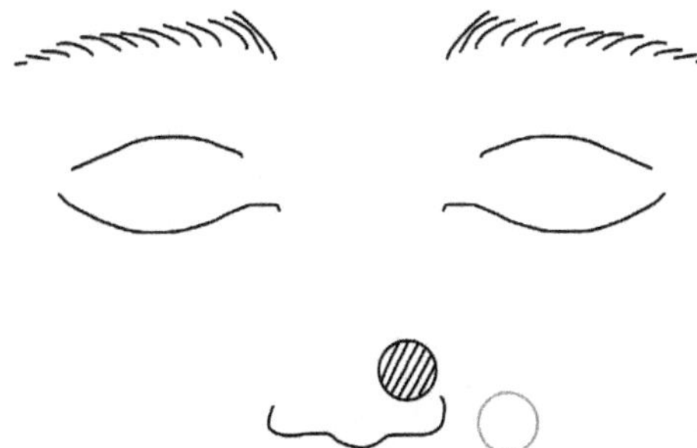

1. Mark out a suitable donor that is,
- 10% bigger than the defect
- has enough laxity to allow direct closure
- at a site that will hide the scar well (i.e. NLF)

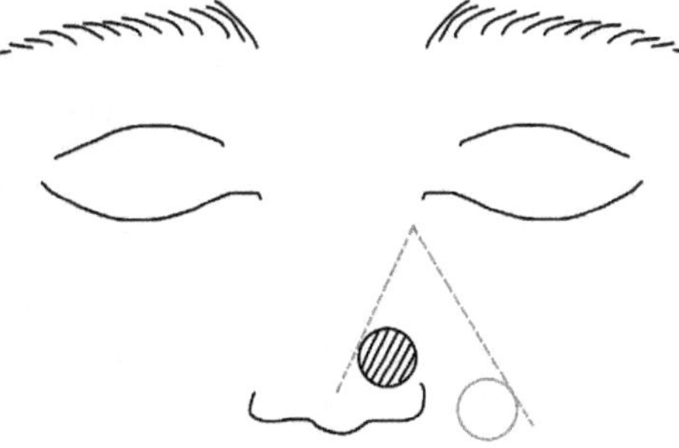

2. Draw tangents from either, which meet at the pivot point at an acute angle.

A smaller angle $\Rightarrow$ less risk of dog ear, but
- it may carry the pivot point too high,
- it increases the area sacrificed to allow the flap to sit

Aesthetically, it is best to keep the pivot point below the level of medial canthus.

The balance of these factors will determine the pivot point.

Figure (contd.): Nasolabial transposition flap

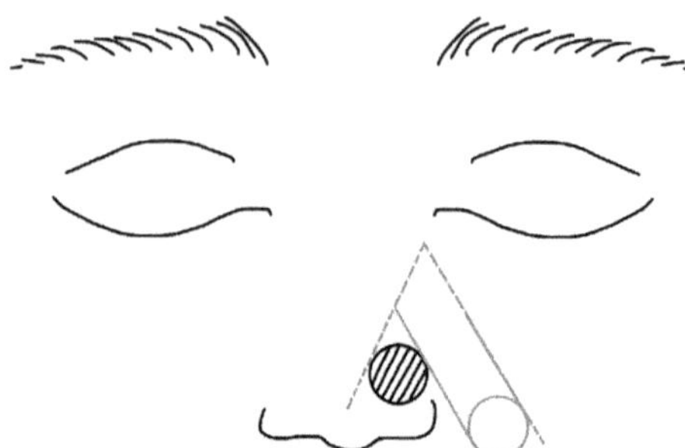

3. Mark and incise the medial tangent of the donor (up to the tangent from the defect)

4. Mark and start incising the lateral incision and raising the flap. Cut as you go, and keep checking how the flap sits in the donor defect.

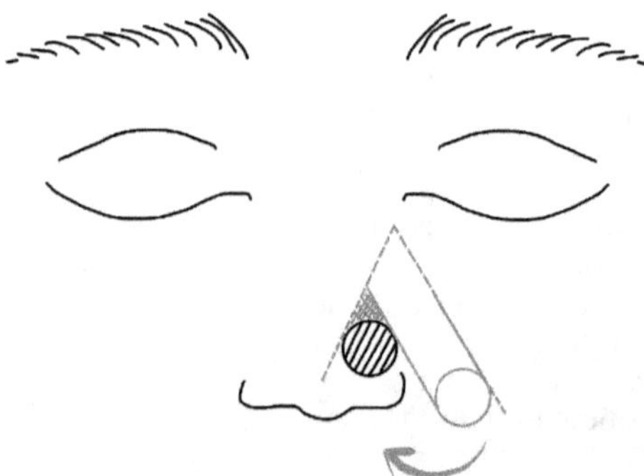

5. Close the donor defect first. The flap should now sit well.

6. Remove the triangular piece of tissue adjacent to the defect, to allow the flap to sit.

NASAL SUPPORT

Hinged septal flap (Millard 1967)	Its an L-shaped flap of part of septum hinged superiorly at caudal end of nasal bones & swung anteriorly (Ref: Figure)
Septal pivot flap (Gillies 1920)	Entire septum is rotated, based inferiorly on septal branch of superior labial artery. Any excess is removed.
Cantilever graft	using bone (eg rib which is fixed rigidly), or rib cartilage (is more pliable)
L - strut	Hockey stick shaped rib graft
Alloplastic	e.g. titanium, vitallium, medpore, but risk of extrusion

Figure: Hinged septal flap

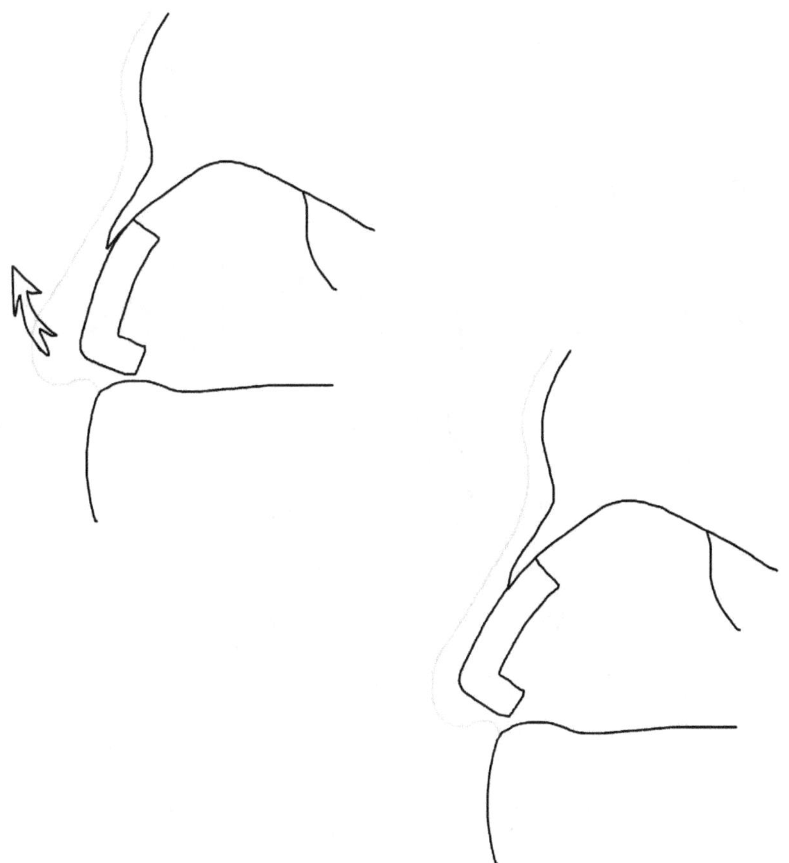

Figure: Septal pivot flap

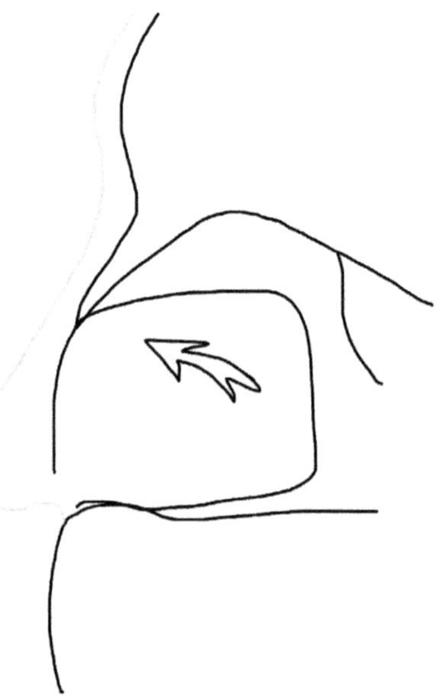

Figure: Cantilever graft

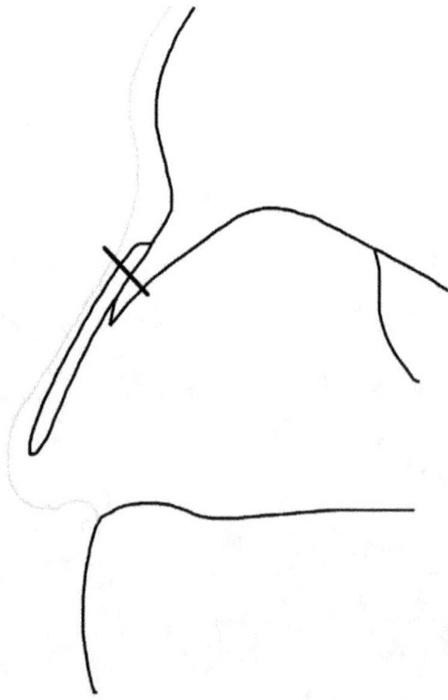

NASAL LINING

SSG	by itself, or to the inside of a forehead flap
Local flap	• Bipedicle mucosal advancement (& allowing donor defect to heal by 2nd intent) works only for small defects • Ipsilateral septal mucoperchondrial flap (Burget & Menick described this variation of the Gillies septal pivot flap) • Contralateral septal mucosa + septum (= "septal door" flap)
Regional flap	• Nasolabial flap (tends to be bulky) • Forehead flap folded inwards (will need a rather long forehead flap. There may not be enough donor site and you may end up going too lateral on the forehead making part of it random pattern)

Cheek recon

Sub-units:
- Suborbital
- Pre-auricular
- Bucco-mandibular

For smaller defects, local random pattern flaps provide a good option, esp. in patients with enough skin laxity. Large defects bordering the nasal aesthetic unit or lid margin can be reconstructed with Mustarde cheek advancement flap.

Figure: Mustarde cheek advancement. It is important to take the incision superiorly just lateral to lateral canthus, to prevent the lateral canthus from being pulled inferiorly as the scar settles. The incision can, theoretically, be carried down to the base of the neck to create a (very) large anteriorly based cervico-facial flap.

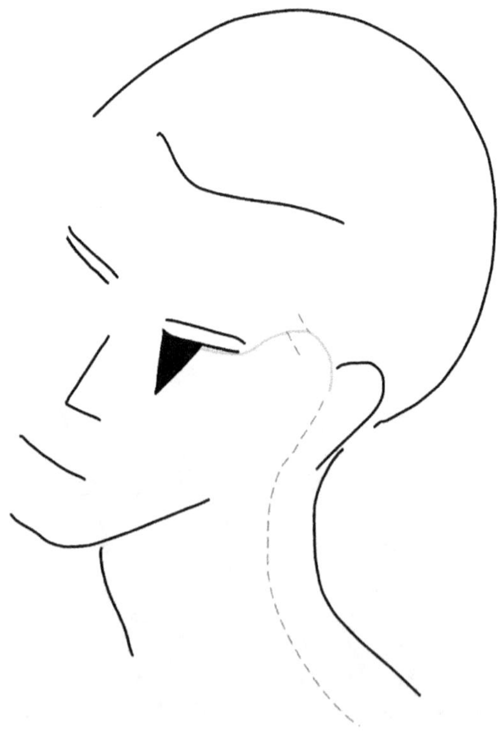

Upper lip recon

< 1/3rd

Central defect	Abbe flap (Ref: Figure)
Lateral defect	Direct closure (if through & through) Peri-alar crescenteric excision (if skin only)
Vermilion intact	Nasolabial flap (Ref: Figure)

Figure: Abbe flap (described 1898)

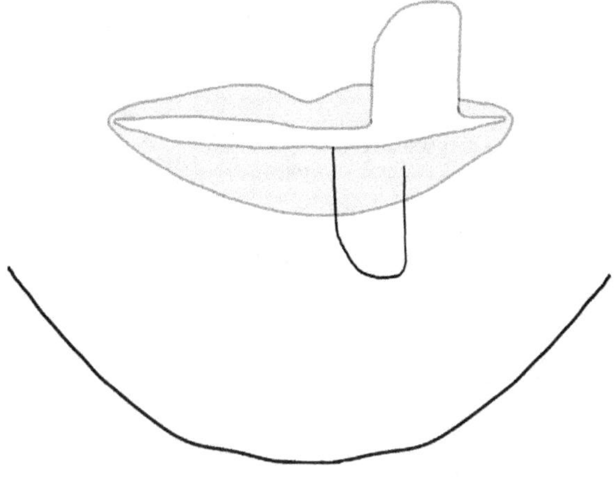

Figure: Nasolabial V-Y advancement flap

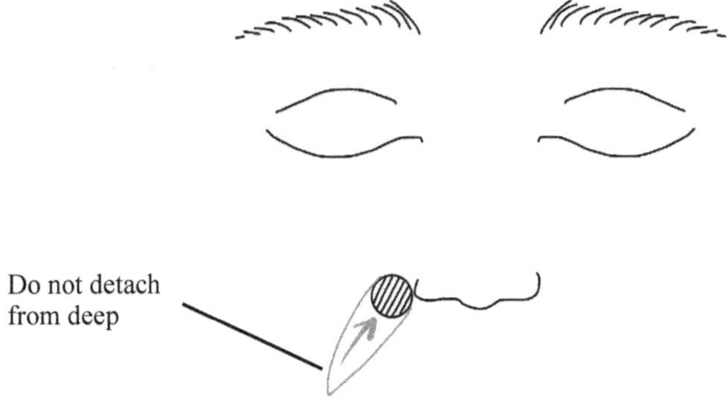

1/3rd-2/3rd

Central defect	Abbe flap +/- peri-alar crescents
Lateral defect	Commissure & philtrum intact: Abbe Commissure involved: Estlander (Ref: Figure)

Figure: Estlander flap

>2/3rd

Sufficient cheek tissue + central defect	Bernard Burrow's flap (Ref: Figure)
Sufficient cheek tissue + lateral defect	Ipsilateral Bernard Burrrow's + contralateral crescenteric excision
Insufficient cheek tissue	Free flap (RFFF + PL sling)

Figure: Bernard Burrows flap

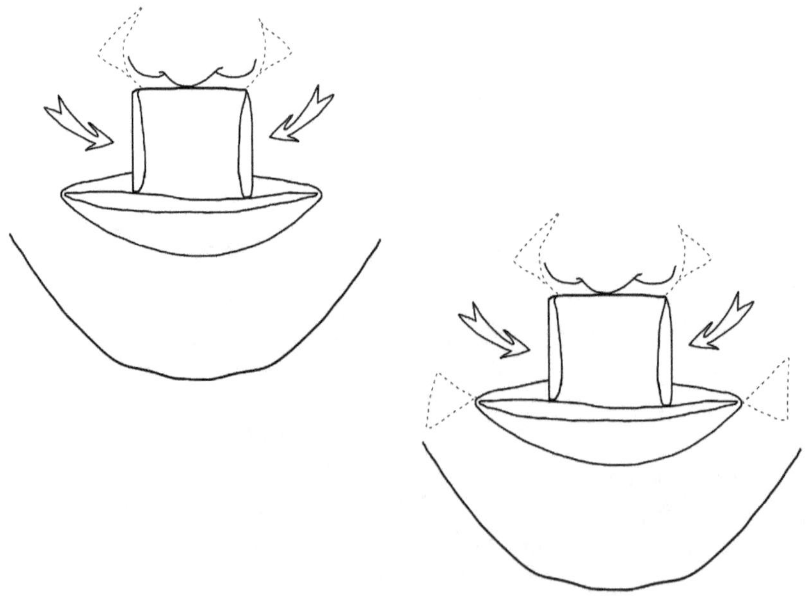

Mucosa of the lower lip/ vermilion

1. Vermilion advancement flap
2. Musculo-mucosal V-Y plasty
3. Bipedicle musculo-mucosal flap (for total vermilion reconstruction)
4. FAMM (Facial artery musculo-mucosal) flap. Can be raised as a superior or inferiorly based flap for intra-oral defects. It consists of mucosa, submucosa, (possibly) buccinator, facial artery branches and its venous plexus.
5. (Tongue flap)

Figure: Inferiorly based FAMM flap

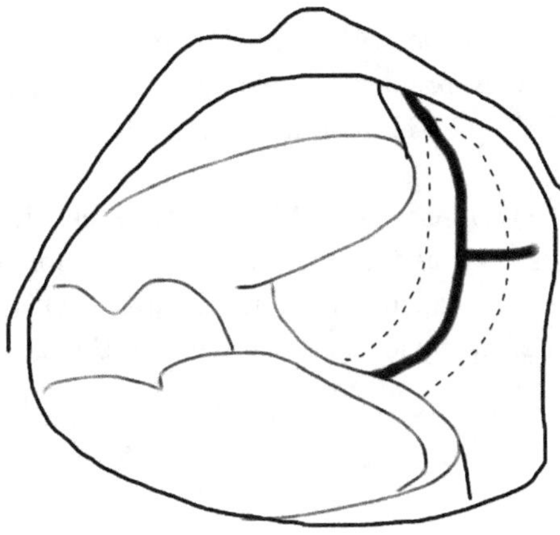

Lower lip recon

<1/3rd:

- Direct closure
- W-shaped excision
- V-shaped excision
- Shield shaped excision
- Single / double barrel

1/3-2/3rd:

- Schuchardt
- Double central reverse Abbe
- Estlander (for <50% defect). Described by Jakob August Estlander, Professor of surgery at Emperor Alexander Univeristy, Helsinki (Ref: Archiv fur Klinische Chirurgie 1872;14:622 reprinted as. Estlander J. *Plast Reconstr Surg.* 42(4):360–4.
- Karapadzic (up to 80%). Described by Miodrag Karapandzic from Belgrade University, then Yugoslavia. n=58, defect size 3.5-7cm for both upper and lower lip defects. Only 13 patients had microstomia. (Ref: Karapandzic M. Reconstruction of lip defects by local arterial flaps. *Br J Plast Surg.* 1974 Jan; 27(1):93–7)
- Step flap

Figure: Schuchardt

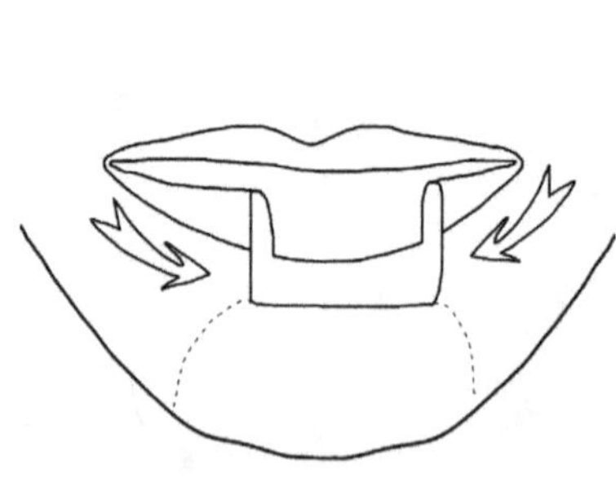

Figure: Estlander flap. Note the flap on the upper lip is smaller in width than the defect, to allow sharing of the tissue deficit between both lips. The vertical height, on the other hand, needs to be matched very well.

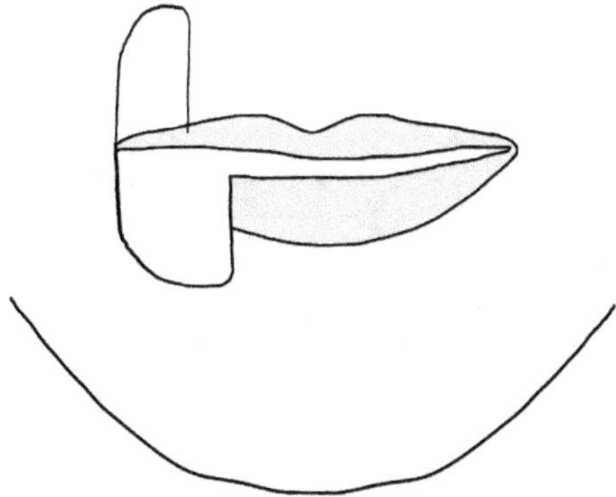

Figure: Karapandzic flap. The nasolabial incision is made first, any facial nerve and artery branches are preserved, tissue rotated medially and then any excess is trimmed off at the NLF.

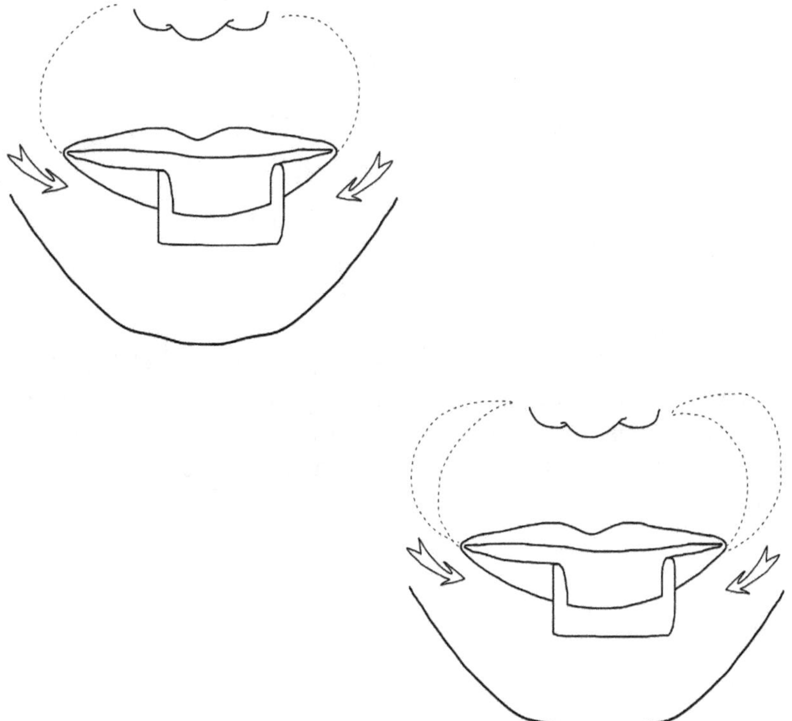

Figure: Step flap. Each "step" breaks the scar and spreads the donor area away from the defect. Once the lateral tissue is advanced medially, usually some excess tissue needs to be trimmed off where it overlaps the chin.

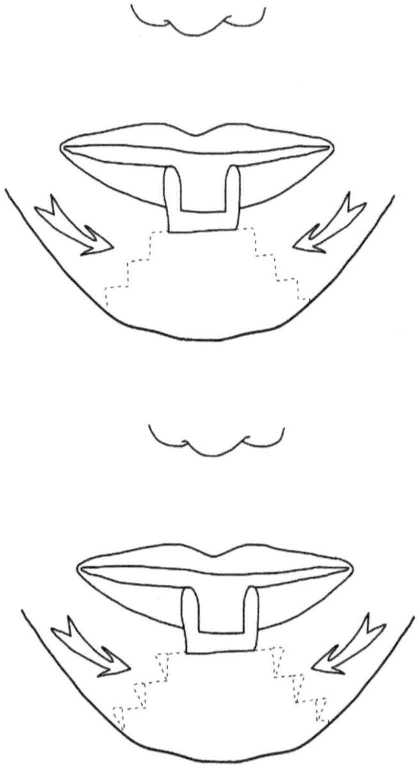

>2/3rd:

- Modified Bernard Webster. Cheek tissue advanced only. Vermilion is reconstructed with a bipedicle mucosal advancement flap. (Ref: Figure)
- RFFF with PL. PL tendon is fixed to maxilla on either side and the flap is folded on either side of it

Figure: Modified Bernard Burrows flap for the reconstruction of lower lip. Nasolabial incisions allow the cheek tissue to be rotated medially. This medial rotation is facilitated by Schuchardt flap at the chin. Once the tissue has been rotated medially, any excess at the incision sited is trimmed.

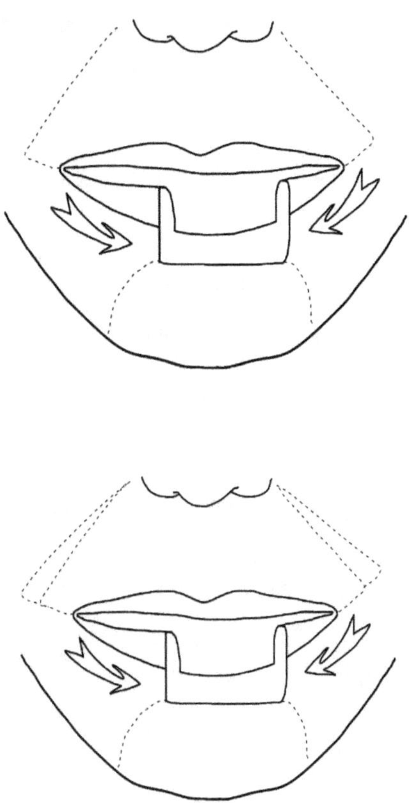

Ear reconstruction

Reference:

Eriksson E & Branemark P. Osseointegration from the perspective of plastic surgeons *Plast Recon Surg*. 1994:93(3);626-37

Helical rim and upper 1/3rd:

Wedge resection	As a triangle, or a star (Ref: Figure)
Anti-Buch (helical rim) advancement	Posteriorly based chondro-cutaneous flap consisting of all of posterior and part of anterior skin & helical rim that is moved superiorly to cover the composite defect
Converse tunnel procedure	Anteriorly based post-auricular skin flap. The defect is sutured edge to edge in an incision made in the post-auricular skin effectively creating a tunnel where a piece of cartilage can be inset and raised later by division of the flap.
Diffenbach post-auricular flap	

Figure: a) Wedge resection, b) Anti-Buch helical rim advancement flap

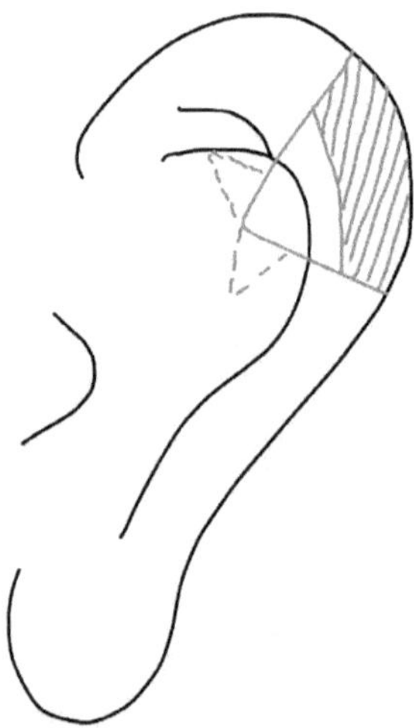
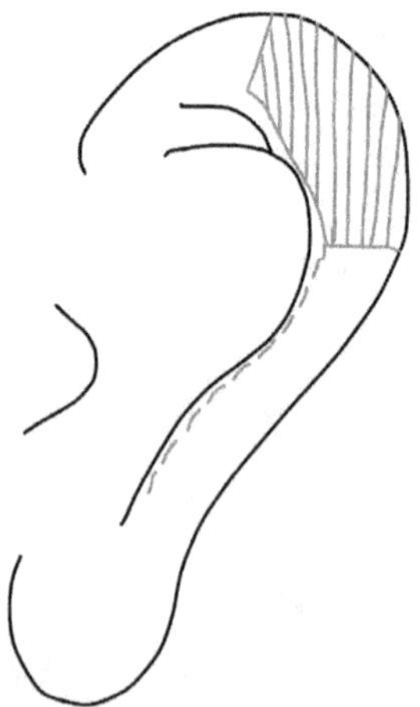

Note, triangular excision of cartilage to allow folding

Middle 1/3rd:

Post-auricular ("Diffenbach") flap. Post-auricular non-hair bearing skin whose dimensions take in to account anterior surface, rim and posterior surface. In 1st stage, the flap is elevated and sutured to the anterior surface. In 2nd stage the flap is divided and posterior surface is addressed.

Anterior conchal defect:
"Revolving door flap". It is a superiorly based flap on post-auricular skin, delivered anteriorly through a cartilage incision and sutured anteriorly. The flap can be divided at 3/52.

Figure: Revolving door flap a) Defect, b) Raising the flap, c) inset

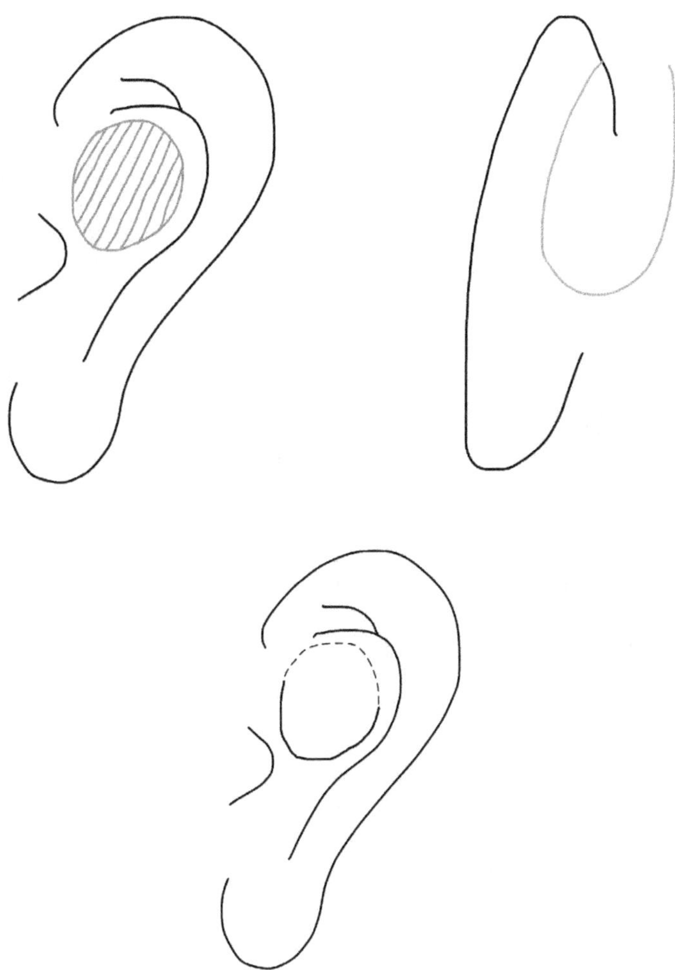

Skin only avulsion:

TPF* + SSG to cover the intact cartilage

*Temporoparietal fascial flap

Total ear reconstruction

Prosthetic
- Stick -on. Simple, cheap but easy to come off as well.
- Branemark osseo-integrated implant (Ref: Eriksson & Branemark)

Autologous
- Nagata technique (classically 4 stage)
- Brent technique (2 stage)

Local flaps practice

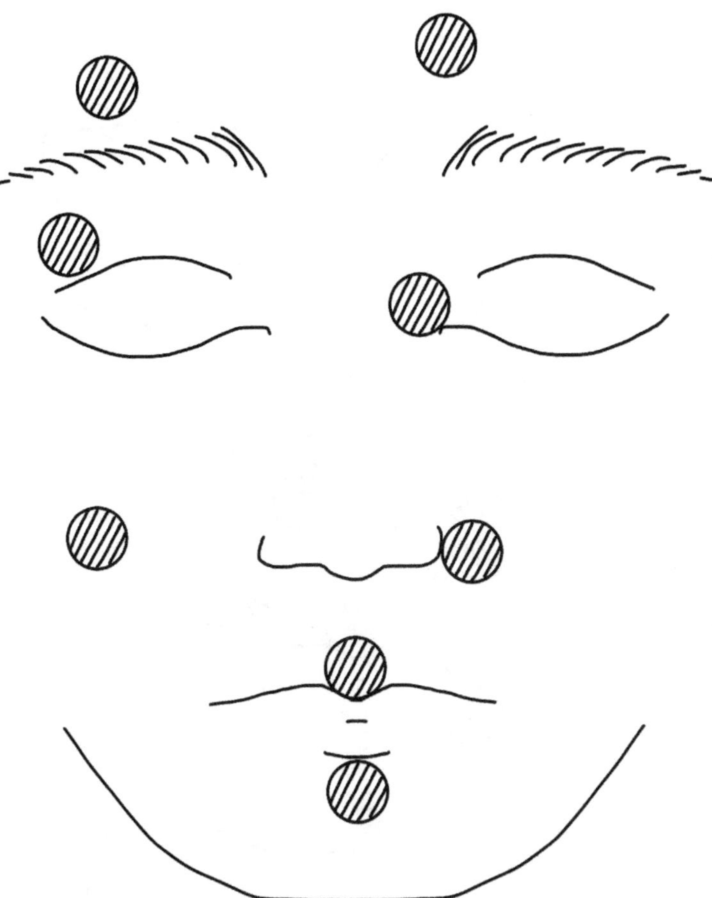

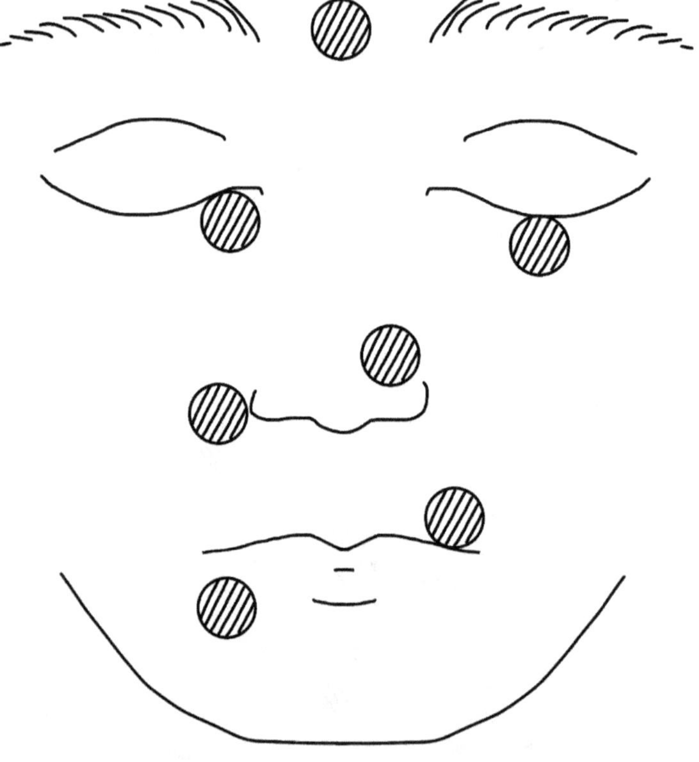

Facial nerve

Ideal recon goal = symmetry in repose and during animation

(In this section 'all caps' roman numerals e.g. VII, XI, XII will refer to cranial nerves of the corresponding number)

Table: Relationship of lesions and deficits

Extratemporal lesion	Ipsilateral motor only
Intratemporal lesion	Ipsilateral motor + lacrimal (tears) + stapedius (hearing) + chorda tympani (taste)

History

Age, occupation
Other PMHx, medications, allergies
History of facial palsy

- What happened?
- How long ago?
- How fast?
- What caused it?

What is troubling the patient at the moment. ("Form, function, psych")

- Eye care. Watering of eye? Infections?
- Oral continence
- Breathing
- Rest of face. Twitching of face? Tears/sweating while eating?
- Problems at work / in social situations. How has the pt adapted?

Examination

LOOK

At rest
At animation, talking, smiling, laughing

- Blink-whether symmetrical
- Movement of forehead, nasolabial fold, commisure
- Look for scars on pre-articular, postauricular areas bilaterally
- Ask for scars on chest, inner thighs, calf

FEEL AND MOVE

- Wrinkle forehead
- Close eyes tight shut, check Bell's phenomenon
- Puff up your cheeks
- Smile, snarl, pucker [know the smile classification]
- Show lower teeth
- Can you hear equally on both sides
- Cottle's test (Ref: Aside)

Aside: Cottle's test/maneuvre (testing the *right* side)

1. Occlude right nostril, ask to breathe from left nostril
2. Pull left cheek laterally and ask to breathe again
3. Is there much difference between 1 & 2?

4. Occlude left nostril & ask to breathe from the right
5. Pull right cheek laterally and ask to breathe again
6. Is there much difference between 3&4? Yes, implies narrowing of the airway at the internal nasal valve (which opened passively by the pull on the cheek)

N.B. Occlude nostril with upward pressure on the nostril, and not with sideways pressure pressure on the ala.

Consider:
- Check Tinel's - if CFNG done.
- Levator function - if lid procedure expected (>10mm excellent, 5-10mm good, <5mm poor)
- Offer Schirmer's (if morphologically prone eye - see section on blephroplasty)

Investigations

- Of cause e.g. CT Head
- Of status of motor end plates, by EMG studies
- Clinical photographs, at rest and at animation
- Videotape

Principles of management

Management will need to address patient's social and functional problems

(PREDOMINANTLY) SOCIAL:

Symmetry at rest and ideally at animation too

(PREDOMINANTLY) FUNCTIONAL:

Corneal exposure

Bilabial speech, drooling

Hearing

Nasal breathing

Any management takes into account
- The cause & duration of the disease
- Patient comorbidities
- Patient's functional demands
- Expected compliance

The principles of management are
1. Manage in a multidisciplinary team (Plastic surgery, ENT, neurophysiology, prosthetics, nurses, clinical psychologist)
2. Protect what the patient has
3. Adapt lifestyle (Ref: Table)
4. Reconstruct / Re-innervate if possible (this depends on the state of MEPs).

Table: Adapt lifestyle

Forehead	Adapt hair style e.g. grow a fringe
Eyes	• Use shades in public • Regular eyedrops • Taping at night
Mouth	Consider *contralateral* BoTnA (Note that the dosage is much smaller than for cosmetic application *and* that there is risk of oral incompetence)

Principles of facial nerve reconstruction

Opinion:

It will be very helpful to read this in conjunction with brachial plexus injury as there are a lot of similarities in the decision making and reconstructive procedures.

MEPs degenerate between 12-18 months, so they need a motor nerve to reach them "before" then. This includes time for operation, healing, Wallerian degeneration and slow nerve growth to reach the MEPs. Hence the idea of operating at/soon after 6 months post-palsy to allow all that to happen. The slowest process i.e. the bottleneck, is the 1mm/day nerve growth, so if a longer donor graft is needed (esp. CFNG), the operation need to be done much sooner.

Probs with all nerve grafts is that they lose 50% axons at every anastomosis. Hence an ideal donor nerve is one with high innervation density(i.e. lots of neurons) and short distance from the MEPs to get maximum axons as quickly as possible to the target.

Situation A - Early repair, MEPs working

Problem	Potential cause	Solution
Both ends available, no gap	Sharp laceration	Immediate direct repair
Both ends available, but there is a gap	Nerve sacrifice in a malignant parotid tumor	Primary nerve graft e.g. using sural nerve
Proximal end available, but no distal end	rare situation Laceration on anterior part of face	Direct neurotisation of the muscles
Distal end available but no proximal end	Excision of acoustic neuroma in petrous temporal bone	Need a nerve to stimulate the muscle (see below)

COMMON PROBLEM

The muscles & their motor end plates are intact but there are no neurons to "fire" them.

SOLUTION

Find some neurons (easier said than done!). An ideal donor nerve needs to be an expendable motor nerve in physical proximity to the recipient facial nerve.

Aside: Options of donor nerves

1. Ipsilateral expendable nerve, usually XII, but sometimes XI, V
2. Contralateral VII (=CFNG)
3. Immediate ipsilateral nerve transfer ("baby sitter") + CFNG

Ipsi- vs contra- lateral donor nerves.
1. Ipsilateral donors, are nerves other than VII.
   - easier to anastomose
   - faster innervation, *but* do not share the same motor function
   - give symmetry at rest *but* mass action on animation e.g. when eating causing social embarrassment
2. Contralateral implies VII only (except e.g. in Moebius)
   - symmetry at rest and potentially with animation
   - *but* takes longer, more operations, needs a compliant patient, and has 2 sites of nerve graft (so 25% axons at best)

Choice 1 - Ipsilateral expendable nerves

A) CHOICE OF IPSILATERAL NERVE

XII is preferred over XI, V (branch to masseter)

Pros (of XII)	Located closeby (for faster reinnervation) High innervation density(more neurons)
Cons (of XII)	Tongue weakness, (Although symmetrical at rest) movements not coordinated with the opposite side, "Jaw winking phenomenon" = face twitching while eating

Ipsilateral XI

- It is far from VII
- Has a different function and
- Leaves a dropped shoulder.

Although classically described, only rarely indicated these days.

Nerve to masseter

- It is located close by, is pure motor and potentially expendable (as there are other muscles of mastication), but
- Needs re-learning

B) OPTIONS TO CONNECT XII

Classic solution 1 (Whole nerve). Take whole of ipsilateral hypoglossal nerve and anastomose (end-to-end) to the facial nerve. Has all the cons as above.

Classic solution 2 (Split XII) Take only part of the hypoglossal nerve (end-to-end) so tongue is not paralysed on one side e.g. 30% of cross section area. The hypoglossal nerve is split longitudinally as far as needed to mobilise it adequately and make a tension free anastomosis with CN VII.

Newer solution (Jump graft) The micro-anatomy of hypoglossal (in contrast to that of e.g. radial or median nerves) consists of fascicles twined in a helix, so any longitudinal split sacrifices a lot more neurons than if these neurons were in longitudinal fascicles.

As a solution, if you make a small split in hypoglossal (to allow end-to-side neurorrhaphy). This won't damage as many neurons, but it doesn't have enough play in it to reach VII. The solution is to use a nerve graft (usually of sural nerve) to bridge this gap. So the donor XII still has a 30% end-to-side anastomosis [with the sural nerve graft] but since the split in the nerve is not carried proximally, it does not sever as many neurons.

The problem with this approach is that at every anastomosis, you lose up to 50% of neurons. So with 2 anastomosis, the best number of neurons reaching the facial nerve are 25% of the donor. This is where the high innervation density of the donor XII is helpful, so even with loss of neurons a significant number will still reach the target.

The phrase "jump graft" is a slant on starting an unresponsive car battery with a jump lead from a "donor" car battery to help start the current flow.

> **Opinion:**
>
> There are better donors than CN XII, esp. in a fit and well motivated patient.

Choice 2 - Contralateral facial nerve graft* (CFNG)

* There is no point in using contralateral XII or XI as donors in isolated unilateral facial nerve palsy

1-2 (contra-lateral) buccal/zygomatic branches are taken for anastomosis to a nerve graft placed across the upper lip. The distal anastomosis is at, or lateral to, the level of lateral canthus on affected side where VII can be located.

Procedure:
- 1st stage = sural nerve graft
- Preauricular incision on good side
- Coapted to buccal branch to zygomaticus or to risorius (usu. 3-4 branches found)
- Subcutaneous tunnel across upper lip using a small catheter
- Nerve graft left at preauricular area on paralysed side
- 2nd stage @6-12 months

Pros (of CFNG)	Its the only solution that offers a chance for symmetry at both rest and animation
Cons (of CFNG)	• Sacrifices at least part of a healthy nerve. • Not easy to coapt on the injured side. • Takes time to grow to the other side, hence patient factors and compliance issues can be important. • Unpredictable (depends on who you ask) • Lower innervation density w.r.t. XII • Needs 2 anastomoses, so lose more neurons than a single coaptation site.

Choice 3 - Halt denervation for now + find a proper nerve (Baby sitter + CFNG)

A "Baby sitter" nerve graft is any ipsilateral nerve transfer for facial nerve while waiting for a CFNG. Pro = It stops the denervation clock, while the re-innervation from the contralateral VII can proceed at its pace.

Whether it is Choice 1, 2 or 3 - all these procedures need to get the motor neurons to the MEPs before they degenerate. In acute situations it is easy to know, but esp. 10-12 months after VII deficit (from whatever cause), the state of MEPs may not be fully known. Clinically, loss of MEPs is indicated by fibrillations (fine involuntary muscle twitch) and fibrillation potentials on EMG. Hence the importance of EMG at that stage.

Situation B- Late repair MEPs not working

Issue = There are no motor end plates to make the muscles contract. So your options are:

1. Find a local muscle which doesn't depend on CN VII, i.e. muscle transfer of a nearby uninvolved muscle, which has both a good nerve and viable motor end plates and muscle fibers.
2. Free muscle transfer with its nerve, which is plugged in to a donor nerve (as above)
3. A kind of a failsafe procedure that offers symptomatic benefit but with minimal overhead

The first two are dynamic procedures (which offer movement and ideally symmetry in both repose and on animation), and the last is a group of static procedures (which at best, offer symmetry at rest) e.g. muscle transfer of temporalis/ masseter.

The management depends upon the zone of face, and upon patient's functional problems and comorbidities. These may be static or dynamic procedures. All static procedures aim to make the patient symmetrical at rest (which usually needs some initial overcorrection to allow for tissue laxity).

Dynamic procedures aim to make the patient symmetrical at animation (mostly for nasolabial fold correction). But since the MEPs have degenerated, our options are,

(a) use a muscle NOT supplied by VII (in which case trigeminal supplied temporalis & masseter are available), or if we want coordinated movement
(b) free muscle transfer + CFNG i.e. we need to provide both a muscle (to replace the one vector of movement) AND a donor nerve.

(c) although free muscle transfer with donor from XII/V/XI is theoretically possible it puts the patient through a big procedure without the hope of symmetry at animation.

The following procedures are ipsilateral, unless specified otherwise.

FOREHEAD

Usually comprises balancing procedures

Non-surgical. Contralateral BoTnA injection

Surgical. Browlift.

- Endoscopic browlift, esp in young
- Melon slice browlift, from just above the eyebrow (in older patients)
- Elliptical excision around a horizontal rhytid (in older patients with prominent frown lines)

EYE

The vast majority of procedures are static procedures.

Upper lid options:

- Gold weight(only works when pt upright, so needs night time care +/- taping)
- (Permanent) tarsorrhaphy, which partly closes the palpabral fissure, so the patient needs less effort to close the rest.

Figure: Lateral tarsorrhaphy. The commonest suture is a double ended 6/0 polypropylene (or equivalent). A small roll of non-adherent dressing (e.g. Jelonet) is needed to prevent the fine suture from cheese wiring through the thin skin of the lid margin.

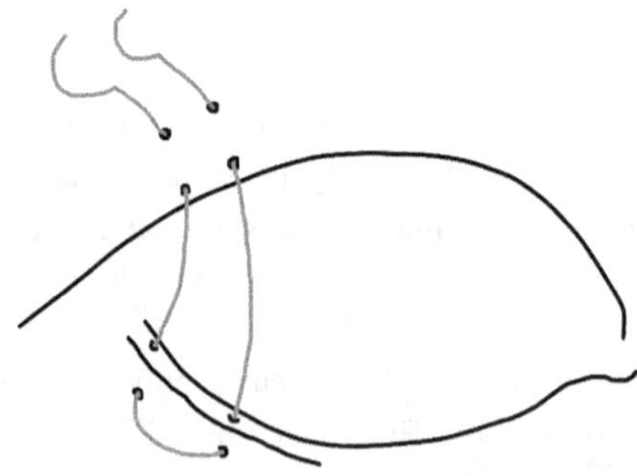

Lower lid options:

1. Canthopexy
2. Canthoplasty (usually with a tarsal strip). Lower lid tarsal plate is exposed at its lateral 5mm (or so) and a mattress suture is passed using a double ended needle and fixed at an appropriate point at the lateral orbital rim. Fixation id done by burring a hole (while protecting the globe!) and passing the suture through it.
3. Tarsal strip +/- Palmaris longus tendon graft
4. Kunht-Zymanowski procedure (horizontal lid shortening, Ref: Figure), direct pentagonal excision, tarsal strip +/- PL tendon sling & canthopexy/ canthoplasty

Figure: 'Kuhnt-Szymanowski' procedure, involves eccentric excision of the anterior and posterior lamellae to achieve a horizontal lid shortening effect. a) Skin and orbicularis incision, b) tarsus and conjunctival excision, c) final scar

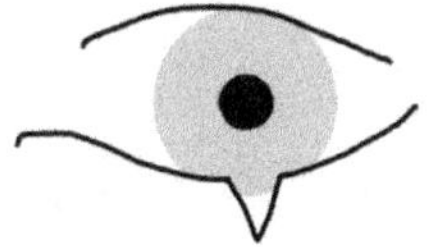

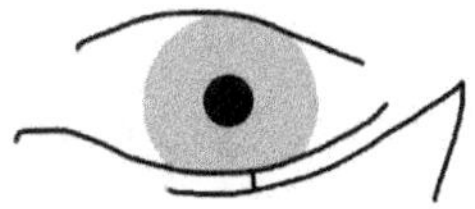

As dynamic procedures, microvascular transfers have been described as well.

> **Aside: Canthopexy vs canthoplasty**
>
> Pexy involves anchoring the lid to the periosteum of the lateral orbital rim which may not be long lasting. Plasty involves anchoring the lid by a suture through a hole drilled in the lateral orbital rim and is longer lasting- of course it involves drilling the rim very close to the orbit).

NOSE

Spreader graft to increase the internal nasal valve angle (between the septum and the lower margin of ULC). The donor may be a nasal septal or chonchal cartilage.

UPPER LIP / NASOLABIAL FOLD

(Nonsurgical option i.e. contralateral BoTnA may not be a good option due to increased risk of bilateral oral incompetence)

Static procedures

- Facelift (but is not permanent),
- Fascia lata sling,
- Multi vector suspension sutures

Dynamic procedures

What is needed is a thin muscle that can act in several vectors of pull. Muscles like serratus anterior, pectoralis minor or gracilis fit the bill. The main target is the nasolabial fold or the angle of mouth.

- Regional muscle transfer, temporalis muscle (Labbe procedure), Masseter transfer
- Free muscle transfer + CFNG

LOWER LIP

Contralateral BoTnA (in depressor labii) can achieve symmetry at rest (risk of oral incompetence, esp with high doses). These may need to be repeated every 3-6 months.

If the results are satisfactory, transection of contralateral depressor labii can provide long term improvement in corner of mouth.

Assessment of facial nerve function & recovery

HOUSE-BRACKMAN SCALE

It grades the degree of facial nerve paralysis by adding scores for superior movement of mid eyebrow and lateral movement of angle of mouth.

Patient is given a score of 1 for every 0.25 cm movement (to a maximum of 1 cm = 4 points). Total scores are interpreted as a grade from I - VI, which correlate with %age function of facial nerve on that side.

SUNNYBROOK SCORE

Referred to as the Sunnybrook Facial Grading System, it is a composite score of resting symmetry, symmetry on voluntary movements and synkinesis. Ref: Table [The complete scoring system is available free online at http://sunnybrook.ca/uploads/FacialGradingSystem.pdf]

Table: Elements of Sunnybrook scoring system for facial nerve function. Each of the following are scored and compared to the normal side

	Features assessed	**Score**
Resting symmetry score	Eye, NLF & mouth	from 0 to 2
Symmetry on voluntary movement	Forehead wrinkle Gentle eye closure Open mouth smile Snarl Lip pucker	1 (unable to initiate movement) to 5 (movement complete)
Synkinesis	Forehead wrinkle Gentle eye closure Open mouth smile Snarl Lip pucker	0 (none) to 3 (disfiguring synkinesis)

Composite score =

voluntary movement score
minus resting symmetry score
minus synkinesis score

Misc.

MECHANISM OF DRY EYE:

Cant blink, so tear film evaporates

MECHANISM OF EYE WATERING:

Orbicularis oculi controls lacrimal drainage by its attachment to the lacrimal sac.

Orbic not working $\Rightarrow$ no removal of tears

How will you manage the patient

1. Have a detailed discussion to understand their current problems. What is their main concern? Is it morphological or psychological? Is it present all the time or in certain situations only? How motivated is the patient and how compliant they have been in past (and with what management)? This will help you individualise your management
2. Make sure that all non-operative measures are in place.
3. Escalate management gradually and in steps, keeping in mind patient compliance.
4. When operating, "bet on a winner" i.e. go for low morbidity procedures which predictably improve the patient's function e.g. tarsal strip, tarsorrhaphy

Skin cancers & sarcoma

Skin cancers

CORE KNOWLEDGE
UK guidelines for management of BCC, SCC and MM
SLNB for MM
Giant hairy naevus
Spitz nevi

APPROACH TO PATIENT - HISTORY
Age, occupation, hobbies, who is at home
Medical issues and allergies
Use of "blood thinners" i.e. aspirin, warfarin, clopidogrel (and newer agents like rivaroxaban)
Family history [remember Gorlin's syndrome*]

Duration, changing appearance (size, shape, colour)
Symptoms like itching, bleeding
Fitzpatrick type
History of sun exposure or sunburn (either as occupation or in childhood. e.g. served in North Africa / Middle east, construction worker, mailman, railway engineer)
Previous history of skin cancers
H/O immunesuppression (DM, organ transplantation, HIV)
Exposure to radiation (e.g. for a previous BCC, or H&N CA)

APPROACH TO PATIENT - EXAMINATION
Site, Size
Fixity to underlying structures, laxity of adjacent tissues [think direct closure vs local flap /graft
Any other similar lesions in the area
Regional lymph nodes

*Gorlin's syndrome (autosomal dom.) is associated with frontal bossing, palmar pits, ondontogenic cysts(on OPG), bifid ribs(on CXR),calcified falx(on CT) +/- learning difficulties. Since it is autosomal dominant, it is important to know for counselling.

XP (Xeroderma pigmentosum, autosomal rec.) shows excessive photo damaged skin with multilple BCCs & SCCs.

APPROACH TO PATIENT - TREATMENT

Your management takes into account the site, size & the definition of clinical margins

EXPECTED CLINICAL QUESTIONS

- Types of BCCs, risk factor for BCCs, guidelines,
- BCC margins, evidence
- If excised, how many are still +ve? who described it?
- Involved margin, what to do? who described it?
- How would you reconstruct with flap, nose tip/dorsum/ala/sidewall, medial canthus, glabella, forehead, cheek, pinna

- Referral criteria for LSMDT [These are 1) suspect lesions, or 2) after diagnosis of stage Ib onwards if SLNB is available, or stage IIb onwards if SLNB is not available]
- Minimum dataset for micro
- Prognostic factors (BT, ulceration, mitosis)
- Breslow thickness, definition
- Evidence for WLE
- Follow up
- AJCC classification, incl difference between 2002 & 2009 classifications
- SLNB controversy
- Recent trials / results
- Who should do block dissection
- Indications for pelvic dissection
- Describe a block dissection
- Adjuvant treatments (ILI, ILP, Interferons, RT)
- MM & pregnancy
- BK mole syndrome
- Lentigo maligna
- Congenital giant hairy nevus

RECOMMENDED PAPERS

Guidelines:

1. Morton CA, Birnie AJ, Eedy DJ. British Association of Dermatologists' guidelines for the management of squamous cell carcinoma in situ (Bowen's disease) 2014. *Brit J Dermatol*. 2014 Feb;170(2):245–60.
2. Telfer NR, Colver GB, Morton CA. Guidelines for the management of basal cell carcinoma. *Brit J Dermatol*. 2008 Jul;159(1):35–48.
3. Marsden JR, Newton-Bishop JA, Burrows L, Cook M, Corrie PG, Cox NH, et al. Revised UK guidelines for the management of cutaneous melanoma 2010. *Brit J Dermatol*. 2010;163(2):238–56.

Classic Trials:

4. Veronesi U, Cascinelli N, Adamus J, et al. Thin stage I primary cutaneous malignant melanoma. Comparison of excision with margins of 1 or 3 cm. *N Engl J Med.* 1988 May 5;318(18):1159-62. Erratum in: *N Engl J Med* 1991 Jul 25;325(4):292

5. Khayat D, Rixe O, Martin G, et al. French Group of Research on Malignant Melanoma. Surgical margins in cutaneous melanoma (2 cm versus 5 cm for lesions measuring less than 2.1-mm thick). *Cancer.* 2003 Apr 15;97(8): 1941-6

6. Cohn-Cedermark G, Rutqvist LE, Andersson R, et al. Long term results of a randomized study by the Swedish Melanoma Study Group on 2-cm versus 5-cm resection margins for patients with cutaneous melanoma with a tumor thickness of 0.8-2.0 mm. *Cancer.* 2000 Oct 1;89(7):1495-501

7. Karakousis CP, Balch CM, Urist MM, et al. Local recurrence in malignant melanoma: long-term results of the multiinstitutional randomized surgical trial. *Ann Surg Oncol.* 1996 Sep;3(5):446-52

8. Thomas JM, Newton-Bishop J, A'Hern R et al.; UKMSG BAPS & Scottish Cancer Therapy Network. Excision margins in high risk melanoma. NEJM 2004;350(8):757-66

Update, new trial, review:
9. Hayes AJ, Maynard L, Coombes G, et al.; UKMSG BAPRAS, and the Scottish Cancer Therapy Network. Wide versus narrow excision margins for high-risk, primary cutaneous melanomas: long-term follow-up of survival in a randomised trial. *Lancet Oncol.* 2016 Feb;17(2):184-92

10. Morton DL, Thompson JF, Cochran AJ et al. Final Trial Report of Sentinel-Node Biopsy versus Nodal Observation in Melanoma. [MSLT-1]. *NEJM* 2014;370(7):599-609

11. Sladden MJ, Balch C, Barzilai DA, et al. Surgical excision margins for primary cutaneous melanoma. In: The Cochrane Collaboration, editor. Cochrane Database of Systematic Reviews [Internet]. Chichester, UK: John Wiley & Sons, Ltd; 2009 [cited 2016 Feb 20]. Available from: http:// doi.wiley.com/10.1002/14651858.CD004835.pub2

12. Gillgren P, Drzewiecki KT, Niin M. 2-cm versus 4-cm surgical excision margins for primary cutaneous melanoma thicker than 2 mm: a randomised, multicentre trial. *Lancet.* 2011;378:1635–1642

BCC(s) / similar skin lesions

You are likely to see an ageing patient with extensive photo damaged skin with (some or all of) lentigines, dyschromia, solar elastosis, actinic keratosis and surrounding telengiectasia. (Ref: Table).

Lentigine	Small brown plaque esp. on sun exposed skin of the elderly
Dyschromia	Alteration in the skin colour
Solar elastosis	Yellow discolouration & skin thickening from elastin deposition
Actinic keratosis	Scaly , dry thickened patches on sun exposed skin

Figure: BCC algorithm / evidence tree (summarised from Telfer et. al. 2008)

<u>100 patients</u>
<2cm size: 3mm clinical margin → 85% clearance
4-5mm clinical margin → 95% clearance [*Wolff & Zitelli 1987*]
[*Breuninger* 1991]
Morpheic: 3mm clinical margin → 66% clearance
5mm clinical margin → 80% clearance [*Breuninger 1997*]

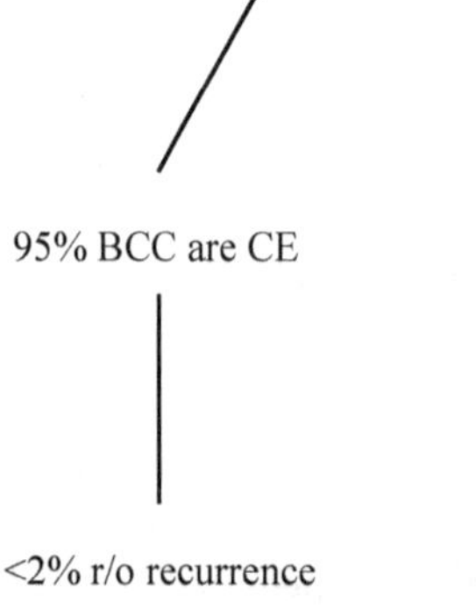

95% BCC are CE

<2% r/o recurrence

4.7 BCCs are incompletely excised

- Histologically, 45-55% 've tumour on re-resection [*Griffiths 1999*]
- Clinically only 1/3rd will recur
  - r/o recurrence = 17% if only lateral margin involved
  - chance of recurrence = 33% if only deep margin is involved [*Liu 1991*]

INDICATIONS FOR RE-EXCISION
- Mid-face(i.e. high risk)
- Deep margin involvement
- Aggressive histology

MODES OF RE-EXCISION
- Re-excision with 5-10mm margin [*Burg 1975*]
- Mohs' Micrographic surgery (MMS)

Mohs' micrographic surgery (MMS)

MMS is a surgical technique which combines staged resection with comprehensive margin control to achieve high excision rates for locally invasive cancers (>98% for primary, >95% for recurrent).

INDICATIONS
Related to site, size, histology of primary, poorly differentiated clinical margins, recurrent, peri-neural/peri-vascular invasion.

It was described by Frederick Mohs in 1944 as a staged process where the tumor bed was painted with zinc paste and patient recalled few days later for the next stage of the surgery.

PROCEDURE
Contemporary Mohs' excision is carried out by a dermatologist with specialist interest in MMS. It is usually a local anaesthetic procedure where the bulk of tumour is removed initially (if it hasn't been done so in a previous operation) with an appropriate clinical margin and sent for histology with a marker suture [so nothing different so far].

Then the Mohs' surgeon marks out a further margin (the first "Mohs' layer") all around the excision. This margin can vary between 2-5mm (depending on tumour characteristics and its site). The incision for the Mohs' layer is made at a 45 degree angle slanting towards the tumour centre. This bevel facilitates "squashing" the specimen later.

Carrying that all around, results in a thin ring of tissue with skin on one side and a bevel-in on its peripheral margin. If this tissue were to be sent to the lab as such, the histopathologist would be unable to identify its location or orientation. Worse still, they will not be able to pass that information to the surgeon.

So the Mohs' layer is divided by the Mohs' surgeon into smaller pieces in theatre.
1. To keep track of location, the surgeon draws a map of the Mohs' layer, both on the lab request & on the op note (Ref: Figure). Each piece is labelled in a numerically ascending order. This will help in localisation of each specimen, but not its orientation
2. To help orientation, the margins on each piece are marked with ink. Three colours are sufficient to allow complete orientation. The now-separate tissue pieces which were adjacent on the patient are coloured with the same ink.

This helps in identification of their location (w.r.t. adjacent tissue pieces) as well as orientation. The ink colour is recorded on the maps as well.

The tissue pieces are then transferred into Moh's "cartridges" which are special enclosures for the tissue (and appropriately labelled). In the lab, each of the pieces is pressed firmly onto a flat surface so that both the deep surface and the bevelled-in margin are "squashed" in to one plane. This allows visualisation of both the deep and peripheral margin on the same slide and rapid reporting of the results.

Figure: Mohs' map, top view. Individual pieces are numbered in ascending order. The resulting pieces are coloured so that adjacent margins on different pieces have the same colour. (G=green, R=red, B=blue).

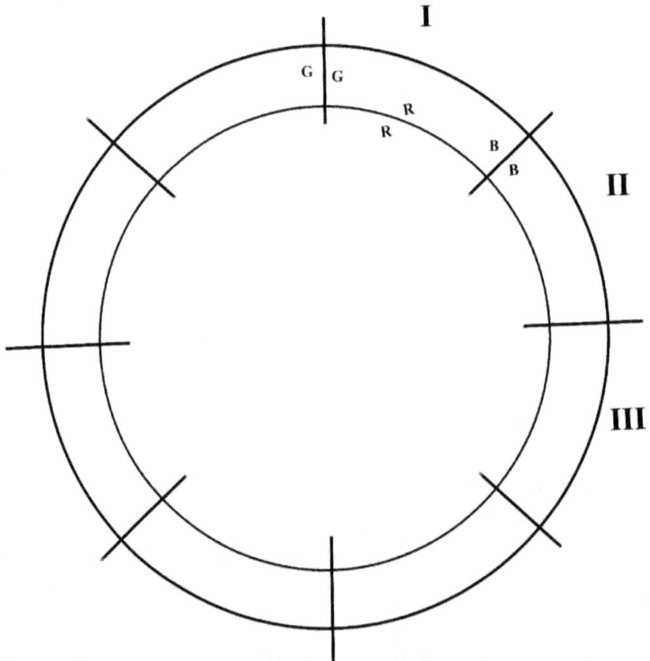

The Mohs' map can have more information drawn on it as well e.g. location of any clinically suspect areas, un-related moles.

Examination of Mohs' excision requires special preparation in the lab as well that needs to be planned in advance.

Figure: Side view of a Mohs' specimen before and after it is flattened in the Mohs' cartridge (only for illustration- this picture is not drawn as part of the Mohs' map).

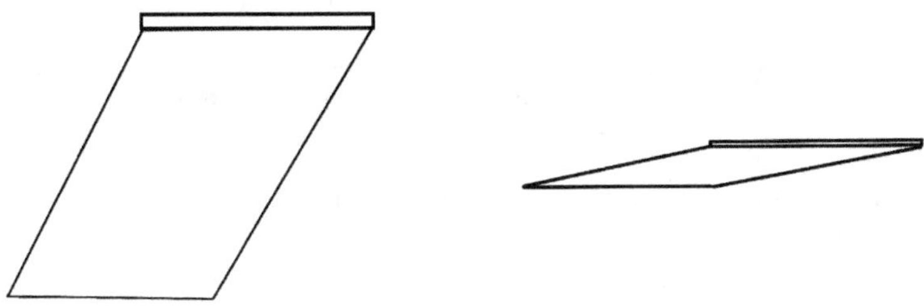

Indications for radiotherapy

1. Primary treatment of high risk disease, if patient is unwilling or unsuitable for surgery.
2. Adjuvant treatment for incompletely excised high risk BCCs

Contra indications to radiotherapy

1. Gorlin's syndrome
2. Radio recurrent BCCs

SCC

It is a malignant tumour arising from stratum spinosum of the epidermis or its appendages. Risk factors include chronic ultraviolet light exposure, sun damaged skin, fair skin, albinism, xeroderma pigmentosum.

Aetiology

- de novo,
- Previous exposure to ultraviolet/ionising radiation, arsenic,
- Chronic wounds,
- Pre-existing lesions e.g. Bowen's disease.

High-risk groups for developing SCC

1. Fair skin (Fitzpatrick I > II > III) esp. with sun damage
2. Skin conditions, e.g. albinism, XP
3. Systemic conditions, e.g. leukaemia, lymphoma
4. Immunocompromised e.g. after renal transplantation
5. Chronic wounds, ulcers. (Marjolin's original description was SCC in an unhealed burn scar after 20 years).
6. Pre-existing lesions e.g. Bowen's disease

Histopathology minimum dataset

The following information should be the minimum part of any histopathology report. Many of these are prognostic factors too.

1. Histopathology subtype
2. Degree of difference erection
3. Depth
4. Dermal invasion level
5. Peri-neural / vascular invasion
6. Excision margins, both peripheral and deep

Factors affecting metastatic potential

1- SITE

Lowest risk	SCC arising in sun exposed sites (except lip / ear)
	SCC lip
	SCC ear
	Non-sun-exposed areas
Highest risk	Areas of radiation or burn injury, chronic ulcers or Bowen's disease

2- SIZE,

>2cm dia.$\Rightarrow$ 2x↑LR, 3x↑mets.

SCC diameter	r/o LR	r/o Mets
< 2cm	7%	10%
> 2cm	15%	30%

3- DEPTH AND LEVEL OF INVASION

SCC depth of invasion	r/o mets
<2mm	rarely metastatic
2-4mm	6-7%
>4mm or Clarke level IV	45%

4- HISTOLOGICAL DIFFERENTIATION

Broder's grade3 & 4 $\Rightarrow$ 2x↑LR, 3x↑mets.

Aside: Broder's grading system
Grade 1: Well differentiated
Grade 2: Moderately differentiated
Grade 3: Poorly differentiated
Grade 4: Anaplastic

Evidence for clinical excision margins

Reference: Broadland & Zitelli 1992

TO ACHIEVE 95% CLEARANCE IN A PRIMARY SCC

4mm margin for:

- <2 cm dia. lesion
- Well differentiated
- Low-risk

6mm margin for:

- >2 cm dia. lesion
- Moderate/poorly differentiated
- Extending to subcutaneous tissue
- On ears/lip/scalp/eyelid/nose

[Note that some of these are histologic features and will not be available at primary excision]

Prognosis

That is related to host factors and tumour factors.

HOST FACTORS

Immunosuppression

TUMOR FACTORS

- Site
- Size in three dimensions i.e. Gross size, histological depth and level of invasion
- Degree of differentiation and histological subtype
- Rate of growth
- Recurrent disease
- Aetiology

Malignant Melanoma

Suspicious black mole somewhere

(Although "exceptions" occur frequently) you are likely to see a melanocytic lesion (on arm/back/abdomen) of a fair skinned individual. This lesion may be symmetrical/asymmetrical, with well/ill-defined borders, homogenous/irregular pigmentation, with or without ulceration.

The steps of management (after history & examination, and if you suspect it to be a melanoma) are :

1. Obtain tissue diagnosis, with a 2 mm excision biopsy, and if +ve, escalate to a 2WW target (in UK only),
2. Local skin MDT(LSMDT) discussion,
3. Wide local excision with appropriate margins, based on the Breslow thickness (& reconstruction)
4. Consider sentinel node biopsy,
5. Regular surveillance for an appropriate length of time [5 or 10 years, see below].

If there is suspicion of an enlarged regional lymph node, perform an (*urgent!*) fine needle aspiration (FNA) and if positive, arrange for an urgent staging CT scan*, and refer to LSMDT where the surgeon's [that is you] recommendation is for a block dissection.

A negative FNA sample does not rule out melanoma. If the node is still clinically suspicious, repeat FNA and if that too is negative, open biopsy will give a definitive answer. [All of these need to be on an urgent basis].

Opinion:

The reason to do a block dissection is local control (to prevent a festering wound due to inexorable growth of melanoma) and to reduce/remove the known tumour load (so there is less likely to seed melanoma deposits systemically). A block dissection cannot prevent micrometastases that may have passed that nodal basin already.

---

* if clinical suspicion is high enough, CT can be requested while awaiting FNA result, to minimise time for definitive management.

Referral criteria for LSMDT

1. Suspect lesions, or
2. After diagnosis of
     A. stage Ib onwards if SLNB is available, or
     B. IIb onwards if SLNB is not available)

MEMBERS OF LSMDT

Derma-, Histopath-, Oncologist (clinical & radiation), Plastic surgeon, radiologist, CNS, Clinical psychologist, Vascular surgeon.

Types of malignant melanoma

1. Superficial spreading (SSMM), which may be in radial growth phase (RGP), or vertical (VGP)
2. Nodular (NM)
3. Lentigo maligna melanoma (LMM), which develop in a pre-existing lentigo maligna
4. Desmoplastic
5. Other types (equine type, spindle cell etc)

MINIMUM DATASET FOR MICROSCOPY

Royal College of Pathologists (RCPath) has published a national minimum data set for reporting MM (https://www.rcpath.org/profession/publications/cancer-datasets.html)

Prognostic factors (of primary MM)

1. Breslow thickness (BT). Distance from the granular layer of epidermis, to the deepest nest of melanoma cells, measured with a micrometer & reported to the nearest tenth of a millimetre. It is the single biggest prognostic indicator for melanoma.
2. Ulceration. This is because the thickness of an ulcerated melanoma cannot be accurately assessed.
3. Mitosis. More mitoses suggest higher malignant potential
4. Regression. Similar to the consideration in ulcerated melanomas, the thickness of a regressed lesion cannot be accurately judged.

AJCC Classification for MM

(Reproduced with permission from Edge SB, Byrd DR, Compton CC, eds. AJCC Cancer Staging Manual. 7th ed. New York, NY.: Springer, 2010)
Ref: https://cancerstaging.org/references-tools/quickreferences/documents/
melanomasmall.pdf

T Classification	Thickness	Ulceration status / Mitoses
Tis	NA	NA
T1	1.00	a: Without ulceration AND mitosis $< 1/mm^2$ b: With ulceration OR mitoses $\geq 1/mm^2$
T2	1.01- 2.00	a: Without ulceration b: With ulceration
T3	2.01-4.00	a: Without ulceration b: With ulceration
T4	> 4.00	a: Without ulceration b: With ulceration

N Classification	No. of metastatic nodes	Nodal metastatic basin
N0	0	NA
N1	1	a: micrometastases b: macrometastases
N2	2-3	a: micrometastases b: macrometastases c: intransit mets/ satellites without
N3	4+ metastatic nodes OR matted nodes OR in transit mets/satellites with metastatic nodes	

M Classification	Site	LDH
M0	No distant mets	NA
M1a	Distant skin, subcutaneous, or nodal metastases	Normal
M1b	Lung metastases	Normal
M1c	All other visceral mets	Normal
	Any distant mets	Elevated

AJCC STAGING FOR MELANOMA

Clinical Staging				Pathologic staging			
Stage 0	Tis	N0	M0	**Stage 0**	Tis	N0	M0
Stage IA	T1a	N0	M0	**Stage IA**	T1a	N0	M0
Stage IB	T1b	N0	M0	**Stage IB**	T1b	N0	M0
	T2a	N0	M0		T2a	N0	M0
Stage IIA	T2b	N0	M0	**Stage IIA**	T2b	N0	M0
	T3a	N0	M0		T3a	N0	M0
Stage IIB	T3b	N0	M0	**Stage IIB**	T3b	N0	M0
	T4a	N0	M0		T4a	N0	M0
Stage IIC	T4b	N0	M0	**Stage IIC**	T4b	N0	M0
Stage III	Any T	$\geq$ N1	M0	**Stage IIIA**	T1-4a	N1a	M0
					T1-4a	N2a	M0
				Stage IIIB	T1-4b	N1a	M0
					T1-4b	N2a	M0
					T1-4a	N1b	M0
					T1-4a	N2b	M0
					T1-4a	N2c	M0
				Stage IIIC	T1-4b	N1b	M0
					T1-4b	N2b	M0
					T1-4b	N2c	M0
					Any T	N3	M0
Stage IV	Any T	Any N	M1	**Stage IV**	Any T	Any N	M1

Micrometastases are diagnosed after sentinel lymph node biopsy and completion lymphadenectomy (if performed). **Macrometastases** are defined as clinically detectable nodal metastases confirmed by therapeutic lymphadenectomy or when nodal metastasis exhibits gross extracapsular extension.

Clinical staging includes microstaging of the primary melanoma and clinical/radiologic evaluation for metastases. By convention, it should be used after complete excision of the primary melanoma with clinical assessment for regional and distant metastases.

Pathologic staging includes microstaging of the primary melanoma and pathologic information about the regional lymph nodes after partial or complete lymphadenectomy. Pathologic Stage 0 or Stage IA patients are the exception; they do not require pathologic evaluation of their lymph nodes

OVERVIEW OF THE STAGING

[This is not an alternative to the classification, but once you know the classification, a descriptive method may be easier to recall than thinking "Breslow thickness 1.8mm non-ulcerated with 3 +ve nodes & no distant mets" mean "T2a,N2b, M0" then wondering what stage it is (IIIB in fact)].

Stage	Summary description	Note
Up to stage II (i.e. Stage 0 through IIC)	Both clinical & pathologic staging share the same TNM categories	
Stage III A	Non-ulcerated primary AND micromets (up to 3)	This situation can only happen with SLNB
Stage III B	*Either* ulcerated primary OR macromets up to 3 OR isolated in-transit mets/ satellites (without +ve nodes) i.e. only one of these should be true	So pt. may have: • Ulcerated pri & micromets • Non-ulcer. pri & macromets • Non-ulcer. pri & in-transit/ satellite mets.
Stage III C	ulcerated primary AND macromets up to 3	
Stage IV	Distant mets (cutaneous/ visceral) OR elevated LDH	

Evidence for WLE = 5x trials

Table: Summary of evidence from major MM trials. Ref: Hellman & Devita

Trial	N	BT (mm)	Margins (cm)	LR	DFS	OS
Veronesi,Cascinelli et al. NEJM 1988 (WHO melanoma progress trial no. 10)						
"WHO trial"	612	0-2	1 vs 3-5	<1mm= none with 1cm 1-2mm= LR with 1cm (not signif.)	-	No difference
Khayat el al. Cancer 2003 (French cooperative surgical trial)						
"French trial"	337	0-2	2 vs 5	-	No diff @10yr (85% vs 83%)	No diff @10yr (87% vs 863%)
Cohn-Cedarmark et al. Cancer 2000 (Swedish cooperative trial)						
"Swedish trial"	989	0.8 - 2	2 vs 5	<1% overall	No diff (rel. hazard for 2cm margin=1.02)	No diff (rel. hazard for 2cm margin=0.96)
Karakousis, Balch et al. Ann Surg Oncol 1996 (Intergroup melanoma trial)						
"Intergroup trial"	740	1-4	2 vs 4	0.4% 0.9% 2.1% 2.6%	No diff @10yr 70% (2cm margin) 77% (4cm margin)	-
Thomas, Newton-Bishop et al. (British Assoc. of Plastic Surgeons/ Melanoma Study Group trial) NEJM 2004						
"BAPS/ MSG trial"	900	≥2	1 vs 3	locoregional (=local+ intransit+ nodal) more with 1cm margin (HR=1.26, p=0.05)	-	Similar (trend to better survival with 3cm margin, but not significant)

* 2016 update of UK MSG trial did not report on locoregional recurrence, but found better melanoma specific survival in 3cm group. Note **Gillgren et al**. (n=932) have shown that for >2mm thick MM, there is no difference in 5yr survival whether you do 2cm or 4cm margin excision (65% vs 65%).

Implications of the WLE trials

WHO TRIAL

For T1 (i.e. <1mm Breslow)	No recurrence with 1cm WLE of T1 (i.e. <1mm) melanoma => 1cm WLE is the standard for T1 MM
For T2 (i.e. 1-2mm Breslow)	Slightly high r/o LR with 1cm WLE (though not significant) leaves the debate open

FRENCH & SWEDISH TRIALS
- 5cm WLE has not added benefit => 2cm WLE is adequate for T2

Combine this with T1 result from WHO trial, tells you that 1cm WLE for T1 & 2cm WLE for T2 is adequate

INTERGROUP MELANOMA TRIAL
- Time to LR & median survival after LR, are unaffected by margin

Supports 2cm margin as adequate, for everything in 1-4mm range

BAPS/MSG TRIAL
Is the only "classical" trial to include T4 (i.e. >4mm thick) melanomas.

It was originally designed to detect LR only, but due to very small numbers, trial design was modified to include locoregional recurrence. This gave marginal value of significance (p=0.05) in favor of 3cm WLE for >2mm melanoma. This trial is the reason UK guidelines suggest a 3cm WLE for >2mm thick melanoma (against all other in the world).

Follow up
- Every 3 months for first 3 years, then (further f/u only if primary > 1.0mm)
- Every 6 months for next 2 years, then give the patient the option of,
- Once a year for the next 5 years (for a total of 10 year follow up)

Opinion:

The reason for this follow up is hidden in the survival curve (Ref Balch AJCC classification JCO 2010) where most recurrences are seen soon after the primary excision, so the follow up is designed to detect those. (Note that Stage 3A does better than 2B, which was possibly a rationale hoped for SLNB in improving survival).

SLNB & associated controversy

PROCEDURE

SLNB is a procedure for surgical staging of node-negative primary melanomas by intraoperative lymphatic mapping and biopsy of first echelon lymph node(s) at the time of WLE. It is a way to identify the first (one/set of) lymph-node to which a melanoma drains, so these nodes can be removed for detailed histopathological examination while sparing the nodes draining other areas of skin.

First described by Cabanas in 1977 for penile cancer. First described for melanoma by Morton (Arch Surg 1992).

The procedure consists of lymphoscintigraphy using technetium 99 injected on the morning of surgery in radiology. The gamma radiation from Tc-99 is detected by handheld probes. The detection of first echelon lymph nodes is also facilitated by the use of vital blue dye (up to 1 ml of) which is injected intradermally at the site of primary, few minutes prior to incision. Detection of a lymph node which is both "hot" (i.e. high gamma count) and "blue" (i.e. has the vital blue dye) makes it a sentinel lymph node. Rate of identification of sentinel node with blue dye alone is 87% whereas with combined blue dye & Tc-99 is up to 99% (Ref, Gershenwald et al. JCO 1998)

REFERRAL CRITERIA FOR SLNB

Stage 1B, i.e.
- <1mm BT with ulceration
- 1-2mm without ulceration

SOURCES OF ERROR

1. More than one "sentinel" nodes as dye transits to many nodes
2. Node found is hot, but not blue (or vice versa). Usually in a watershed area where the Tc-99 & vital blue dye have been injected at slightly different places
3. No sentinel node detected, if dye fails to enter any node (needs to be mentioned in the consent process)

The 15-25% of all SLNB procedures show a +ve SLNB. Note that 2-4% SLNB procedure are false negative.

Hardly anything has sparked such passion and controversy in cancer management that SLNB for melanomas has! The following are the arguments by each camp.

THE "AGAINST" CAMP - PROF MEIRION THOMAS

- There is no therapeutic advantage to SLNB. Because SLNB removes disease load, so the nodal mets take longer to recur. Thus the increased DFS (in MSLT-1, see below) is merely a by-product of trial design.
- A proportion of +ve SLNBs are false +ve. Not all tumour deposits are destined to cause disease and may lie dormant or be overcome by immune system.

THE "FOR" CAMP - PROFS CHARLES MORTON & JOHN THOMPSON

- Therapeutic advantage does not have to be the end point e.g. UK BAPS/MSG trial [ironically first authored by Prof. Thomas] did not show a survival difference between 1 vs 3cm margins, and only showed improvement in loco-regional control (and that too, after trial design adjustment).[FYI, in the 2016 update of the UK MSG trial, loco-regional recurrence has been excluded from data analysis].
- Reasons for offering SLNB are
    i.   Prognostic = main argument
    ii. Decreases r/o nodal involvement at CLND
    iii. Decreased r/o surgical complications [scraping the barrel here, imho]
- Identifies the 20% patients (of intermediate thickness MM) which have microscopic nodal mets. The alternative would be for all patients to have CLND only or SLNB only.
- Offers the patient (who has been detected +ve on SLNB) a chance to be enrolled for clinical trials (currently it is MSLT-2 from the surgical perspective).

CURRENT RATIONALE FOR SLNB

1. UK MM guidelines - prognostic indicator
2. Negative SLNB comforts low risk patients
3. Positive SLNB allows eligibility for trials which may be of benefit

MSLT 1 trial

1. REASONS FOR SETTING UP MSLT 1

Ref: https://clinicaltrials.gov/ct2/show/NCT00275496

Primary outcome: whether WLE + SLNB +/- CLND affects overall survival

Secondary outcome: morbidity of SLNB, DFS, distribution of recurrences

2. MSLT 1 DESIGN
Figure: MSLT 1 design

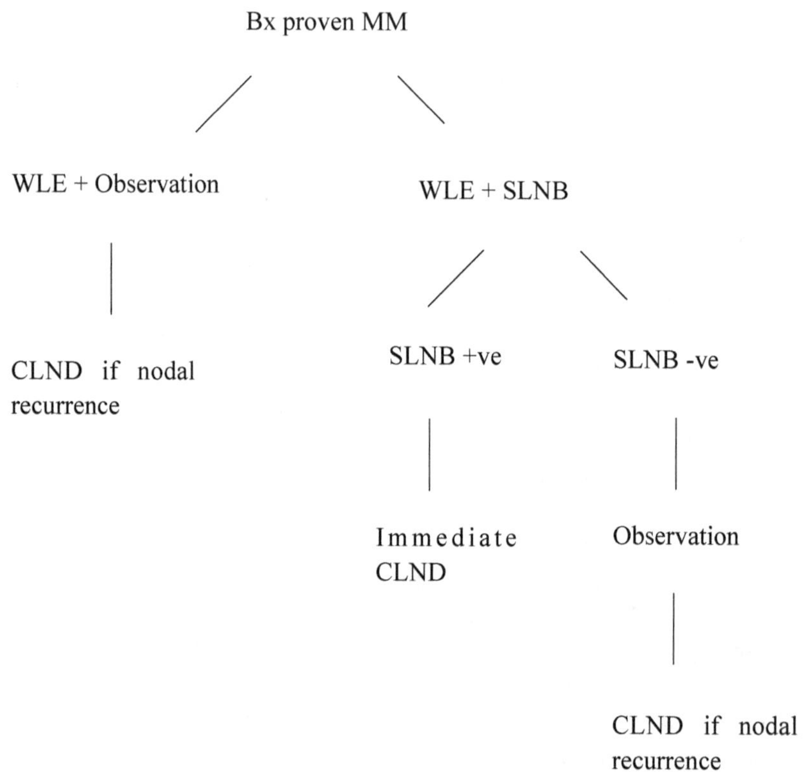

3. MSLT 1 RESULTS
Observation limb:
- ↑ #of nodes at CLND
- ↑ r/o lymphoedema post CLND

SLNB & Immediate CLND limb:
- ↑ DFS (i.e. ↑ melanoma-specific survival)

- No difference in 10yr survival
- Improved melanoma specific survival in SLNB negative subgroup (Ref: Table)

Table: Melanoma specific survival (in MSLT 1)

	SLNB +ve	**SLNB -ve**
Intermediate thickness MM	62%	85%
Thick MM	48%	64%

[Therefore a negative SLNB is reassuring for the patient that all *known* disease has been removed with the caveat that it does not change *how long* they live for]

4. ISSUES WITH MSLT 1 RESULTS
- Classification of intermediate thickness melanomas as 1.2 to 3.5mm
- Seemingly high proportion of "lost to follow up" or "died from other causes" in SLNB group.

MSLT 2 trial

1. REASONS FOR SETTING UP MSLT 2
Is it necessary to do CLND in every +ve SLNB? since only 8-12% of CLND (after a +ve SLNB) have nodal involvement (8% if examined with HE stain, 12% with special techniques).

2. MSLT 2 DESIGN

Biopsy proven primary MM
(BT>1.2mm OR ulcerated, any BT)
<u>AND</u> SLNB +ve

Observation with serial ultrasound   Immediate CLND

SLNB after a previous WLE

Clinical concern is that once WLE is done, it is no longer possible to identify the sentinel node that drains that area of skin.

Evidence = Evans et al. Ann Surg Oncol 2003
- n=76, where SLNB was performed after a previous WLE
- 99% success rate in SLNB [but this "sentinel node" is of the area of skin far away from the primary]
- Mean yield = 2.0 SLN / patient
- 15% = overall +ve SLN rate, on histo
- 4% = risk of MM in SLN negative basin

Block dissection for melanoma

WHO SHOULD DO A BLOCK DISSECTION
A surgeons who does at least 15 "blocks" per year [though there is no evidence behind this number]

INDICATION FOR A BLOCK DISSECTION
Known disease in the nodal basin (tissue diagnosis is usually by FNAC)

INDICATIONS FOR PELVIC DISSECTION
There is not much of a consensus. Prof. Balch at BAPRAS' Advanced Educational Course (2010) said that there is argument to say that every "inguinal" dissection should be an "ilio-inguinal" dissection.

Queen Elizabeth Hospital Birmingham Skin MDT indications are
- >3 inguinal nodes, or
- >3cm disease, or
- inguinal canal involvement

EORTC (European Organisation for Research & Treament of Cancer) Melanoma Group practice review paper (Testori et al. 2013):
> Surveyed 75 centres (predominantly european centres) and 65% do an ilio-inguinal dissection when SNB is +ve for macro-mets. [There is more data in this paper but it confusingly talks about 3 entities, ilio-inguinal dissection, deep inguinal dissection and superficial inguinal dissection without offering any distinction between the first two].

Describe a block dissection

Informed consent

GA, position, prep & drape

Identify landmarks

Incision, centered on disease

Identify boundaries

Start peeling off

Preserve important structures (Ref: Table)

Remove specimen, mark & send for histo in formalin

Washout with water

Hemostasis

Drains

Closure

Postop intructions (check bloods, drains out strategy, followup for wound review/histology/followup)

Table: Important structures that should be preserved if not directly involved in disease

Nodal basin	Important structures
Axilla	Cephalad: Branches of axillary artery & associated veins. (Brachial plexus is well covered within its fascial layer) Anteriorly: Medial pectoral nerve (usually sacrificed in dissection) Posteriorly: Thoraco-dorsal n/vasc. bundle Deep (along chest wall): Long thoracic nerve
Groin	Superiorly: Superficial inferior epigastric vessels Medially: Saphenous vein Centrally: Sapheno-femoral junction, branches of superficial femoral artery

For neck dissection, you would be expected to know the boundaries and contents of the triangles. If you have not seen many, then a good description is MacCammon & Shah, Operative techniques in Otolaryngology 2004; 15:152-9.

Adjuvant treatments

(ILI, ILP, Interferons, RT)

MM & pregnancy

Very little evidence base about the effects of MM in pregnancy

Management of patient with numerous atypical moles

This is no UK consensus.

1. RISK

- Estimates vary as to the risk of development of melanoma and somewhere around 1:10k nevi *per year* develop into melanoma.
- Positive family history (as well as numerous atypical moles), confers an almost 100% lifetime risk of melanoma.
- de novo melanomas account for 30-70% of cases

2. MANAGEMENT

The strategy is melanoma prevention by sun protection and routine skin examination, ideally q3/12 (visible inspection +/- digital photography +/- dermoscopy).

The issue is that,
- we don't know if it increases survival in this patient group, although we hope that catching it early would mean catching it at low Breslow thickness,
- visual inspection is inadequate to diagnose all melanomas.

RECOMMENDATIONS OF MANAGEMENT

1. Bergman W, van Voorst Vader PC, Ruiter DJ. [Dysplastic nevi and the risk of melanoma: a guideline for patient care. Nederlandse Melanoom Werkgroep van de Vereniging voor Integrale Kankercentra]. Ned Tijdschr Geneeskd. 1997 Oct 18;141(42):2010-4. Dutch
2. NIH Consensus conference. Diagnosis and treatment of early melanoma. Jama. 1992;268:1314–9

Lentigo maligna (LM)

Premalignant condition which presents as a flat uniform colored macule with well defined edges, usually on the cheek of a patient in their 60s & 70s. Can be from a few millimeters to a few centimeters in size. Its progression into melanoma is not very well defined, but areas of variegated colour are concerning.

Management of lentigo maligna consists of either
- Watch & wait (including pt education about warning signs), or
- Excision (one stage or serial, depending on the size of the lesion), or

- Incision biopsy of any darker patches within a large LM [this is the *only* indication for an incision biopsy in a suspicious melanocytic lesion. Otherwise, all suspected melanomas should have an excision biopsy. Ref Marsden et al].

Any bleeding/itching/ulceration should raise immediate concern of progression to melanoma (& a biopsy). A melanoma developing in an LM is called Lentigo Maligna Melanoma (LMM). #ConfusingTerminology

Congenital giant hairy nevus

These are rare disfiguring lesions present at birth with associated risk of malignant melanoma and neuro-cutaneous melanosis. Typically it is a baby presenting with a large disfiguring melanocytic lesion covering trunk, arms, legs &/or back. Incidence is approx. 1:20k

HOW BIG IS A "GIANT"?
The definition of "giant" has no consensus. It is variously reported as >20cm, >2%TBSA(outside H&N), >1% in H&N or those that cannot be excised in one operation (Ref: Arneja & Gosain CME: Giant congenital melanocytic nevi, PRS 2007; 120(2): 26e-40e) #ConfusingTerminology

Similarly, the risk of conversion to melanoma is not well quantified either. The numbers range from 2-90%, but it is certainly high enough to justify treatment.

HISTORY
Important points to note in the history are:
- Duration,
- Distribution,
- Recent changes esp. lumpiness, itching, bleeding,
- Seizures / Normal developmental milestones

Neurologic involvement is diagnosed on an MRI scan, usually by a neurologist/paediatrician. Signs and symptoms may include developmental delay, seizures and hydrocephalus. Because of multiple specialties involved in their care, these babies are best managed in a tertiary care paediatric centre where all specialties involved in their care are likely to be present under one roof.

Complications include,
1. Irritating symptoms like nodularity, itching, hypotrichosis
2. Psychosocial dysfunction secondary to aesthetic appearance
3. Prolonged treatment with the risk of surgical complications

4. Malignant transformations of cutaneous lesions
5. Extracutaneous melanocytic deposits causing seizures and malignant transformation.

EXAMINATION

Among other things, note:
- Size and distribution
- Coarse, thick hair growth
- Areas of lumpiness / ulceration / bleeding (either trauma or development of melanoma, always consider a biopsy)
- Is the child's interaction appropriate for their age (developmental milestones)

PRINCIPLES OF MANAGEMENT

- Early management to minimise transformation into malignant melanoma. It depends upon the age of presentation, size of lesion & its site.
- Multidisciplinary approach. Dermatologist for regular examination, early plastic surgery input, paediatricians & general practitioner. Neurologist if needed child psychologist

INDICATION FOR TREATMENT

- Excision of established melanoma,
- Prophylactic excision to decrease risk,
- Symptom control,
- But also,
    - aesthetic improvement,
    - psychosocial well-being,
    - maintenance of function

TREATMENT OPTIONS - NONSURGICAL

Within the first few weeks of life, based on the premise that melanocytes are more superficial at his stage and will migrate deeper overtime.

1. **Curettage of epidermis and upper dermis.** Heals in 10-14 days with little complications. Not recommended on scalp for risk of alopecia
2. **Dermabrasion / Versajet™**, possibly effective up to 1 year (5% r/o infection, 15% HT scarring)
3. **Chemical peels (using Phenol)**. IT Jackson et al. (PRS 2000; 105(1):1-11) have described their experience of using chemical phenols peels. Interestingly, the average pt. age was 3.8 years.

(Lasers have also been described but there is an inherent danger in providing large amounts of focussed energy to a pre-malignant lesion).

TREATMENT OPTIONS - SURGICAL

1. **Serial excision**, if expected to be excised in 3 stages or less (6 months apart)
2. **Tissue expansion & excision**, if serial excision will take >3 stages (i.e. aim to minimise the number of operations that the pt will have)
3. **Excision & reconstruction with skin substitutes & SSG**, have also been described

Stuff that no one tells you!

Spitz nevi

Rapidly growing symmetrical melanocytic lesion in a young child/adolescent whose clinical behaviour can vary from completely benign ("typical Spitz nevus") to frankly malignant("Spitzoid melanoma"). It typically looks like a brown/black or pink well circumscribed nodule on the cheek but its histopathology and clinical course are very difficult to correlate.

First described as "juvenile melanoma" by Sophie Spitz in 1948 as a case series, it was originally considered benign. Although Spitz originally described it as a benign lesion but at least one child in her series died of metastatic melanoma and similar histologic appearances were found in adult patients too, underlining the diagnostic challenges even at the outset.

MANAGEMENT DILEMMAS

- How to counsel parents & child
- Local management
- Surveillance & followup

SAFE MANAGEMENT

Frank detailed discussion with parents that,

- This is something that has an uncertain behaviour.
- Many of these lesions behave as "simple moles" but we can't be sure which ones will be the miscreants
- You are managing it as a team of specialists (MDT) and if needed will refer to another (even more) specialist team.
- There is/isn't an evidence *at this point in time* that this particular lesion is cancerous
- The safest way forward is management & surveillance as the worst case scenario (urgent excision, MDT discussion, regular followup).
- To contact GP / surgeon urgently if there is a sudden change in the lesion or any lump in the nodal basins.

LOCAL MANAGEMENT

After clinical diagnosis, complete excision with up to 5mm margin is sufficient. There is no evidence to support a further WLE in benign cases. Of course, if there is a feature suggestive of malignant melanoma it needs to be managed as such.

Considering the complexity of decision making, have a low threshold for further specialist referral.

MDT DISCUSSION

Not every histopathologist is comfortable with Spitz nevi so consider referring the histopath slides to a specialist. I'm not aware of any formal guidelines for management of Spitz nevi.

SURVEILLANCE

Regular self examination and followup as a melanoma is probably the safest approach. i.e. every 3 months for 3 years, then 6 months for another 2 years. Consider yearly f/u beyond that for 5 years (for a total of 10 years).

Actinic Keratosis (AK)

These are common pre-malignant lesions that occur on sun exposed areas, especially in Fitzpatrick 1 & 2 skin types and are related to cumulative sun exposure.

PRESENTATION

Red/pink/brown papules with scaly surfaces usually on scalp, forehead, face or back of hands.

CLINICAL BEHAVIOUR

- Spontaneous regression, up 25% regress over one year (but of these 15% recur)
- Persistence
- Progression to invasive SCC, with 6-10% risk at 10 years (60 to 65% SCCs arise from previous AKs)

TREATMENT

1. Cryotherapy

   67% lesion response rate/patient, 94% good or excellent cosmetic outcome (Thai et al. Int J Dermal 2004, 89 pts, 421 lesions). Hence a good option for solitary lesions

2. 5% Flourouracil (5FU, *Efudix*) xBD for 2-4/52 (manufacturer recommendation).
   - 80% reduction in number of lesions,
   - 94% clearance at two weeks
   - 98% clearance at four weeks (Berman B, Amini S et al. 2009)
     86% reduction in number of lesions if using 0.5%FU (likely due to increased patient compliance)
     SE = blotchy red angry looking rash (can be bad enough for patient to stop treatment) which is worse with 5% than with 0.5% formulation.

3. 5%IMQ (Imiquimod, *Aldara*) 2x/week for 16 weeks (manufacturer's recommendation)
   - 45-85% clearence -> 10% recurrence @12 months, 16% recurrence @18 months (Stockfleth et al. 2002)
   - SE = erythema, edema, ulcerations, blisters
   - Not licensed for use above the clavicle (i.e. in head and neck)

4. 3% diclofenac gel (*Solaraze*) xBD for 2-3/12 (Rivers et al. 2002)
   - 60% improvement
   - Useful if patient less compliant to 5FU or Aldara

5. Photodynamic therapy (PDT) with ALA (alpha hyroxy levulinic acid) has been described as well

Rates of sustained clearance of AK at 12 months (Krawtchenko et al. Br J Derma 2007)
   - Cryo = 4% (less side effects, but quick and easy)
   - 5FU = 33%
   - IMQ = 73% (most clearence, but longer treatment and side effects)

Aside: Cryotherapy

Cryotherapy is the application of sub-zero temperature for treatment of clinically benign lesions. Cryogen is liquid nitrogen at *minus*160 Celsius if delivered from a C-tip cryogun. The duration of application is generally 7 seconds and the tissue damage is done when it thaws after freezing. Cryo works better without scabs on the surface.

One method of application is to freeze the lesion completely and then count to 7 seconds while topping up any areas that want to thaw. Alternatively, you can start counting from the moment of first contact.

DFSP

Rare soft tissue sarcoma which is locally aggressive but has low malignant potential.

PRESENTATION

It presents as a solitary, usually asymptomatic plaque with blue/violet hue
- Mid to late 30s
- males = females
- usually @ trunk

Risk of local recurrence(LR) is proportional to the adequacy of the surgical margin.

TREATMENT
- WLE
- MMS
- Rarely (e.g. in advanced cases), RT / chemo with Imatinib

Ref: Meguerditchian et al. Am JCO 2009. n=48, single institution

	WLE	MMS
n	28 (2cm margin)	20 (2 layers)
LR @4yr	4%	zero %

Ref: Paradisi et al. Cancer Treat Rev 2008. n=79, literature review

	WLE	MMS
LR @5yr	13	zero

Protocol at LSMDT in QEH Birmingham = 1cm WLE & MMS of the margin

Merkel cell CA

Rare and aggressive tumour of neuroendocrine origin. The cell of origin is Merkel cell which is derived from neural crest and functions as a slowly adapting mechanoreceptor. (It differentiates as a part of Amine Precursor Uptake & Decarboxylation, APUD system).

PRESENTATION
Rapidly growing, firm, flesh coloured dome shaped papule on sun exposed skin.

DEMOGRAPHICS
- 2 x ↑ ♂
- 20x ↑ caucasians
- Average age @diagnosis = 70yrs
- 1/3rd occur in H&N

Increased risk (up to 100x ↑ than baseline) if h/o PUVA therapy for psoriasis. MCC confers increased risk of multiple myeloma, non-Hodgkin's lymphoma(NHL) & chronic lymphocytic lymphoma (CLL).

COURSE
Very high risk of LR, regional/distant mets

Poor prognostic factors
- male gender
- 65yr+ age
- >2cm size
- Trunk
- Nodal / distant disease on presentation

STAGING
1) MSKCC staging system. Allen et al. JCO 2005 (n=250, over 30 years)

Stage	Criteria	5yr survival
I	<2cm	81%
II	>2cm	67%
III	Nodal spread	52%
IV	Distant mets	11%

AJCC staged MCC in 2010 (http://www.cancer.gov/types/skin/hp/merkel-cell-treatment-pdq#section/_45).

2) AJCC Classification

(Reproduced with permission from Edge SB, Byrd DR, Compton CC, eds. AJCC Cancer Staging Manual. 7th ed. New York, NY.: Springer, 2010)

T Classification	Description
TX	Primary tumor cannot be assessed
T0	No evidence of primary tumor (e.g., nodal/metastatic presentation without associated primary)
Tis	*In situ* primary tumor.
T1	Maximum tumour size ≤2 cm
T2	>2 but ≤ 5 cm
T3	>5 cm
T4	Primary tumor invades bone, muscle, fascia, or cartilage.

N Classification	Description
NX	Regional lymph nodes cannot be assessed.
N0	No regional lymph nodes metastasis.
cN0	Nodes negative by clinical exam[1] (no pathologic node exam done)
pN0	Nodes negative by pathologic exam.
N1	Metastases in regional lymph node(s).
N1a	Micrometastasis[2]
N1b	Macrometastasis[3]
N2	In transit metastasis[4]

M Classification	Description
M0	No distant metastasis
M1	Metastases beyond regional lymph nodes
M1a	Metastases to skin, subcutaneous tissues, or distant lymph nodes
M1b	Metastasis to lung
M1c	Metastases to all other visceral sites

[1]Clinical detection of nodal disease may be via inspection, palpation, and/or imaging.
[2]Micrometastases are diagnosed after sentinel or elective lymphadenectomy.
[3]Macrometastases are defined as clinically detectable nodal metastases confirmed by therapeutic lymphadenectomy or needle biopsy.

[4]In transit metastasis: a tumour distinct from the primary lesion and located either (1) between the primary lesion and the draining regional lymph nodes or (2) distal to the primary lesion.

Stage	T	N	M
0	Tis	N0	M0
IA	T1	pN0	M0
IB	T1	cN0	M0
IIA	T2/T3	pN0	M0
IIB	T2/T3	cN0	M0
IIC	T4	N0	M0
IIIA	AnyT	N1a	M0
IIIB	AnyT	N1b/N2	M0
IV	AnyT	AnyN	M1

TREATMENT OF PRIMARY
3cm WLE / MMS (no difference between them)

NODAL MANAGEMENT
70% risk of nodal spread @2yrs

ELND - no trials

SLNB - up stages 1/3rd of patients (Gupta et al. *Arch Dermatol* 2006)
- +ve SLNB => 3x ↑ r/o recurrence
- +ve SLNB + adjuvant therapy → 50% 3yr survival
- +ve SLNB without adjuvant therapy → zero% 3yr survival

ROLE OF RADIOTHERAPY
RT to Primary site *and* nodal basin, for
- large tumors
- locally unresectable tumours
- +ve regional nodes

Sebaceous CA

Mixed adnexal tumour with a variable site of origin, histologic growth pattern and clinical presentation. 75% periocular (from Meibomian glands), 25% elsewhere (H&N, trunk, salivary glands, genitalia)

PRESENTATION

Slow-growing painless nodule, or chronic diffuse blephroconjunctivitis

DEMOGRAPHICS

↑ Asians

2x ↑ ♀

7-9th decade

Associated with radiation exposure and Muir Torre syndrome

COURSE

↑ r/o LR & mets

- direct extension eg via lacrimal duct
- lymphatic
- hematogenous (to lungs, liver, brain, parotid)

MANAGEMENT

WLE with 5-6mm margin

- 36% LR @5yr
- 18% mortality @5yr

WLE + MMS

- 11% LR

AFX (Atypical FibroXanthoma)

AFX is a locally aggressive but rarely metastasising spindle cell tumour on head and neck of sun exposed individuals (usually in their 70s) on trunk and extremities of younger patients (usually in their 30s). Incidence is the same in both genders.

PRESENTATION

Rapidly growing dome shape papule/nodule, covered with thin epidermis, on actinically damaged skin of a fair complexion individual +/- ulceration

DIFFERENTIAL DIAGNOSIS

Pyogenic granuloma, SCC, BCC, amelanotic melanoma, MCC

MANAGEMENT

WLE or MMS

Table: Difference between WLE and MMS in management of AFX (Ref: Davis & Brodland, Dermatol Surg. 1997)

	WLE	MMS
n	25	19
Recurrence	12% @6yrs	Zero %
Mets	4%	Zero %

Management protocol at LSMDT in QEH Birmingham:
1cm WLE and MMS of the margin

Aside: Historical note

Previously both AFX & MFH were considered different presentations of the same malignancy with AFX being superficial sarcoma (with low/intermediate r/o mets) and MFH a deeper sarcoma (with increased risk of mets). The 2002 WHO classification mandated cell line origin for classification of sarcomas making MFH an obsolete term, versus "undifferentiated pleomorphic sarcoma NOS"

MFH (Malignant FibroHistiocytoma)

It is a soft tissue sarcoma, which is histologically either an undifferentiated pleomorphic sarcoma or a myxofibrosarcoma.

DEMOGRAPHICS
Usually in elderly
10% in H&N

PRESENTATION
Progressively enlarging skin colour or subcutaneous nodule, usually solitary & up to 50% may have distant metastasis at presentation (usually to lungs).

DIFFERENTIAL DIAGNOSIS
SCC, BCC, Amelanotic melanoma

MANAGEMENT
Surgical excision + RT

PROGNOSIS
Prognosis is poor with 30-35% mets *after* surgery

Angiosarcoma (AS)

Uncommon, aggressive and usually fatal neoplasm of vascular endothelium. 2-3x ↑ common in females.

TYPES
- "Idiopathic" cutaneous AS. 50-6-% of cases
- Lymphedema associated (=Stewart-Trevez syndrome)
- Radiation induced
- Epitheloid

1) Cutaneous Angiosarcoma
Presents as violet/red ill-defined patch on central face/forehead/scalp. Has a tendency to bleed and ulcerate. It has high metastatic potential to viscera. Prognosis is poor with 50% mortality @15months.

2) Lymphedema associated Angioscarcoma
Initial description by Stuart & Trevez in six patients (many years) after mastectomy.
- 5% risk @five years post mastectomy.
- Presents as violet black nodule over the brawny edema.
- Carries poor prognosis & low survival

3) Radiation induced Angiosarcoma
After RT for benign or malignant conditions

4) Epitheloid angiosarcoma
Rare type. Likely on lower limb

MANAGEMENT
Surgical excision with wide margins
Consider amputation of extremity, if no distant involvement
Chemo/Radio as palliation

Effects of radiation

Figure: UV radiation types and their wavelength ranges

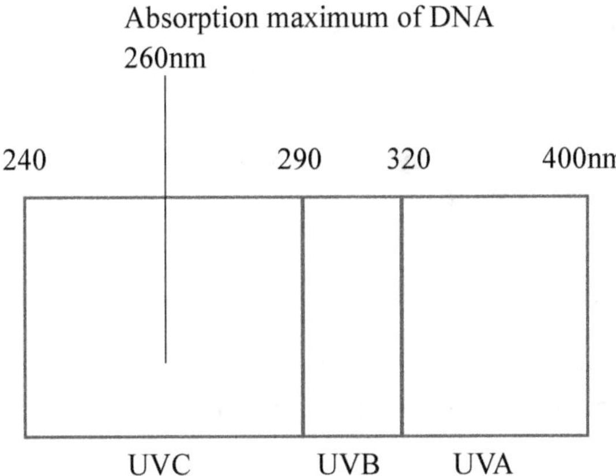

Tanning beds in adolescent:
- At least 1.4x ↑ risk of MM
- 2x ↑ risk of MM, if >10 sessions

UVC is absorbed by ozone, but is the most damaging to DNA (as DNA absorption maximum is 260nm). UVB & UVC → pyrimidine dimers & other photoproducts → link adjacent pyrimidines → bend the helix → interference with DNA replication & RNA synthesis. The characteristic DNA mutation induced is C:G to T:A, and inactivation of p53 tumour suppressor gene.

Figure: Cell cycle

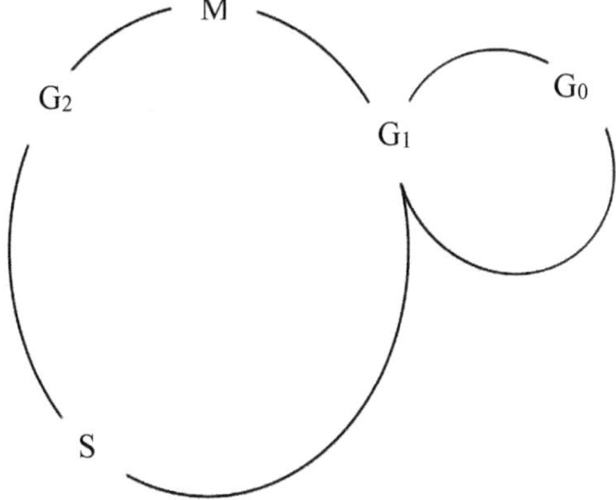

Major mechanism of radiation damage:

Cells in S-phase (Ref: Figure) have already initiated DNA synthesis and have no choice but to carry on (i.e. divide or die). If the DNA polymerases can't remove a damaged segment of DNA (Ref: Aside, DNA repair pathway), they are replaced by more tolerant polymerases which allow damaged DNA to go on replicating and letting the cell divide ("Tolerance mechanism").

Aside: DNA repair pathway = Nucleotide Excision Repair pathway (NER)

This pathway includes
1. proteins that recognise DNA damage,
2. nucleases that excise that DNA strand,
3. DNA polymerases to synthesise new DNA, and
4. DNA ligase that join the new DNA to the 'backbone'

Sarcoma

CORE KNOWLEDGE
Principles of management
Organisation of sarcoma MDT

APPROACH TO PATIENT - HISTORY
(see below)

APPROACH TO PATIENT - EXAMINATION
Appropriate examination of the swelling (site, size, tenderness, fixity, distal neurovascular status of the limb and hepatomegaly).

APPROACH TO PATIENT - MANAGEMENT
Make sure you refer the pt to the sarcoma MDT before attempting any tissue diagnosis

The prognostic factors for sarcoma are:
1. Site
2. Size
3. Histological type & grade
4. Surgical margins

EXPECTED VIVA QUESTIONS
- Risk factors e.g. herbicides
- Tissue diagnosis or imaging first, and why
- Grading
- Principles of limb salvage/ recon

RECOMMENDED PAPERS
1. Misra A, Mistry N, Grimer R, Peart F. The management of soft tissue sarcoma. *J Plast Reconstr & Aesthetic Surg.* 2009 Feb;62(2):161–74.

Sarcomas are rare malignant mesenchymal tumours arising from bone or soft tissues. As plastic surgeons, we are only likely to see soft tissue sarcomas. This would (& should) be in a tertiary care centre in a multidisciplinary setting only.

I strongly recommend reading the review by Grimer & Peart (JPRAS 2009) which gives an excellent description of the condition and management. For most part, what follows is the information that I could not find in that paper and had to look elsewhere.

Clinical evaluation

Clinical evaluation of a suspected sarcoma is different form any other cancer in that 1) the oncologic clearance & reconstruction must be planned before any biopsy, and 2) the swelling must be imaged (MRI) before any biopsy is attempted.

1. EXAMINATION

There is no one "typical" presentation of the diverse group of soft tissue sarcomas. Any swelling which is rapidly growing, has evidence of neovascularisation (telengiectasia or prominent veins) or high metabolism (warm to touch without evidence of infection) should raise alarm bells of a soft tissue sarcoma.

If a swelling is
- >5cm in size,
- deep to deep fascia,
- rapidly growing, and
- increasingly painful

there is 85% chance that it is a soft tissue sarcoma (Misra et al. JPRAS 2009). It should be evaluated with an MRI scan, *before* a histologic diagnosis is attempted. This is due to,
- high risk of seeding the biopsy tract
- because edema from the biopsy will make interpretation of a later MRI difficult

The biopsy site has to be planned by the sarcoma surgeons who will do the final excision, as they will need to excise the biopsy tract as well and plan reconstruction.

2. IMAGING

An MRI scan will show the extent of the tumor, tissue planes & compartments that are involved/spared, as well as integrity of neurovascular structures traversing the area (esp. in an extremity).

Once a histologic diagnosis is made, pt. will need a staging CT scan. The commonest sites of sarcoma mets are,

- From extremities, 70% go to lungs
- From retroperitnoeal / visceral, go to liver
- Lymph node mets are uncommon (<4%) except in a some childhood cancers

3. BIOPSY OPTIONS

There is more than one _wrong_ way to biopsy a suspected sarcoma. Hence imaging before biopsy makes a lot of difference.

Biopsy type	
Incisional	Not recommended
Tru-cut	Standard practice, as a good core sample can be obtained. This should only be done by the sarcoma surgeon.
FNAC*	Cannot help you grade the tumor effectively and hence not useful to plan surgery. Not recommended
Excisional	Never a good idea as it risks contamination of surrounding tissues. Not recommended

*technically it is a cytology, and not a biopsy ;)

For sarcomas, tissue diagnosis is only part of the story and management is affected more by tumour grading.

Grading

Features useful in histological grading of sarcomas are:

- necrosis,
- mitosis,
- pleomorphism,
- differentiation,
- cellularity

Different grading systems lay different emphasis on each of these characteristics.

No single grading system is best for all sarcomas, either because some histological types cannot be graded well or that definitive grading may be logistically impossible for very large tumors (e.g. >1kg). Because of this limitation, "high grade" sarcoma may be defined slightly differently in each centre.

Systems of grading

	Source	Reference
4 stage system		(Broders)
3 stage system	NCI (national cancer institute)	Costa et al. Cancer 1994
	French Federation of cancer centers (FNCLCC)	Trojani et al. Int J Cancer 1984
2 stage system	Memorial Sloan Kettering Cancer Centre (MSKCC)	

1. TROJANI GRADING SYSTEM

Histologic characteristic	Score
Tumor	Score 1: 0-9/10hpf
	2: 10-19/10hpf
	3: 20+/10hpf
Necrosis	Score 0: No necrosis
	1: 1-50% necrosis
	2: >50% necrosis
Differentiation	Score 1: like adult tissue
	2: Sarcoma of a definitive histologic type
	3: synovial / embryonal / undifferentiated sarcomas

Total score:

2 or 3 $\Rightarrow$ Trojani grade 1

4 or 5 $\Rightarrow$ Trojani grade 2

6 though 8 $\Rightarrow$ Trojani grade 3

Inter-observer agreement on Trojani grading (Ref: Devita and Hellman)
- 60-75% on grade
- 60-75% on histo type

Sarcoma staging

1. AJCC CLASSIFICATION 2010

(Reproduced with permission from Edge SB, Byrd DR, Compton CC, eds. AJCC Cancer Staging Manual. 7th ed. New York, NY.: Springer, 2010)

It excludes GIST, desmoid, Kaposi, infantile fibrosarcoma
It adds staging for angiosarcoma, extraskeletal Ewing's, DFSP

Stage	Grade*	Tumor**	Node	Mets
I A	GX - G1	T1a-1b	N0	M0
I B	GX - G1	T2a-2b	N0	M0
II A	G2-3	T1a-1b	N0	M0
II B	G2	T2a-2b	N0	M0
III	G3	T2a-2b	N0	M0
	G any	any T	N1	M0
IV	any G	any T	any N	M1

* Grading is by Trojani 3 stage system
** T1 is <5cm & T2 is >5cm, either can have a suffix 'a' (if tumour is superficial to deep fascia), or 'b' (if tumor is deep).

SIZE

AJCC has specified that 5cm is an arbitrary limit to help dichotomise patient population. Other than that, it holds no special value and that the size should be treated as a continuous variable.

DEPTH

Depth is relative to the deep fascia of the trunk or extremity. A superficial tumour is located entirely in the subcutaneous plane without any extension through the muscle fascia or in to the muscle.

GRADING

Traditionally AJCC favoured a 4 tier grading system, but currently uses the 3 tier FNCLCC (i.e.Trojani) grading system. Since grading is an important part of disease staging & management planning in sarcomas, it s important to ensure adequate specimen for an accurate grading. A sample from a small number/ volume of core biopsies can be non-representative e.g. if it show low grade tumour.

2. SARCOMA STAGING (ENNEKING)

Enneking stage	Grade	Site	Mets
I A	G1	T1	M0
I B	G1	T2	M0
II A	G2	T1	M0
II B	G2	T2	M0
III A	any G		Regional
III B	any G		Distant

T1 = Intra-compartmental, T2 = Extra-compartmental
G1 = low grade, G2 = high grade

Excision

Types of sarcoma excisions may be,
1. Incomplete, usually from an attempted biopsy of a lesion "not" recognised as a sarcoma. (Aside: "Whoops" procedure)
2. Marginal, again usually from removal of a "lipoma"
3. Wide
4. Radical

Aside: The "Whoops" procedure

An operation where a subcutaneous swelling is removed as a "lipoma" but histology confirms it as a sarcoma.

Due to its wide catchment area, the West Midlands sarcoma tertiary care centre (based at the National Orthopaedic Hospital in Birmingham) sees enough of these for this category to be recognised as a separate entity. It facilitates communication between specialties that a biopsy has been performed whose incision and dissection may lie outside the ideal approach for removal of such a lesion and that this potentially seeded tract will need to be removed at the time of definitive surgery. It also identifies that an imaging scan will show artefacts.

Ideally you want a radical excision for sarcomas, but this may violate tissue planes and remove n/vasc. structures. This is esp. a problem on limbs, where major vessels or nerves may lie close to the tumour, and so limb salvage may need to be considered. The surgical plan (within the sarcoma MDT) takes into account (in addition to histologic type, grading, size and location) whether a tumour free plane may be found adjacent to these structures (hence the need for a good quality, free from biopsy artefact MRI & a specialist radiologist).

If there is doubt about a clear margin (either preop, intraop or at histology) then radiotherapy (&/or chemo) may be considered.

If the neurovascular structures in the limb are clearly involved, then the next question is how much function the pt will have in that limb if these are removed with the tumour. If the expected function is very little, then amputation will need to be considered. This is never an easy decision, and needs to balance
- Expected survival after amputation,
- Expected function after amputation,
- Risk of recurrence if these structures are preserved intraop followed by postop radiotherapy, alongside
- Pt wishes

Even if the tumour in not on the limbs, all biopsy methods potentially seed the biopsy track. These biopsy tracks need to be removed at the time of definitive excision. Anticipating this problem, the sarcoma surgeon needs to plan biopsy with the definitive approach and reconstruction in mind.

The complexity of this decision making is precisely the reason for having a sarcoma surgeon, a plastic reconstructive surgeon, clinical and radiation oncologists, specialist nurses as well as histopathologist and radiologist under the same roof at the same time - the sarcoma MDT.

Magnetic resonance imaging (MRI)

MRI is an imaging modality that uses strong magnetic fields and radio frequencies to visualise anatomical structures in detail by looking at the subatomic particles called protons.

Protons have an inherent ability to align themselves with an external magnetic field (due to a quantum mechanical property called "spin"). How well the protons align is related to the strength of the magnetic field.

This alignment, once achieved, is disrupted by a radiowave of appropriate frequency* causing the protons to wobble like a top ("precession") as they absorb the energy from that radiowave. When this radiowave is switched off, the protons want to get back into their alignment and release the absorbed energy as a new radiowave of the same frequency. The strength of the emitted radiowave is proportional to the number of protons in a small volume (called a "voxel", a slant on the word 'pixel').

The time it takes for the protons to realign themselves is related to the **T1 relaxation time**, which is unique for each tissue (although affected by the external magnetic field).

Protons aligned together by the external radiowave affect each other as well ("spin-spin interaction") and recovery from this effect is related to the **T2 relaxation time**. This time interval is unique to each tissue as well, but is not affected by the external magnetic field.

T1 images are better at showing anatomy while T2 show pathology. STIR images utilise a specific technique to suppress the signal from fat allowing improved images in the vicinity of fatty tissue. Similarly FLAIR technique allows suppression of signal from fluid & is used mainly to suppress CSF signal for better CNS views.

*Larmor frequency

Congenital

Vascular anomalies

CORE KNOWLEDGE
Classification
Difference between hemangiomas and malformations
Concerns
Management principles

APPROACH TO PATIENT - HISTORY
How old is the baby?
When did it appear?
- Parents may not remember exactly, so spend a bit of time exploring

Progression with time
Is it isolated? or are there more vascular anomalies / other congenital anomalies
- Always consider syndromic conditions
- >5 hemangiomas => 20% r/o visceral hemangiomas esp intra-hepatic

Any complications, pain, bleeding, change in size when the baby cries, or with dependancy.
- Ask the parent to *carefully* move the baby around so that the lesion is dependant

Developmental history
Family history
Parental concerns

APPROACH TO PATIENT - EXAMINATION
Confirm the site and size of the lesion
Are there any signs of complications? e.g. bleeding, scab
Consider the risk of functional problems
Consider the risk of psychosocial problems
Look for other similar lesions by examining the rest of the baby

APPROACH TO PATIENT - TREATMENT
Treatment principles are
1. Minimise physical complications
2. Alleviate psychosocial distress
3. Avoid overly aggressive procedures

Exact treatment depends on the specific diagnosis (see below)

EXPECTED CLINICAL QUESTIONS

In practice you may see a baby's face showing a large vascular anomaly on e.g. a cheek/ tip of nose / eyelid. Or it may be a large vascular anomaly on limb / torso / peri-anal area, covering a certain percentage of body surface area.

Make sure to think through and express your concerns about any obvious functional problems expected (e.g. deprivational amblyopia, breathing difficulty etc), but it is unwise to commit to a specific diagnosis at least until you have taken the history.

- Classification of vascular anomalies
- Classification of vascular malformations
- Schobinger classification
- Phases of haemangioma
- Indications for propanolol
- Indications for other treatments
- Options of treatment if first line does not work
- Contents of treatment agents (e.g. Onyx, Ethibloc, OK432)
- Complications

RECOMMENDED PAPERS

1. Mulliken JB, Glowacki J. Hemangiomas and vascular malformations in infants and children: a classification based on endothelial characteristics. *Plast Reconstr Surg.* 1982 Mar;69(3):412-22
2. Beck DO, Gosain AK. The Presentation and Management of Hemangiomas *Plast Reconstr Surg.* 2009 Jun;123(6):181e – 191e.
3. Gampper TJ, Morgan RF. Vascular anomalies: hemangiomas. *Plast Reconstr Surg.* 2002;110(2):572–85.
4. Jackson IT. The challenge of large vascular malformations. *European J Plast Surg.* 2009 Feb;32(1):1–9.
5. Liu AS, Mulliken JB, Zurakowski D, Fishman SJ, Greene AK. Extracranial Arteriovenous Malformations: Natural Progression and Recurrenceafter Treatment *Plast Reconstr Surg.* 2010 Apr;125(4):1185–94.

Classification of vascular anomalies

The current classification is from 1996 by ISSVA (International Society for Study of Vascular Anomalies). It is based on the description by Mulliken & Glowacki (PRS 1982) but with some additions.

A. Tumors
1. Infantile Haemangiomas*
2. Congenital haemangiomas**
    RICH
    NICH
3. Rare forms
    Kaposiform hemangioendothelioma

B. Malformations
1. Fast flow, with arterial component
2. Slow flow
    Venous
    Capillary
    Lymphatic

* Infantile Haemangiomas, are true endothelial tumors
** RICH, are present at birth but involute rapidly afterwards. NICH, as the name suggests, do not involute.

Infantile haemangioma

It is a tumour of vascular endothelium that characteristically appears soon after birth, grows rapidly (out of proportion to the body growth) for 12 to 18 months, then regresses spontaneously over several years and finally involutes into a fibrofatty mass.

It is one of the commonest congenital anomalies affecting up to one in 10 babies A commonly quoted figure is that 30% regress by two years, 50% by five years and 70% by seven years of age.

Treatment

A) DO NOTHING

This is especially true for small, isolated lesions which are not cosmetically sensitive. It is still advisable to follow up the baby up regularly especially if the lesion is rapidly increasing, to monitor its growth, anticipate problems (with lesion or with your diagnosis!), address complications and for parent education/ reassurance.

Parents can be quite concerned with the appearance of the lesion and its growth. They'll need reassurance that this is not a cancer and in fact is a very common condition. Parents may want the lesion treated with propranolol nonetheless (esp. if they've been searching internet forums). You may want to explain that treatment with propranolol is up to 18 months and though its risk profile is very favourable, the risks are not zero.

Always consider the very small risk of childhood sarcomas mimicking as haemangioma, especially if you are not in a specialist centre (hence the regular follow up). There have only been approximately 4500 paediatric soft tissue sarcomas reported in the SEER database (http://www.cancer.gov/cancertopics/pdq/treatment/child-soft-tissue-sarcoma/HealthProfessional/page1) between 1975 - 2008.

B) PHARMACOLOGICAL

1) Oral propranolol

Increasingly becoming a de facto standard. A typical dose is 2mg/kg/day in 2 divided doses, for 12-18months. Monitor the baby's BP and BM for first 48hrs in hospital. There is risk of hypoglycaemia, hypotension (e.g. at start of treatment, or after dose increases) and recurrence (esp. if treatment is stopped before the lesions starts to involute).

2) Oral corticosteroids

Used commonly before propranolol was available for this indication. Typical dose is <3mg/kg/day for 4-6 weeks, followed by tapering over 2-3 months. Dose can be up to 5mg/kg/day (but always check with a paediatrician and BNF for children).

30% babies are "clear responders", 30% are "non-responders" & rest are intermediate. There are risks of cushingoid face, GI complaints, irritability etc. but usually resolve when steroids are stopped. Steroids may be considered instead of propranolol e.g. if there are no facilities available to admit the child for monitoring.

3) Chemotherapeutics

Before propranolol, these were the 2nd line treatment (in available centres) after steroids. Vincristine has a 96% response rate. The given dose is half the "oncologic dose" hence systemic side effects are less. But it needs to be administered intra-venously by a paediatric oncologist and has the inherent risk of local extravasation (with ulceration and skin necrosis).

4) Interferon Alpha2a

Mostly of historical significance only. Given for 9-14 months (to avoid rebound growth) it has an associated risk of developmental diplegia (hence an initial neurological exam, which is repeated monthly).

C) SURGICAL

Surgical option is almost never used for actively growing lesions. Previously that was the case because most of these lesions were self-limiting. These days is it is because of the effectiveness of therapy with propranolol.

Residual involuted hemangiomas may be excised later in life for cosmetic reasons.

Complications

1. Endangering, which can imminently compromise life / limb / function
2. Rapid growth, which may compromise function
3. Ulceration & bleeding
4. Cosmesis

High risk conditions associated with location of haemangiomas

1) Haemangioma on upper lid

Deprivational amblyopia,

Inability develop binocular vision,

Astigmatism secondary to the pressure on cornea

2) Haemangioma on nose

Risk of respiratory obstruction as babies are obligate nose breathers for 4-6 months each

3) Preauricular/Parotid area

Conductive hearing loss leading to speech and developmental delay

4) Subglottic lesions

Associated with multiple cutaneous haemangiomas. Increased risk of symptomatic airway involvement. (Don't forget to involve your ENT colleagues).

5) PHACES Syndrome

It is an acronym describing an association of haemangiomas with CNS vascular malformations. (**P**osterior fossa malformation **H**aemangioma, **A**rterial, **C**ardiac, **E**ye, **S**ternal abnormalities)

6) Posterior cutaneous haemangiomas

Risk of spinal-cord anomalies

7) Perineal cutaneous haemangiomas

Risk of imperforate anus, renal anomalies

KASABACH-MERRITT PHENOMENON

It is a consumptive coagulopathy which can be rapidly life threatening. Conceptually, it can be thought of as a localised form of DIC. It needs urgent *medical* management preferably in a specialised centre (usually with steroids).

Vascular malformations

These are aberrant collection of microscopically normal structures.

History, examination and management principles are still the same as above. These cases are managed in a team approach with input from paediatrician, paediatric cardiologist, interventional radiologist, GP and healthcare visitor.

Management algorithm

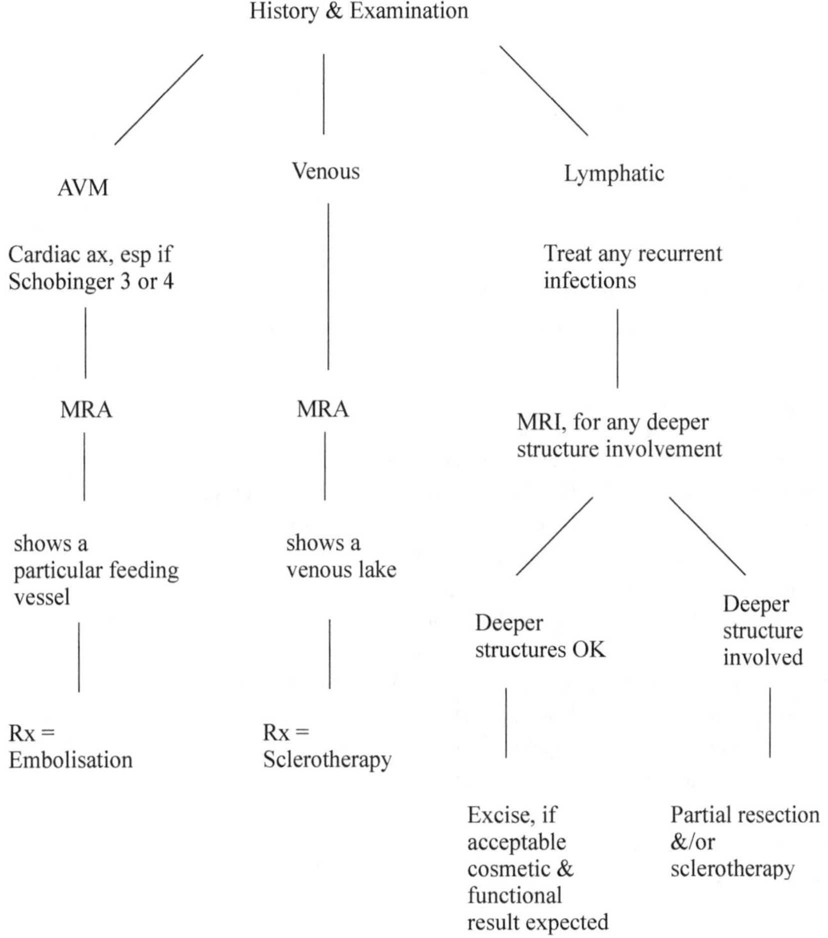

AVM

DIAGNOSIS
Mostly on history

EXAMINATION
Visible pulsations
Palpable thrill
Bruit

CLASSIFICATION (SCHOBINGER)
1. Quiescent
2. Growing
3. Tissue destruction (bleeding, or ulceration)
4. High output cardiac failure

TREATMENT
Embolisation +/- surgery

Embolisation route: trans-arterial or percutaneous
Embolising agent: coil / beads / absolute alcohol / "Onyx".

Aside: Onyx™

Onyx™ is used more frequently in H&N AVMs. It consists of ethylene vinyl co-polymer (EVOH) dissolved in DMSO (dimethyl sulphoxide) with suspended micronised Tantalum (as a contrast for flouroscopy). Once injected in the AVM, the DMSO solvent escapes in blood, causing the EVOH copolymer & Tantalum to precipitate (from outside in) over about 5 minutes.

It comes as two formulations, Onyx18 (6% EVOH, that has lower viscosity) and Onyx34 (8% EVOH) and looks like a grey toothpaste-like material. Its good penetrance makes it better than other embolising agents to travel to the nidus.

It is quite expensive (approx £5k) and there is risk of extrusion (though it heals over time).

Venous malformations

HISTORY
Can become firm and painful for a few days (risk of thrombophlebitis)

Get bigger with trauma, puberty, pregnancy

EXAMINATION
Engorges with dependency

TREATMENT
1. Sclerotherapy by an interventional radiologist. Contrast is injected in the malformation, which typically looks like a "bunch of grapes", then sclerosant is injected until the swelling is palpably hard. Patient is admitted overnight for iv fluids to prevent renal failure.
2. Surgery, for any residual disease provided acceptable cosmesis and functional result can be obtained.

Lymphatic malformations

Slow-growing, painless but prone to recurrent infections

CLINICAL CLASSIFICATION
Macrocystic: single cyst in one plane. Rx = surgery / injection with sclerosant.

Microcystic: hundreds of small cysts which infiltrate normal tissues, hence can't be injected and any primary surgery will likely be extensive. Rx = Bleomycin

TREATMENT OPTIONS
1) Sclerotherapy
2) Bleomycin. Works well by injection "around" the area and has good penetrance
3) Surgery for any residual disease (provided acceptable cosmesis and functional result can be obtained).

Sclerosants
1. STD: Sodium Tetra Dacyl sulphate comes as "Fibrovein" (in 0.2%, 0.5%, 1% & 3% strengths).
2. Ethibloc: alcoholic solution of corn protein ("Zein") which has thrombogenic and fibrogenic properties
3. OK432: Lyophilised mixture of Group A Strep pyogenes treated with Benzyl penicillin. Comes as "Pacibanil", given as 0.2ml injection and can be repeated.

Capillary malformations

Incidence approx. 1:1000 population

TREATMENT

1) Laser, PDL (295nm), or KTP lasers have 1-1.5 mm penetrance
2) Surgery, for debulking

STURGE WEBER SYNDROME

Capillary malformation over trigeminal nerve distribution (usu. forehead and cheek) with associated intra-cranial malformation (r/o epilepsy and developmental delay).

PORT-WINE STAIN (PWS)

Not to be confused with Cafe-au-lait patch of neurofibromatosis

Cleft lip & palate

CORE KNOWLEDGE
Embryology
Epidemiology
Management principles
Associated syndromes
Repair techniques
Patient pathway
Counselling

APPROACH TO BABY - HISTORY
Diagnosis may be made on a

- prenatal ultrasound (needs a good instrument, favourable lie of foetus and a skilled operator),
- at birth (by parents or paediatrician), or
- later in life (especially sub-mucous cleft palate, which commonly presents to GP/paediatrician as "delay in speech development")

INITIAL CONTACT WITH PARENTS
1. Congratulate parents
2. Counsel family
    Rapport, history (baby's development, FHx)
    Ideas, expectations and concerns
3. Evaluate
    Cleft starting with theory
    Associated syndromes
    Comorbidities
4. Introduce MDT. Nurses, cleft surgeon, geneticist, clinical psychologist, ENT/max fax
5. Discuss feeding and growth
6. Discuss timeline for surgery (Lip@3/12, Palate 6-9/12, Dental 8-12yr)

Additionally for Pierre Robin syndrome, admit the baby for:
7. 48hr saturation monitoring
8. Weight gain chart
9. Parental education, BLS training & competencies (e.g. NPA insertion & care)

APPROACH TO PATIENT - EXAMINATION
Cleft lip

Cleft palate

> Examin baby's palate in the "cleft position" with parent and doctor sitting opposite with knees almost touching. Baby's torso is on parent's lap and head in doctor's lap. The baby is held by the parent from shoulders and torso. Position yourself to allow gentle extension of baby's neck to allow visualisation of the cleft. [It is very important to explain this manoeuvre to the parent before you attempt it]

APPROACH TO PATIENT - TREATMENT
See below

EXPECTED CLINICAL QUESTIONS
Expect to see a picture of the baby showing a right/left complete/incomplete unilateral cleft lip and/or palate. You should be comfortable describing the condition you see.

Draw the markings for a unilateral cleft lip repair [Plenty of practice].

Counselling

RECOMMENDED PAPERS
1. Fisher DM, Sommerlad BC. Cleft Lip, Cleft Palate, and Velopharyngeal Insufficiency *Plast Reconstr Surg.* 2011 Oct;128(4):342e – 360e.
2. Johns DF, Rohrich RJ, Awada M. Velopharyngeal Incompetence:: A Guide for Clinical Evaluation. *Plast Reconstr Surg.* 2003 Dec;112(7):1890–8.
3. Liau JY, Sadove AM, van Aalst JA. An Evidence-Based Approach to Cleft Palate Repair *Plast Reconstr Surg.* 2010 Dec;126(6):2216–21.
4. Stal S, Brown RH, Higuera S, Hollier LH, Byrd HS, Cutting CB, et al. Fifty Years of the Millard Rotation-Advancement: Looking Back and Moving Forward *Plast Reconstr Surg.* 2009 Apr;123(4):1364–77.
5. Liau JY, Sadove AM, van Aalst JA. An Evidence-Based Approach to Cleft Palate Repair. *Plast Reconstr Surg.* 2010 Dec;126(6):2216–21.

6. Eurocleft Part 1- Principles & study design CPCJ 1992
7. Eurocleft Part 2- Craniofacial form & soft tissue profile CPCJ 1992
8. Eurocleft Part 3- Dental arch relationships CPCJ 1992
9. Eurocleft Part 4- Assessment of nasolabial appearence CPCJ 1992
10. Eurocleft Part 5 - General discussion n conclusion 1992 CPCJ
11. Bongaarts DutchCleft 2004 Nov CPCJ
12. Mars GOSLON Yardstick to ax dental arch 1987 CPJ
13. McCance Sri Lankan CLP model analysis CPCJ 1993

Embryology

Lip = 4-8/40
Palate = 7-10/40

NOMENCLATURE

Primary palate = anterior to incisive foramen = Palatine process of maxilla
Secondary palate = posterior to incisive foramen = hard palate posterior to incisive foramen & all of soft palate

Stats needed for counselling

	CL / CLP	CP
Epidemiology	1:1000 overall 1:750 Caucasian 1:500 Asian 1: 2k African	1:2000 No variation with race
	M : F = 2:1	more in females
	L : R : bilat = 6 : 3 : 1	
	CLP : CL = 2 : 1	
	3% syndromic	
The risk of cleft in next baby		
One child affected	4%	2%
One parent	2-4%	2-4%
One parent AND one child	7%	7%
One child AND +ve FHx (but normal parents)	14-17%	15%
Associated syndrome		

	Van der Woude:
	  AD
	  Lip pits (=accessory salivary glands)
	  +/- syndactyly
		Down's

		Trisomy 13
		Stickler

	CL / CLP	CP
		Pierre-Robin sequence VCF = DiGeorge = 22q11 deletion CHARGE

TRISOMY 21 (DOWN SYNDROME)

Affects approximately 1:700 live births, babies have characteristic facial features and variable degree of learning difficulties. The condition is associated with congenital heart defects and hypothyroidism.

TRISOMY 13 (PATAU SYNDROME)

Affects approximately 1:10K live births, the baby has an extra 13 chromosome. It is associated with CNS and ocular malformations, CL/P, polydactyly and severe learning difficulties.

STICKLER

Risk of retinal detachment, cardiac and sensorineural problems

VCF

Also called DiGeorge / 22q11 deletion syndrome

Affected system	Consequence	Notes
Cardiac abnormalities	Abnormally medial positioned carotids	Risk of damage in (posterior/ lateral) pharyngeal flap surgery
Abnormal face	Flat long expressionless face, +/- Downslanting palpebral fissures & epicanthal folds, +/- Pinched nasal tip	D/D with Mobius syndrome
Thymic aplasia		
Cleft palate		
Hypocalcaemia		

CHARGE

It is an acronym for **C**oloboma of eye, **H**eart defects, choanal **A**tresia, growth **R**etardation, **G**enital, **E**ar anomalies and hence the need for MDT management.

PIERRE-ROBIN SEQUENCE (PRS)

= micrognathia + relatively large tongue (causing glossoptosis) + wide U-shaped cleft palate.

It is called a 'sequence' because there is one causative factor which results in a cascade of abnormalities. The palate develops from bilateral pillars which assume a horizontal position in 7-8th week of gestation. A smaller size (rudimentary) jaw interposes the developing tongue between this process and physically prevents the palatal shelves (usually the left one, which develops a week after the right) from assuming their normal position. This results in the wide U-shaped cleft palate.

After birth, the baby is at risk of obstructing their airway by the tongue which is *relatively* larger than the airway. (Note that in absolute terms, the main problem is the small mandible which cannot position the tongue in the right place. The base of tongue is retro-positioned and the baby may not be able to keep his airway open).

Eventually the babies "grow out of it" as the size of the airway gets better and the baby has more strength and control of their musculature. But until that happens, the baby needs protection of their airway and a means to feed. A small airway and a cleft palate makes it difficult for many of these babies to breathe and feed at the same time.

Management of PRS varies between different centres. The following practice is from the Birmingham Children Hospital's cleft team. All babies are admitted (for at least 48 hours) for,

1. Continuous oxygen saturation monitoring
2. Monitoring of weight gain
3. Parental education, training and assessments for feeding, basic life support, NPA insertion and care.

The baby may be able to maintain their oxygen saturation lying supine. If they can't, then try nursing them on their side. Since they cannot feed while on their side, an NG is appropriate. If the baby desaturates with NG and lateral nursing, then they need an NPA.

Some centres have tried early operative interventions with distraction osteogenesis of the mandible, glossopexy, tracheostomy and there is no consensus on management.

Note PRS is an exception to what used to be called "Back to Sleep" public campaign on parental guidance that babies should always sleep on their backs to prevent risk of SIDS. Nowadays it is called "Safe to Sleep campaign".

Classifications

It is no one universal classification of cleft lip/palate. Most people would use elements of more than one classification to describe a given situation at hand.

1) Descriptive
Probably the most commonly used of all classifications. This involves a detailed description of each element in the cleft lip/palate.

2) Kernahans. Cleft of primary palate including lip, or cleft of secondary palate

3) Kernahan's stripped-Y (1971)
It is a pictographical representation of various components of cleft (Ref: Picture). Degree of stippling is proportional to the amount of cleft. Crosshatching means submucous (cleft palate) or microform (lip) condition.

Figure: Pictographic representations of CLP

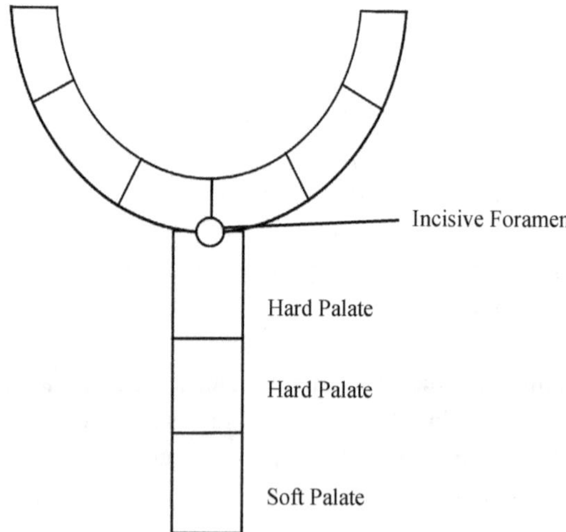

4) LAHSHAL (Kreins 1989)

It is a palindrome representing lip, alveolus, hard palate and soft palate, starting from the right lip. Capital letter represents complete cleft.

- Lower case represents incomplete left
- Hyphen (-) represents structure is not involved
- Asterisk (*) represents microform

Table: Examples of usage of LAHSHAL classification

LAHSHAL	Description
LAHS	Complete right unilateral cleft lip, alveolus, hard and soft palate
...S...	Complete soft palate cleft
...s...	Incomplete soft palate cleft
......l	Left incomplete cleft lip

Features of cleft lip

1) Orbcularis oris, levator labii, nasalis
- Disruption of continuity, orientation & quality of muscles
- Muscles run parallel to cleft margin and insert in alar base/columella/intra-dermal.

2) Decreased vertical lip height

3) Alveolus and nasal floor are open (in CL)

4) Pre-maxilla is rotated

Features of cleft nose

1) Hypoplastic maxilla i.e. the foundation of the nasal pyramid is retruded
2) Alar base displacement - cephalad and posterior
3) LLC subluxed
4) Hypoplasia of alar dome, making it wide and floppy on the affected side
5) Lack of overlap between ULC and LLC
6) Shortened columella

Table: Summary of CL/P repairs

	CL	CP
Timing of repair	3/12 repair, No RCT, but "10 weeks, 10lb, Hb = 10" which allows • Parent education • Parent-child bonding • Child to gain weight • Treating team to identify other congenital anomalies • Decreased anaesthetic risk	6-9/12 No
Type of repairs	Straight line = Rose-Thompson	

	Quadrangular flap = Le-Mesurier (Features: Cupid's bow created from lateral lip + 90deg Z-plasty. Problems: violates Cupid's bow, results in a long lip)	Hard Palate
		 1) Von Langenbeck
		     Bilateral bipedicled mucoperiosteal flap based on greater palatine artery +/- lateral relaxing incision
		     Concerns: Can result in a short palate & VPI by removing periosteum over growing centres
		 2) V-Y push back (Veau-Wardill-Kilner)
		     Unipedicle mucoperiosteal flap + V-Y advancement + anterior areas left to granulate
		 3) Vomerine flap
		     Can be combined with either of above techniques, in case of wider clefts

	Triangular flap = Tennison-Randall (Feature: Z-plasty at vermilion)	Soft palate 1) IVVP (**I**ntra **V**elar **V**elo **P**lasty), involves aggressive dissection & reconstruction of muscles and mucosal layer in the midline, popularised by Sommerlad 2) Furlow repair Double z-platies in opposite directions on oropharyngeal and nasopharyngeal sides of the soft palate. It lengthens soft palate and re-orients the LVP
	Rotation-Advancement = Millard's "cut-as-you-go"	

	CL	**CP**
	Options for wider clefts • pre-op taping • lip adhesion • orthodontic appliance	
Salient complications	Long lip Short lip Prominent scar Notching of lip	Fistulae: up to 50%, esp in wider clefts Midfacial growth retardation Airway obstruction secondary to bleeding postop VPI: Inappropriate incomplete closure of soft palate against posterior pharyngeal wall during speech

Marking a rotation advancement flap

1. Point 1, deepest point of Cupid's bow (this will be the eventual midline)
2. Point 2, highest point of Cupid's bow on normal side
3. Point 3, highest point of Cupid's bow (medial cleft side) is marked so that it is the same distance from 1 as is point 2.

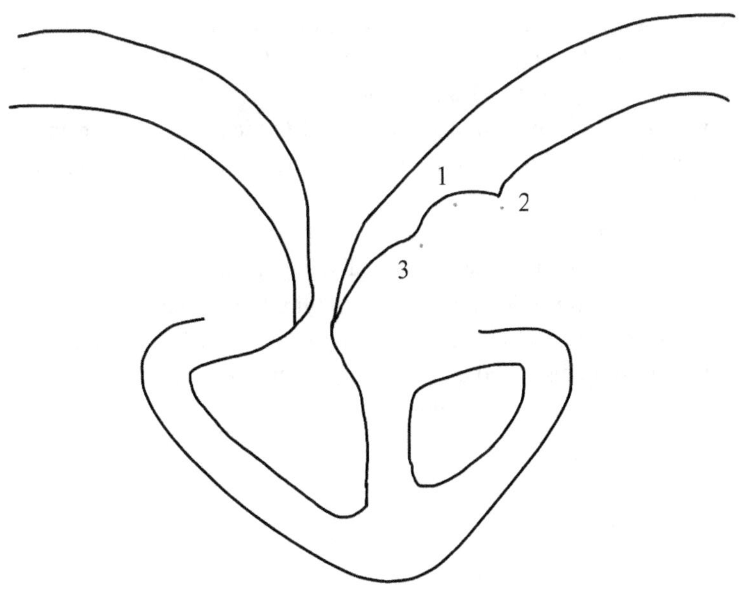

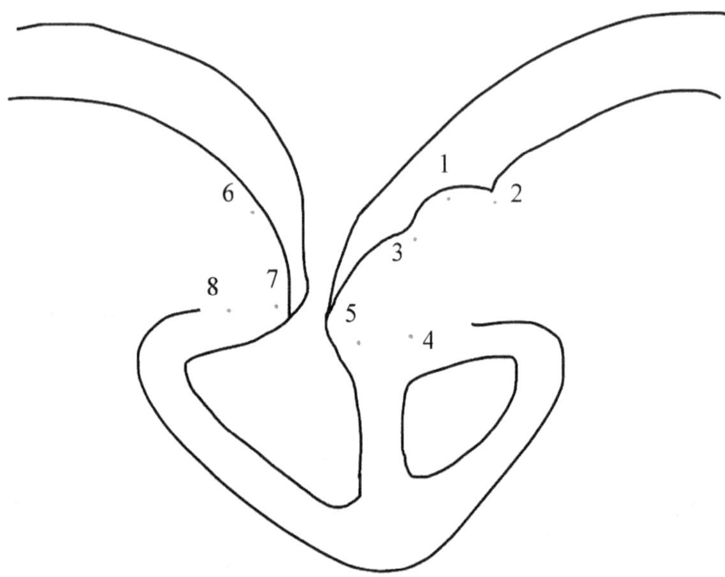

Figure (*contd.*): Marking for a rotation advancement flap

4. Point 4, base of columella at medial crus of LLC, normal side.

5. Point 5, base of columella at medial crus of LLC, cleft side. Double check that 4 & 5 are equidistant from midline.

6. Point 6, most suitable point of white roll (which will become the highest point of Cupid's bow) on lateral cleft side. Suitability is judged by a combination of,
    - thickest vermilion
    - vermilion same thickness as on medial cleft side
    - good quality vermilion (as opposed to thin, fibrotic band like)
    - same distance from its lateral commissure as point 2 (most reliable)

7. Point 7, most medial good quality skin just outside nasal sill

8. Point 8, variable point (see below)

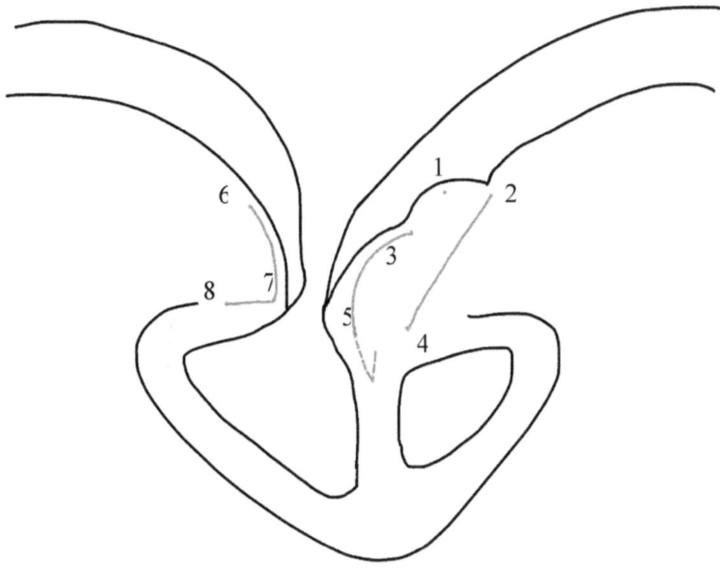

Figure (*contd.*): Marking for a rotation advancement flap. Draw lines,

- between 2 & 4, is the height of philtral column on the normal side (this is what we aim to recreate on medial and lateral cleft sides)
- a curved line between points 3 & 5, which will form the medial "pillar" of the cleft side philtral column. The curve should be the same length as line segment 2-4. Often it isn't, whereby the curve can be extended *onto* the columella for a short distance and (if still short) can be brought down again. The catch is that, a) none of the extension should cross the midline and b) the higher you take the incision on the columella, the less projected nose you will end up with.
- between 6 & 7, that is then carried over horizontally towards the alar base to point 8. This will form the lateral "pillar" of the cleft side philtral column. Therefore, point 8 is chosen so as to make the segment 6-7-8 the same length as 2-4, which should be the same as the curve 3-5 (and any extension there of).

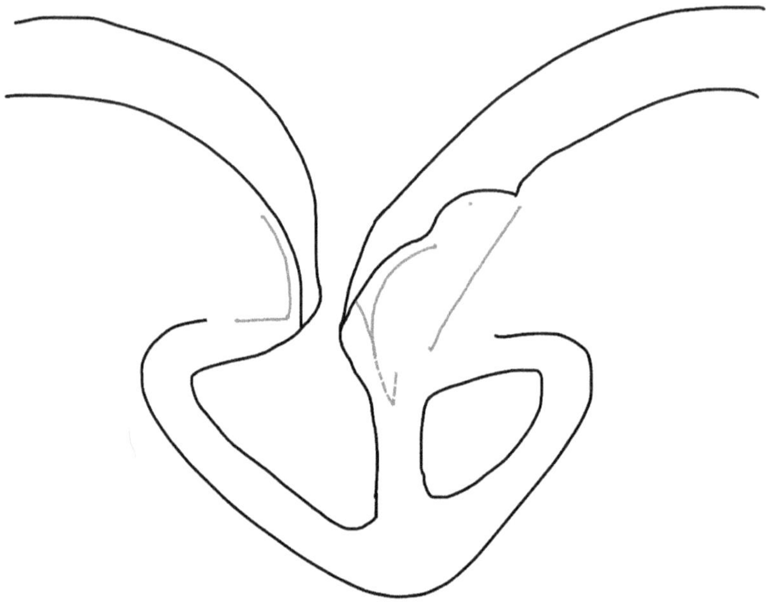

Figure (*contd.*): Marking for a rotation advancement flap.
Finally the C-flap is marked at the unused skin on medial cleft side. This flap will be transposed to create the nasal sill.

Evidence

Early repair vs late lip. Not much
Ref: Eurocleft, Dutch cleft (Boongarts et al.) & SriLankan studies (McCance et al.)

Cleft palate repairs

VON LANGENBECK REPAIR

It consists of bilateral bipedicle flaps, supplied prediminantly by the greater palatine artery (Ref: Figure). The medial defect is closed preferentially, while the secondary defects (laterally) are allowed to heal secondarily.

Larger clefts cannot be reliably closed with a one stage technique, in which case muco-periosteal flaps from the vomer ('vomerine flaps') are used for a staged repair.

Figure: VonLangenbeck repair

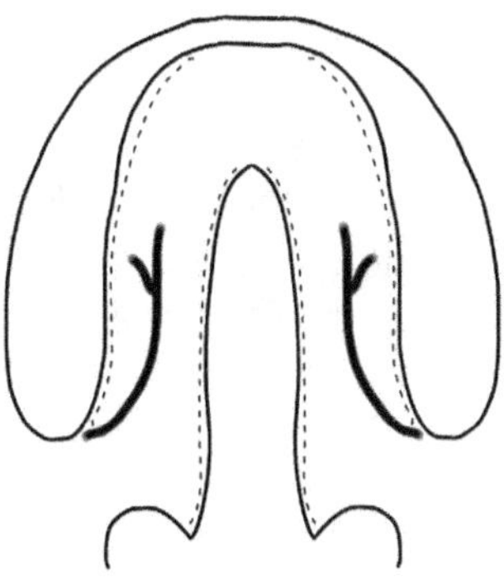 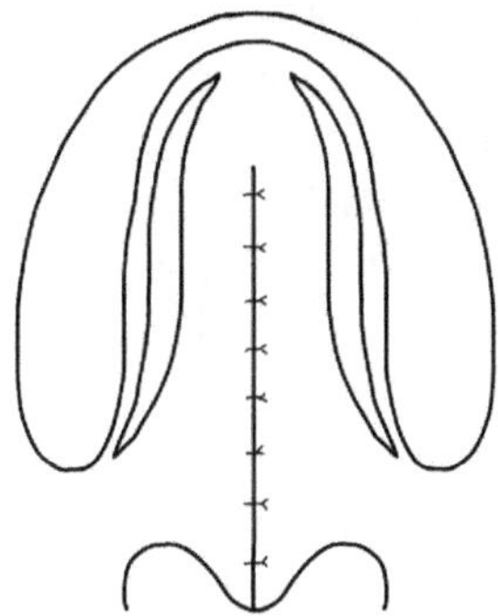

IVVP

Perhaps the most common soft palate repair technique in UK is IVVP (intra-velar veloplasty), described by Sommerlad. It involves aggressive dissection of the levator in an attempt to re-establish its continuity.

FURLOW

Re-repair of soft palate, especially to gain length, is commonly by Furlow's double opposing Z-plasty (Ref: Figure). The opposing Z-plasties are in the oral and nasal layers. Levator is dissected as part of the posteriorly based flap in either layer.

Figure: Furlow double opposing Z-plasty. a) Incision on the oropharyngeal surface, b) incision on the nasopharyngeal surface

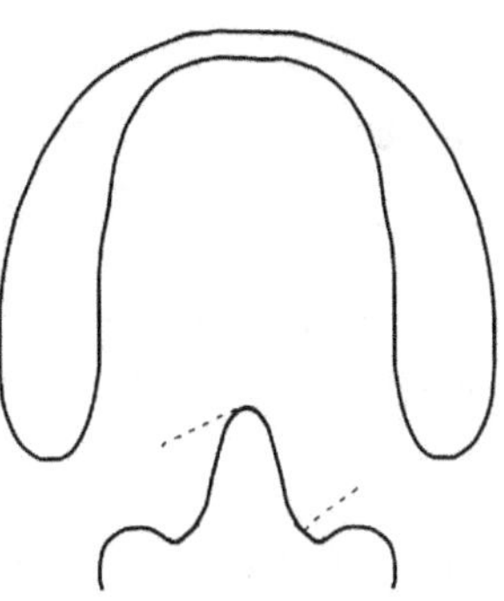 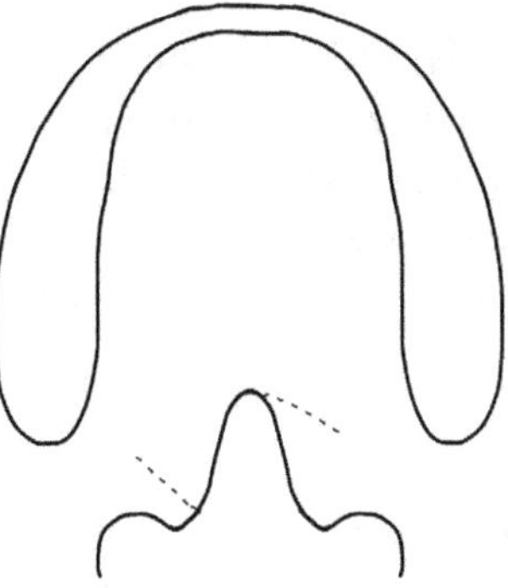

VPI

It is the inappropriate or incomplete closure of soft palate against posterior pharyngeal wall during speech. Clinically it manifests as

- hypernasality - excessive nasal twang
- nasal emissions - excessive air flow out of the nostrils
- facial grimacing - use of facial muscles in an attempt to control air flow during parts of speech
- compensatory articulation - attempt to pronounce by producing sound from a different area
- nasal substitution
- sibilant distortion

Figure: Anatomy of soft palate, note there are complementary muscular slings that contribute to velopharyngeal function (Levator & tensor superiorly, Palato-glossus & -pharyngeus inferiorly)

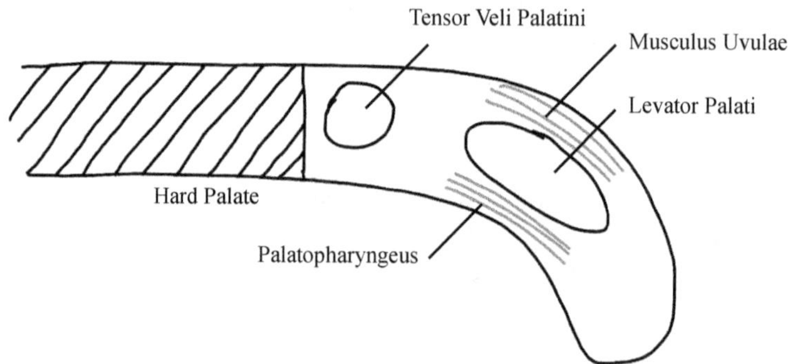

Diagnosis

1. Lateral video fluoroscopy, which allows dynamic visualisation of movement of soft palate during speech
2. Nasendoscopy in 6-7 years old cooperative child
3. Multiview video fluoroscopy (Lateral, frontal and basal views) can be performed but involves higher dose of radiation and does not add much to the information

Submucous cleft = Bifid uvula + midline notching of hard palate (at junction with velum) + zone pellucida (white line in midline of soft plate due to separation of muscles) +/- epithelial pearls

Management

Rule out functional problem: speech assessment by a speech therapist

1. Palate lengthening: Palate re-repair / Furlow
2. Augmentation of posterior pharyngeal wall, which may be static or dynamic.
   A. Static
      - augmentation with grafts - but risks extrusion and migration
      - posterior pharyngeal flap (Ref: Figure)
   B. Dynamic

Follow up

Follow up in combined cleft clinic (Plastics cleft surgeon, geneticist, psychologist, specialist nurse) +/- ENT/MaxFax
- q3/12 in first year,
- then @ 2 years,
- 2x follow-up, 3yrs apart (i.e. up to 8 yrs age)
- 3x follow up, 2yrs apart (i.e. up to 14yrs age)

Additional follow up:
Hearing assessment & Speech and Language assessment for palate repairs @ 1.5yr & 3 yrs of age.

It is important input from maxillofacial surgeon when secondary dentition is about to erupt. The cleft side canine tooth usually comes through the alvelolus and the child may need alveolar bone grafting just before it happens.

ENT input, as the soft palate muscles are not working and cannot do the normal function of aiding the drainage of middle ear via the eustachian tube. This places the child at high risk of recurrent middle ear infections and effusions with resulting distress, hearing loss, psychosocial and educational problems.

Geneticist, who can discuss with parents about the risk of further children having similar condition and help identify hereditary syndromic conditions. This is helpful both for counselling and to involve other specialities as needed, to anticipate and mitigate systemic problems.

Figure: A) Posterior pharyngeal flap B) Hynes C) Orticochea pharyngoplasty

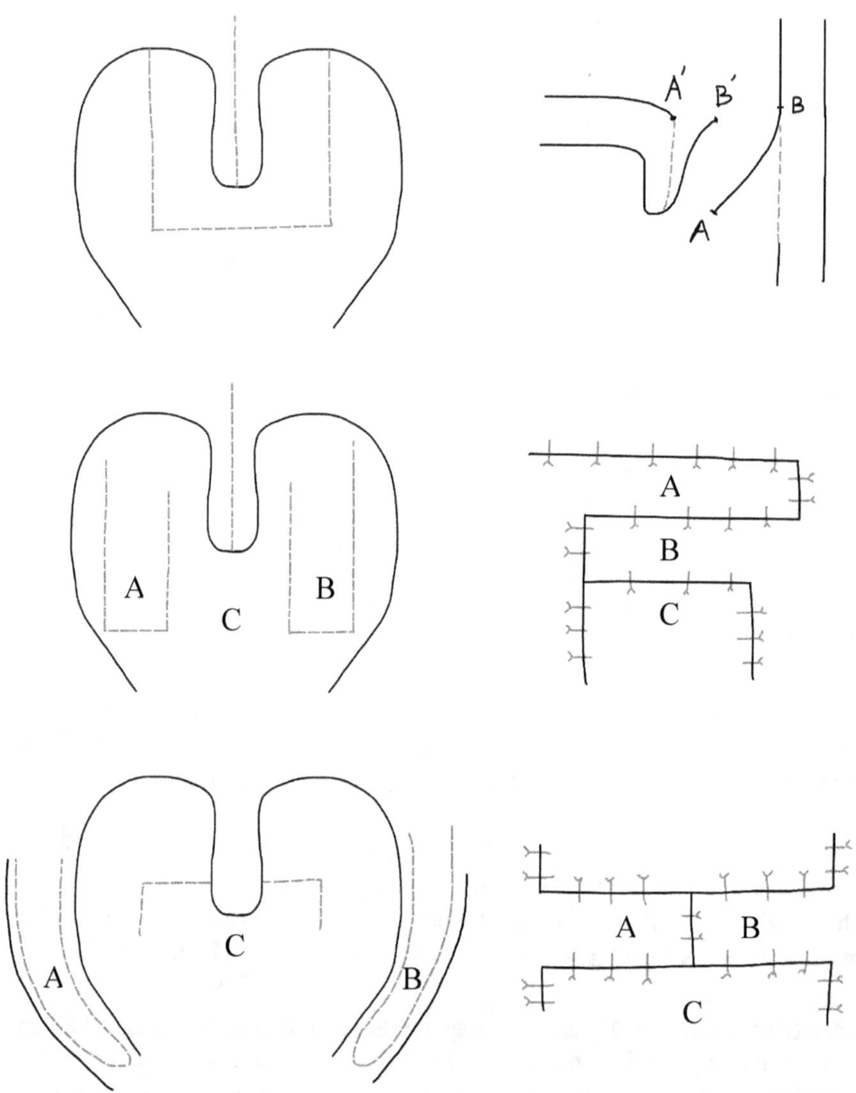

Craniofacial

CORE KNOWLEDGE
Embryology
Classification of craniofacial anomalies
Principles of management
Indications for operative treatment
Timing of operative treatment
Craniosynostosis
HFM
Microtia

APPROACH TO PATIENT - HISTORY

General
Age
Whether only child? Are they fit and well?
Developmental history:
> To include antenatal/pregnancy/delivery. development
> Growth & development

Medical issues/congenital anomalies

Specific
When was the deformity initially noted?
Is it getting better/worse?
Specific systemic symptoms

Airway	Problem breathing? Snores when asleep?
Eye	Recurrent eye infections?
ICP	Irritable, especially in the morning? Tense/bulging soft spot (fontanelle), vomiting?
Neuro-developmental	Achieving milestones?

Which paediatrician and other specialties are involved in care (and how often)

APPROACH TO PATIENT - EXAMINATION

LOOK	Describe what you see...
Shape of skull (from front, side & top)	Trigono- / scapho- / brachy- / turribrachy-cephaly, or parallelogram
Ears	symmetrical / low set / microtia
Orbits	symmetrical / prominent eye
Midface	hypoplasia
Nose	root / tip deviated
Cheeks	symmetrical / retruded on one side
Chin	in midline / deviated

FEEL	
Anterior fontanelle	open / closed (usually closes 9-18/12 age)
Posterior fontanelle	open / closed (usually closed by 6/12 age)
Any palpable ridge of bone	
SCM	[Remember it pulls the ipsilateral occiput]

Try to assess neck movements by e.g. a finger snap, or a toy

Don't forget to:
- Check for limb abnormalities
- Ask for known cardiac abnormalities

APPROACH TO PATIENT - TREATMENT
Strictly within a specialised team comprising
A) Surgical members
- Craniofacial plastic / max-fax surgeon (or both)
- Neurosurgeon
- ENT, if needed

B) Medical specialties
- Geneticist
- Clinical psychologist

- Pediatrician
- Ophthalmologist

C) Non-doctors
- Specialist nurses
- Prosthetist

Principles of management of syndromic craniosynostosis are to consider,
1. Airway
2. Vision
3. Hearing
4. ICP
5. Nutritional support
6. Correction of deformity
7. Support of social development

Note that the management in childhood is centred on **crisis prevention** (airway, eyes, ICP, neurodevelopmental delay etc). In contrast, management in adulthood is geared towards **definitive correction** of deformity (osteotomies, distraction osteogenesis, soft tissue procedures and final adjustment).

EXPECTED CLINICAL QUESTIONS
- Craniosysnostosis (definition, types, associated syndromes)
- Functional problems with craniosynostosis
- Principles of management
- Signs of raised ICP
- Monroe-Kelly doctrine
- Identification and management of airway compromise
- SAT / OMENS/ Pruzansky classifications
- Clinical section (microtia, HFM, Mobius). Patient may be from any age group.
- Tanzer's classification
- Associated middle/internal ear problems
- Embryology (unlikely in clinical but certainly in MCQs)
- Specialties involved in management of a case

Opinion:

Do not expect to make a spot diagnosis of every craniofacial condition imaginable (esp. under stress of being examined!). Most of these conditions are rare and unlikely to be seen in general plastic surgery clinic. You should still be competent to spot an abnormality, know that it needs referral to the nearest specialist centre and be able to describe it to a colleague for referral.

RECOMMENDED PAPERS

1. Tessier P. Anatomical classification facial, cranio-facial and latero-facial clefts. *J Maxillofac Surg.* 1976 Jun;4(2):69-92.
2. Vento AR, Mulliken JB. The OMENS classification of hemifacial microsomia. *Cleft Palate Craniofac J.* 1991;28(1):68-76
3. Horgan JE et al. OMENS-plus: Analysis of craniofacial and extracraniofacial anomalies in hemifacial microsomia. *Cleft Palate Craniofac. J.* 1995;32: 405
4.
5. Persing JA. MOC-PS(SM) CME Article: Management Considerations in the Treatment of Craniosynostosis *Plast Reconstr Surg.* 2008 Apr; 121(Supplement):1–11.
6. Forrest CR, Hopper RA. Craniofacial Syndromes and Surgery *Plast Reconstr Surg.* 2013 Jan;131(1):86e – 109e.
7. Gougoutas AJ, Singh DJ, Low DW, Bartlett SP. Hemifacial Microsomia: Clinical Features and Pictographic Representations of the OMENS Classification System. *Plast Reconstr Surg.* 2007 Dec;120(7):112e – 120e.
8. Fan K, Kawamoto HK, McCarthy JG, Bartlett SP, Matthews DC, Wolfe SA, et al. Top Five Craniofacial Techniques for Training in Plastic Surgery Residency *Plast Reconstr Surg.* 2012 Mar;129(3):477e – 487e.

9. Pruzansky, S. Not all dwarfed mandibles are alike. *Birth Defects* 1: 120, 1969.
10. Kaban, L. B., Moses, M. H., and Mulliken, J. B. Surgical correction of hemifacial microsomia in the growing child. *Plast. Reconstr. Surg.* 82: 9, 1988
11. David DJ, Mahatumarat C, Cooter RD: Hemifacial microsomia: A multisystem classification. *Plast Reconstr Surg.* 80:525–535, 1987
12. Vento AR, Mulliken JB. The OMENS classification of hemifacial microsomia. *Cleft Palate Craniofac J.* 1991;28(1):68-76
13. Horgan JE et al. OMENS-plus: Analysis of craniofacial and extracraniofacial anomalies in hemifacial microsomia. Cleft Palate Craniofac. J. 1995;32: 405

14. Brent B. Ear reconstruction with an expansile framework of autogenous rib cartilage. Plast Reconstr Surg. 1974 Jun;53(6):619-28
15. Brent B. Technical advances in ear reconstruction with autogenous rib cartilage grafts: personal experience with 1200 cases. Plast Reconstr Surg. 1999 Aug;104(2):319-34; discussion 335-8
16. Nagata S. Modification of the stages in total reconstruction of the auricle: Part I. Grafting the three-dimensional costal cartilage framework for lobule-

type microtia. Plast Reconstr Surg. 1994 Feb;93(2):221-30; discussion 267-8.

17. Nagata S. Modification of the stages in total reconstruction of the auricle: Part II. Grafting the three-dimensional costal cartilage framework for concha-type microtia. Plast Reconstr Surg. 1994 Feb;93(2):231-42; discussion 267-8

18. Nagata S. Modification of the stages in total reconstruction of the auricle: Part III. Grafting the three-dimensional costal cartilage framework for small concha-type microtia. Plast Reconstr Surg. 1994 Feb;93(2):243-53; discussion 267-8.

19. Nagata S. Modification of the stages in total reconstruction of the auricle: Part IV. Ear elevation for the constructed auricle. Plast Reconstr Surg. 1994 Feb;93(2):254-66; discussion 267-8.

Classifications of craniofacial deformities

Use only to understand the spectrum of conditions. It is NOT required for the exam. (Ref: Whittaker, CPJ, 1981)

I. Clefts
II. Synostoses
III. Atrophy / Hypoplasia e.g. Romberg's
IV. Neoplasia/ Hyperplasia e.g. fibrous dysplasia
V. Unclassified

Whittaker's classification encompasses a diverse variety of clinical cases so its contents have been modified considerably e.g. most surgeons classify CF clefts with either Tessier or Van der Meulen classification, synostoses as syndromic or non-syndromic. There are further classifications of each of the categories e.g. SAT / OMENS /OMES+ classifications for hemifacial microsomia.

Cranio-synostosis

DEFINITIONS
Cephalic index = BPD / OFD x100
i.e. ratio of biparietal diameter & occipitofrontal diameter, max width / max length, expressed as a percentage
- > 81 is brachycephaly i.e. short AP diameter
- <76 is dolichocephalic i.e. long AP diameter

Macrocephaly is head circumference >97th centile
Microcephaly is head circumference <3rd centile

Plagiocephaly means "asymmetric head shape"
Turricephaly is tall head relative to width and height

Summary of non-syndromic craniosynostoses

Condition & incidence	Suture involved	Key features	Notes
Brachy- 1:2.5k	b/l coronal	Short head	Consider as SYDROMIC until proven otherwise
Plagio- 1:4.5k	unilateral coronal	Forehead retropositioned on affected side Raised supra-orbital ridge Laterally positioned lat canthus Nasal root towards affected side Cheek prominent ipsilat Chin deviated away	Bifrontal osteotomies and ipsilateral orbital advancement at 12-18/12 to remove frontal bar
Scapho- 1:8k	sagittal	Long head	Operated @ <6/12 for calvarial remodelling as untreated -> 10-15% r/o raised ICP
Trigonoceph aly 1:10k	metopic	Keel shaped head Palpable ridge Hypotelorism	Normal inter-canthal distance: 18-22mm @birth 25mm @ 5yr age
Lambdoid (rarest)	single lambdoid suture	Flattened occiput ipsilateral	

Summary of syndromic craniosynostoses

Condition & incidence	Inheritance pattern	H&N features	Other features
Apert 1:25-100k	AD	B/L coronal synostosis Turribrachycephaly Midface hypoplasia	Complex syndactyly ("Spade / Mitten / Rosebud")
Crouzon 1:10-25k	AD	B/L coronal synostosis Midface hypoplasia (Marked) exorbitism	No syndactyly
Saetre-Chotzen 1:10k	AD	Uni. coronal synostosis Low set hairline Ear anomalies	Simple incomplete syndactyly

Condition & incidence	Inheritance pattern	H&N features	Other features
Carpenter **1:10k**	AR	Sagittal / bicoronal synostosis Widely separated eyes Hydrocephalus	+/- heart defects
Pfeiffer **1:15k**	AD	Coronal synostosis Midface hypoplasia	Broad thumbs and toes

Positional plagiocephaly versus unilateral lambdoid synostosis

Note that position of the ear serves as a proxy marker for the growth (or lack of growth) at the skull base.

"**P**ositional **P**lagiocephaly has a **P**arallelogram shaped head when viewed from the top"

Figure: a) Positional plagiocephaly, b) Lambdoid craniosynostosis

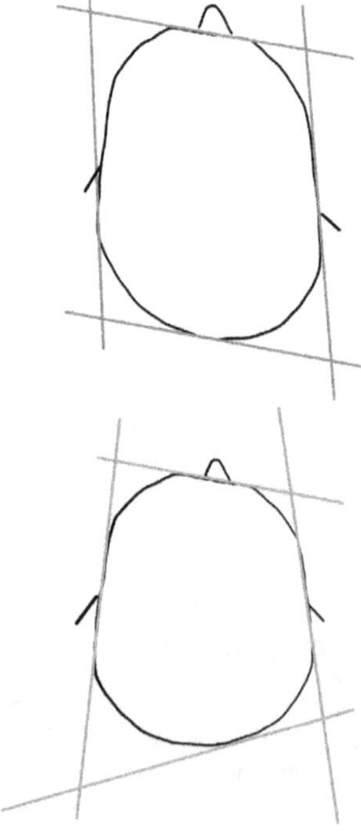

General considerations of management

- ALL management should be done in a specialist centre with a specialist craniofacial team
- Radiological investigations are not done until they impact management
- Indications for CT scan:
    - Confirm fusion of suture,
    - Identify extent of bony abnormality (eg skull base)
    - Associated intracranial conditions (eg hydrocephalus, Arnold-Chiari malformation*)

MONROE-KELLY DOCTRINE

Effectively it states that skull is a fixed volume container with brain, blood & CSF in it - for one thing to expand, something else has to move out.

ARNOLD-CHIARI MALFORMATION

Herniation of part of brainstem (+/- cerebellum) through the foramen magnum, due to raised intra-cranial pressure.

Signs/Symptoms of airway compromise*

Tachypnea
Nasal flaring
Costal recession
+/- noisy breathing

Management of airway compromise

Immediate: Admit, position, NPA +/- trachy
Long-term: mandibular distraction

S/S of raised ICP

Head ache (consider if child is old enough to tell that)
Irritability
Bulging fontanelle
Failure to thrive
"Sun set" sign (is quite late!)
Papilledema

*These can be very subtle in the neonate!

Typical timing of operations

< 1 year:

- FOAR +/- strip craniectomies
- Cranial vault remodelling
- VP shunt for hydrocephalus

Years 3-4:

- LeFort III +/- frontal bone advancement
- Monobloc advancement

Adolescence:

- Jaw surgery
- LeFort I
- Genioplasty

Craniofacial clefts

It is a group of craniofacial conditions that do not respect embryological boundaries and where a variable degree of <u>excess or deficiency</u> of <u>soft tissue and bony elements</u> exists along <u>linear planes</u>.

Classification

Tessier classification
(J Maxillofacial Surg, 1976) is based on the location of the deformity in relation to oral and orbital cavities. CF cleft are numbered based on their location in relation to the oral cavity & orbit. Clefts 0-7 are located around the oral cavity and 8-14 around the orbit. They commonly occur together.

Van der Meulen classification
(PRS, 1983) is based on the concept of a zone of dysplasia in the anatomical area of the deformity e.g. zygomatico-orbital

Some common eponyms

HFM **(Hemifacial microsomia)**	Unilateral #7 cleft
TCS **(Treacher Collins Syndrome)**	Bilateral #6,7,8 clefts
Goldernhar syndrome	HFM + epibulbar dermoids + vertebral anomalies
Nager syndrome	TCS + hypoplastic thumbs + severe mandibular hypoplasia + increased r/o cleft paalte

Microtia, hemifacial microsomia

A typical patient is a child/adolescent with facial deformity on one side, e.g.
- anterior and inferiorly displaced misshapen ear
- a smaller (Rt/Lt) hemi-mandible, with/without an occlusal cant [ask them to smile]
- macrostomia
- chin deviation (to Rt/Lt)

Clinically the first important thing is to be sure is which side is the normal one, and which is the abnormal side. Try determining that from the moment you see the patient and during history taking.

GENERAL HISTORY

How old is the child
Only child? Other siblings, fit and well?
(If school going age) How is the child doing at school
Developmental history
Family history
Parental concerns

SPECIFIC HISTORY

When was this problem noticed
Is there any other problem known/suspected? (Briefly ask about major systems- neurological, GI, CVS, skeletal, urogenital, any other)

Ear

- Did the child pass hearing test at birth?
- Any ear infections since? Needed Grommets? (same side/contralateral)
- Any investigations to check if problem with nerve (conductive vs sensorineural)
- Any aids to help the hearing? (e.g. BAHA)

Eyes

- Eye infections?
- Both eyes close when asleep?

Mouth/facial nerve

- Smile symmetrical? Problem while feeding?
- Any operations on corner of mouth

Mandible

- Is there any metalwork in the jaw? Is any planned? (Distraction Osteogenesis)

Soft tissues asymmetry

EXAMINATION

Describe what you see and do it systematically. One description may be as below. Note the systematic attention to and description of each element as you describe what you see. [You may be asked what condition are you thinking of and how your examination so far fits in to it].

"This is a baby/child with an **asymmetry** of face

Right **ear** is small, low set/anteriorly placed

I can/cannot see an external auditory **meatus** (which makes it anotia/lobular/ conchal/small conchal / atypical ear deformity by Tanzer's classification)

Right **orbit** is abnormal, displaced inferiorly/superior

Eyes are downslanting

or, Eyes/eyelids appeared normal

+/- squint

There is an element of **macrostomia**

Symmetrical **smile**

Scars of macrostomia repair/distraction osteogenesis (DO)

Right **mandible** appears hypoplastic

Minimal/moderate/severe **soft tissue** deficiency"

If old enough, ask the child to open mouth and check occlusal cant. [The space between the two incisors gives you the true midline].

INVESTIGATIONS

It is especially important in children that only those investigations are ordered which impact clinical management, as a CT involves a certain radiation dose and MRI can involve a GA.

- CT head, to assess orbit, mandible and middle ear
- MRI, to determine the course of facial nerve
- Audiometry

	Microtia	HFM	TCS
Epidemio	1:10k 2x ↑ females ↑ Asians (Japanese) & Hispanics R:L:B = 5:3:1 ↑ risk at 4+ pregnancies	1:3.5k-5.6k 3:2 male:female 3:2 right:left 80% unilateral (2nd most common condition after CLP)	1:50k
Embryo	1st & 2nd branchial arches form hillocks	1st & 2nd branchial arches	1st & 2nd branchial arches
Associations	EAC & middle ear abnormalities Hearing defects (80-90% conductive) Syndromes (HFM, TCS, Goldenhar's)		

SYSTEMS OF CLASSIFICATION

Pruzansky classification, originally in 1969, modified by Mulliken and Kaban 1988 (to add subtypes IIA & IIB) is a classification of mandibular hypoplasia.

SAT classification, by David David in 1987 classified **S**keletal, **A**uricular and soft **T**issue components to devise a management algorithm.

OMENS classification, considers **O**rbital asymmetry, **M**andibular hypoplasia, **E**ar deformity, **N**erve (i.e. facial nerve) dysfunction and **S**oft tissue deficiency. The mandibular classification uses the modified Pruzansky system.

OMENS Plus takes account of extra-cranial deformities as well.

MANAGEMENT

Remember the management needs to involve all relevant specialties e.g. general paediatrics, ENT, MaxFax as well as plastics surgery in a specialised centre.

A typical management timeline is as follows (Ref: Weinzweig's Plastic surgery Secrets Plus)

Early	Airway Cornea Feeding Hearing Genetic testing
6-12/12	Commissuroplasty
12-15/12	Hearing assessment (+ palate repair in TCS)
2-4 yr	Neurodevelopmental evaluation Mandibular distraction if Pruzansky III / Obstructive sleep apnea +/- wedge excision of coloboma vs Tripier flap (in TCS)
6-8 yr	BAHA /ear reconstruction Coordinate ear recon & jaw surgery
7-10 yr	+/- orbital repositioning +/- zygoma augmentation Facial animation with gracilis Gold weight for orbicularis
Teens - adult	Dental Orthognathic correction (LeFort I / Bilat sagittal split osteotomies) Genioplasty Soft tissue augmentation

External ear recon options

1) Alloplastic i.e. stick on

2) Prosthetic = osseointegrated implants

3) Autologous

      Brent's technique

      Nagata's technique

BRENT'S TECHNIQUE

Originally 4 stage, (now Brent uses 3-stage, but most people refer to Brent's original description).

Starts at age 6 yrs

1. Framework. Templated from contralateral (normal) ear, on an acetate xray film. Uses contralateral constochondral juction cartilage at 6-8th ribs. Carve the skeleton. Bury under the skin
2. Lobular transposition
3. Elevation of framework
4. Tragus

NAGATA'S TECHNIQUE

2 stage. Starts 10 yrs age. Everything except lobular transposition in stage 1. Lobular transposition only in stage 2.

Complications of autologous

Skin loss, Infection, flap loss (more in Nagata), donor site complications

Cephalometrics

Frankfurt horizontal plane.	Passes through the top of both bony meatuses (porion) and the floor of the left orbit. Note that 3 points r needed to make a plane.
SN line	Centre of sella turcica to nasion (frontonasal suture in the midline)
NA line	Nasion to the deepest concavity on the anterior profile of maxilla
NB line	Nasion to the deepest concavity on the anterior profile of maxilla
SNA	Measures maxillary protrusion. Less means maxilla is retruded (e.g. in CLP).
SNB	Measures mandibular prominence Less means retrognathia, more is prognathism

SNA & SNB judge lateral facial bony profile w.r.t. skull base (which is an invariant, assuming no base of skull malformation).

Relationship between maxilla and mandible
1. Difference between SNA & SNB
2. Occlusion class, which describes the relationship between maxilla & mandible with reference to the relation between their 1st molars. Most caucasian population has class II occlusion, so it is considered "normal" & the other 2 types are called class I or III mal-occlusions.

Note that occlusion class refers to the "back" of the jaw while SNA/B angles refer to the front.

Distraction Osteogenesis (DO)

Distraction osteogenesis is the generation of viable bone by controlled movement of an osteotomised bone segment. After the osteotomy there is a latency period (3-7 days) followed by activation/distraction period (at a set rate for as long as needed) and finally the consolidation period (6-12 weeks, to allow the osteotomy site to heal).

DO was popularised after Ilizarov' experience in 1950s for lower limb lengthening. The distraction is referred to as
1. uni-focal (one osteotomy, to transport one segment),
2. bi-focal (one osteotomy with an existing bone gap, to transport one segments), or
3. tri-focal (two osteotomies with an exiting bone gap, to transport 2 segments).

Prominent ears

Talk to the child!! & talk to the child a lot more than you talk to the parents.

HISTORY
Were the ears noted at birth?
Anything tried soon afterbirth? Since then?
How is his/her hearing? Can she hear well from both ears?
Is the child prone to ear infections?
Any ear operations/grommets?
Apart from appearance, how is it giving trouble
Is the child bothered? (determine if it the ears, parents &/or school that is the reason)

Ever been picked on at school (because of this condition)

Have child's friends mentioned it?

What do the parents and family feel (about the condition and management)?

EXAMINE

Is the hair style trying to cover the ears?

Inspection, from front

One or both ears prominent ("Normal" is considered where in full frontal view, tragus is just visible, with a small amount of conchal bowl, antihelix and helical rim visible close to each other)

Inspect from either side, back as well as the top, to judge the severity of the deformity.

Identify the contribution of each of the following:
1.   Unfolding of antihelix
2.   Prominent conchal bowl (whether the "bowl" is actually large, or a normal side "bowl" has rotated outwards and away from the head)
3.   Prominent lobule

Palpate

The key manoeuvre is to try to tuck the prominent helical rim back and see if that improves the deformity. In case of a prominent concha, there will still be a residual deformity.

Judge the pliability of the cartilage and thickness of skin (Adult cartilage is decidedly stiffer and hence needs more doing to mould it).

Always ask for clinical photographs with clear view of ears and (if needed) child's hair tied back. Ask views from front, from either side and a view each from the top and behind the child (with hair tucked up).

MANAGEMENT

1)   To operate or not?

It is a debatable issue that a) whether it is advisable to operate on the child before they understand (& can participate in) decision making, or b) is it better to operate early and avoid any psychosocial issues altogether.

2)   What age to operate on?

Classical thinking has been to operate around 8 years of age . The argument is that the ear has achieved near-adult proportions, the child is cooperative and understands the reason for the operation. Also, the concept of physical differences is not well rooted by that stage and the child faces little bullying at school. Other surgeons operate early arguing that the child does not need to go through bullying or adverse body image. [Know the arguments and have a stance. Do not sit on the fence].

OPERATIVE PROCEDURE
GA, supine

Choice of incision
1) 1cm posterior to helical rim. Allows for direct visualisation of the antihelical fold
2) (Retro-auricular) sulcal incision. Better hidden, but access may be a bit difficult.

Choice of skin excision
The first choice is between "Yes" or "No". The idea is to remove any excess skin (which is pretty uncommon). Removal of skin plays no part "holding" the position of the ear postop. If excising skin, the next choice is between an oval or a dumb-bell shaped excision.

Choice of dissection
It always preserves the perichondrium. Gault's technique raises an additional fascial flap to cover the sutures at closure.

Choice of cartilage management
1. Anterior scoring (*'Chong Chet'*). Old school surgeons swear by it, but it is less commonly seen these days. It relies on Gibson's principle which states that scoring one side of the cartilage allows release of 'internal stresses' which allow it to bend in the opposite direction. One variation uses a fine drill to abrade the cartilage, making it thinner and pliable.
2. Posterior suturing (*'Mustarde'*). Original technique uses vital blue dye and a green (21G) needle to mark out the points where the sutures will be positioned.

Choice of sutures
Usually non-absorbable e.g. 4/0 prolene although Ethibond and PDS are popular too.

Management of conchal bowl
• Melon slice excision of excess concha, if the size of bowl is large

- Furnas' (concho-mastoid) sutures, if bowl is excessively rotated (i.e. increased concho-mastoid angle).

Choice of skin closure
Continous absorbable (e.g. monocryl) or interrupted absorbable (e.g. vicryl rapide).

Dressings
One that can stay on for 7 days and can come off easily after that.
Head bandage for comfort and to decrease the risk of injury and hematoma.

FOLLOW UP
In dressing clinic at 7 days to remove dressing. Child should be able to shower but with minimal manipulation of the pinna. Most surgeons ask for a head band for 6 weeks. Clinical photos at 3 months.

ALTERNATIVE TO OPERATION = EARLY DX & MGT.
Prominent ears noticed at birth can be potentially managed with a head bandage. Presence of maternal oestrogens is thought to soften the cartilage and it moulds back to a more normal shape. However this "re-moulding" needs to commence within a few days of birth for maximum value.

[In winter BAPRAS 2015, Stevenage unit showed very good results with early moulding using an improvised device made from readily available stock supplies. It is started as soon as possible after birth, certainly within first 3 months of life. The device is used for the same period of length, as was the baby's age at commencement of treatment, i.e. 6 weeks duration if management began at 6 weeks of age]

Hypospadias

It is a congenital anomaly of the male external genitalia, characterised by:
1. presence of a dorsal hood of foreskin
2. abnormally ventral position of urethral meatus,
3. variable degree of ventral curvature ("chordee").

Chordee = abnormal ventral curvature of the penile shaft. Structurally, it is a firm, inelastic band of tissue between the dystopic urethral meatus and the glans, from what otherwise would have been the corpus spongiosum.

CORE KNOWLEDGE
Definition, epidemiology (for counselling parents)
Associations
1-2 repair techniques

APPROACH TO PATIENT - HISTORY
General
How old is the child? Is he the only child?
Any other medical conditions/congenital anomalies known?
Developmental history, conception/pregnancy/delivery
How many siblings are there? Are they fit and well?
Did the father have the same problem?
What are parents' concerns

Specific
What is the current problem?
- Micturating from the wrong place?
- Stream from >1 places?
- Spray?
- Have the parents noticed an erection? Is it straight?
- Have the parents noticed 2 testes? (explain that you will need to confirm that)

Are any other congenital anomalies known? (Worth repeating this question)

APPROACH TO PATIENT - EXAMINATION
[With parents' permission and presence by the bed side. Strongly consider wearing gloves and apron as getting soaked is a known occupational risk]

Penis

Ideally micturating, to look for:

- Flow
- Direction
- Stream
- Ballooning
- Trickling

Location of meatus & its shape

Foreskin

- Present or not
- If present, is there enough preputial skin for a graft adequate for the degree of hypospadias you see
- What are the parents' views on circumcision.

Ventral curvature

Associations

Inguinal hernia

2x testes

APPROACH TO PATIENT - INVESTIGATIONS

- None, if distal hypospadias and is an isolated condition
- USS, if h/o repeated UTIs, or there is proximal hypospadias (to look for structural abnormalities of the proximal renal tract, undescended testis etc.)
- Karyotyping, if testes are not palpable

APPROACH TO PATIENT - TREATMENT

Team approach, esp. if other congenital anomalies are present.

Timing of repair

- 12-18/12 (preferable). Most preschool penile growth is done by 1 yr age. Genital awareness starts around 18/12 age. The child wont remember the surgery, when they grow up. [Note Snodgrass himself repairs these early]
- 3-4 years. ↑ cooperative, no diapers.

EXPECTED VIVA QUESTIONS

- Identify the site of hypospadias
- Classification
- Epidemiology, associations
- Draw a cross section (Ref: Figure)
- Draw the repair that you are familiar with

RECOMMENDED PAPERS

1. Snodgrass WT. Snodgrass technique for hypospadias repair. *Brit J Urol International*. 2005 Mar;95(4):683–93.
2. Bracka A. Hypospadias repair: The two stage alternative. *Brit J Urol*. 1995; 76(S3): 31-41
3. Obaidullah MA. Ten year review of hypospadias repair from a single centre. *Br J Plast Surg*. 2005; 58: 780-9
4. Duckett JW & Snyder H. The MAGPI hypospadias repair in 1111 patients. *Annals Surg*. 1991;213(6):620-5

Figure: Steps of how to draw a cross section. a) draw the corpora, b) deep fascia, c) skin and superficial fascia, d) neurovascular structures

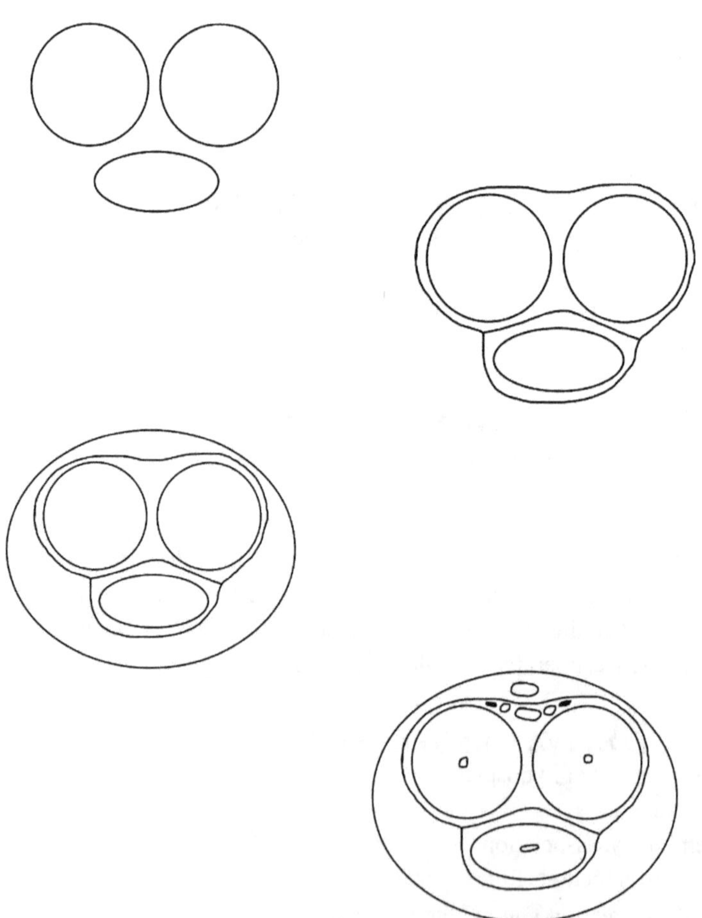

Figure: Cross section of penis. The different layers have been numbered. Note the skin and superficial fascia are depicted with a single line.

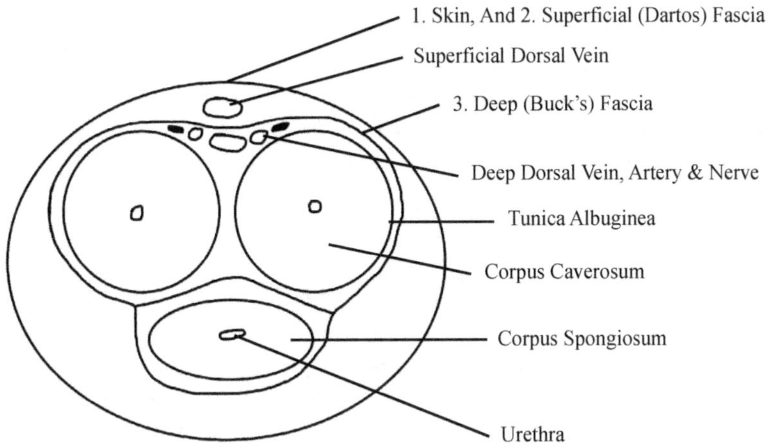

Classification

Descriptive classification based on the position of dystopic meatus, broadly into distal or proximal (half of the shaft). More specifically it may be glanular, coronal, subcoronal, distal shaft, proximal shaft, scrotal or perineal.

Epidemiology

(for parent counselling) Hypospadias is a common congenital anomaly affecting 1:300 live births, ↑ if father is affected or birth after IVF treatment.

Associations

Proximal hypospadias is associated with increased risk of undescended testes, inguinal hernia, proximal urinary tract anomalies and recurrent UTIs.

Choice of procedures

The choice of procedure is dictated by:
1. Position of the dystopic meatus
2. State of urethral plate
3. Degree of curvature (chordee)

The two commonest procedures in UK are those described by Snodgrass and Bracka.

Tubularized incised plate (Snodgrass)

Snodgrass repair is based on the premise that the urethral plate is a highly vascular structure and can heal without appreciable scarring. Hence in tubularised incised plate repair, the urethral plate is incised longitudinally and left unsutured. This acts as a "relaxation incision" to allow the urethral plate to be tubularised around a catheter.

Figure: a) Snodgrass repair, b) close up of the urethral plate incisions

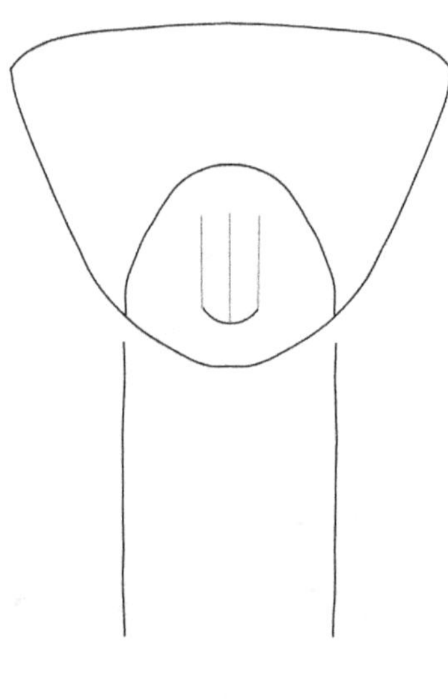

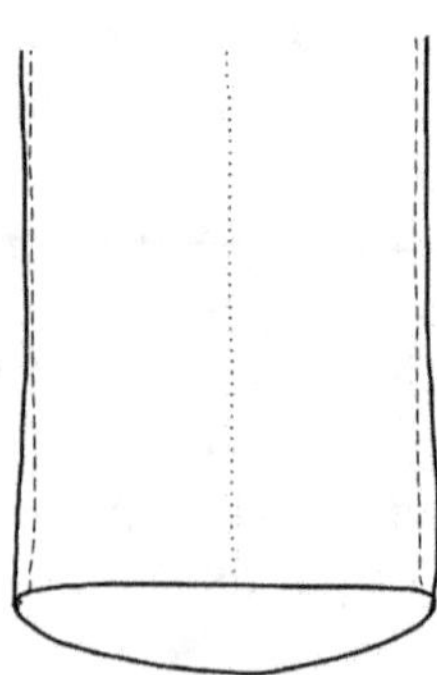

PROCEDURE

Ref: Snodgrass BJUrol. 2005 [A very well illustrated paper!]

Some of the major steps described in this paper are:

1. GA + dorsal penile block
2. Traction sutures in glans (x1) & dorsal hood (x2), 5/0 prolene
3. Circumferential incision proximal to the dystopic meatus (If the baby is *not* circumcised, then carry that incision on to the prepuce)
4. Penile skin is degloved to penoscrotal junction
5. Artificial erection test (Ref: Horton's test)
6. Incise along junction of glans wings and the meatus (i.e. either edge of the urethral plate)
7. Incise midline of the urethral plate (but *not* the glans) and carry it down to corpum cavernosum
8. 6Fr urinary catheter in to the bladder
9. Start tubularization from neo-meatus with 7/0 vicryl → running 2 layer closure
10. Dartos pedicled flap from preputial hood & dorsal shaft, that is button-holed and transposed ventrally. It is only possible if doing a circumcision at the same time.
11. Glansplasty with 6/0 running vicryl

Postop. care:
Sponge bath
Analgesia
Cotrimoxazole
Remove catheter at 1/52

Aside: Horton's test

Tourniquet, 21G cannula, Normal saline
Injected in to corpus cavernosum

Aside: Snodgraft

If the urethral plate is of poor quality (i.e. not very vascular), then urethral plate is incised and a suitable graft added to it ("Snodgraft"). Note that Bracka technique does not rely on urethral plate.

Ref: Bracka BJUrol. 1995 [Another very well illustrated paper]

Procedure - 1st stage

GA + penile block + penile tourniquet
Erection test, urethral sounds of progressively larger diameter (up to 14G)

1. Stay sutures in midline and glans
2. Midline incision from neo-meatus to dystopic meatus
3. Subcoronal incisions to access and release chordee
4. Chordee release with 15blade *up to corpora cavernosa* (+ dorsal plication for any residual chordee)
5. Repeat Horton's test
6. Stay sutures in prepuce and harvest a preputial graft (alternatively buccal mucosal or post-auricular graft that is de-fatted)
7. Inset graft with 7/0 vicryl with a proximal V-shaped extension to avoid narrowing the meatus + quilting
8. Tie over of jelonet and proflavin wool, with 4/0 nylon
9. 8Fr silicone catheter

Postop care:

Home next day on analgesia and co-trimoxazole
Return at day 5 for removal of tie-over [Bracka's description is to do it under sedation, Birmingham Children Hospital do it under GA]

Procedure - 2nd stage

Timing: 6 months later

1. Subcoronal incision to deglove penile skin up to just proximal to original meatus.
2. Tubularization of neo-urethra starting at meatus with 7/0 vicryl.
3. Waterproofing layer, is a proximally based flap of subcutaneous tissue from dorsal hood, transposed ventrally to cover urethral repair.

Postop. care:

Catheterise for 6 days
Cotrimoxazole + analgesia

Other eponymous procedures

1. Mathieu's flip flap

    Uses a rectangular random pattern turnover flap of skin based distally at the dystopic meatus. Being random pattern limits its dimensions and hence the defect that can be reliably covered.

    Figure: Mathieu's flip flap repair. a) Design a distally based skin flap, b) flap turn over and inset

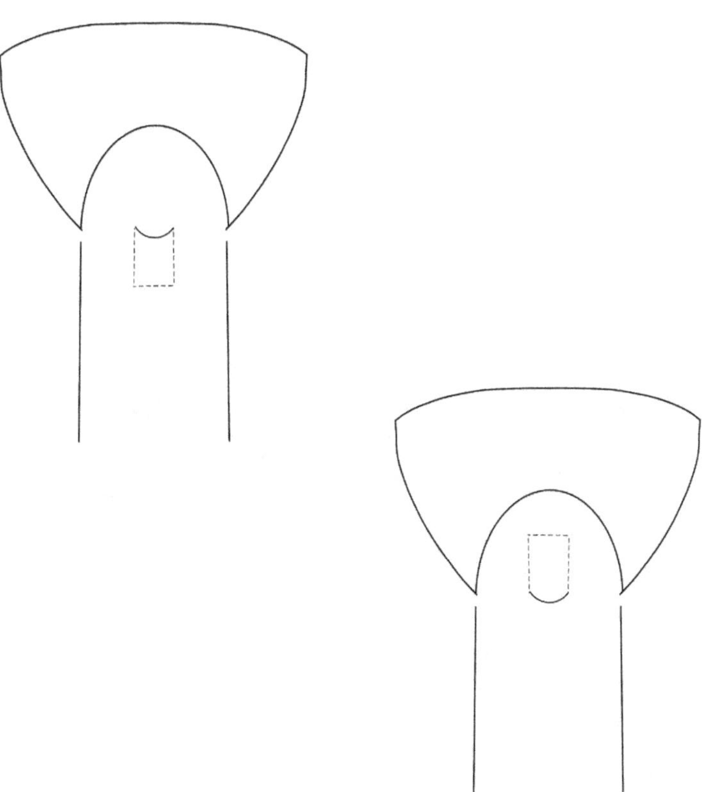

2. MAGPI (**M**eatal **A**dvancement and **G**lanulo**p**lasty)

    Meatal advancement is by a longitudinal incision from the dystopic meatus to the neo-meatus, which creates an elliptical/diamond shaped defect. This defect is the closed transversely [similar in principle to the Heineke-Mikulicz repair in a pyloromyotomy].

Figure: MAGPI repair. a) Vertical incision, b) Intermediate stage, c) closure. Note that the design inherently limits the useful of this technique for only the very distal hypospadias

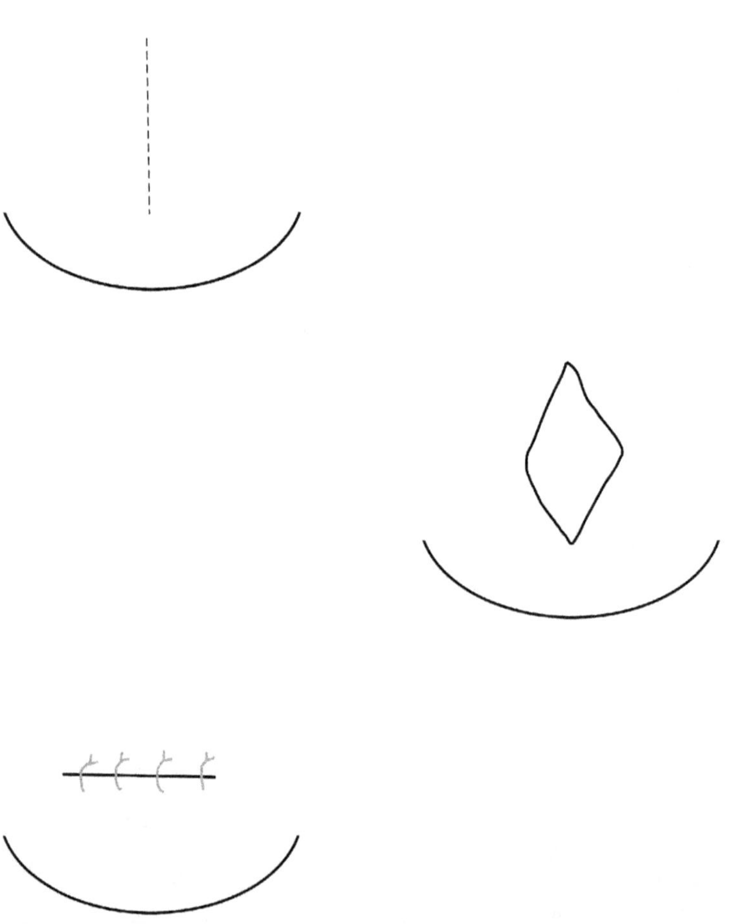

Congenital - Hands

CORE KNOWLEDGE
Swanson's classification
Syndactyly
Radial agenisis
General principles of management

APPROACH TO PATIENT - HISTORY
Child's age
Any abnormality of the other hand/limb
Any abnormality of feet/chest
 Any other congenital abnormality
Developmental history, from conception, pregnancy, delivery
Family history of congenital anomalies
Parental concerns

APPROACH TO PATIENT - EXAMINATION
Examine both hands, both feet, chest wall
Observe the child's motor skills & functional level, whether appropriate for developmental age, any restriction in use (Ref: Table).

Table: Concerns in a congenital hand anomaly

Functional (most important)	e.g. syndactyly of 1st web will decrease grasp and of other webspaces will reduce independant digit movement.
Developmental	eg syndactyly of digit of unequal length will cause tethering and over time ause deviation of longer digit and flexion contracture.
Cosmetic (least important)	altered appearance of hand

APPROACH TO PATIENT - TREATMENT
"Function, Function, Function" - Do not compromise the child's function in order to improve the looks (see below).

EXPECTED CLINICAL QUESTIONS

- Classification of congenital hand anomalies (Swanson's)
- Poland syndrome
- Definitions, principles of management of any congenital anomaly (Poland and syndactlyly are commonest)
- Draw flaps for web space release (4-flap, 5-flap Z-plasty)
- Syndactyly release (Cronin, Buck-Gramcko flaps)
- Apert syndrome (features, classification of Apert hand= Spade/spoon/rosebud)

RECOMMENDED PAPERS

1. Bates SJ, Hansen SL, Jones NF. Reconstruction of Congenital Differences of the Hand. *Plast Reconstr Surg*. 2009 Jul;124(Supplement):128e – 143e.
2. Foucher G, Lora P, Khouri RK, Medina J, Pivato G. Camptodactyly as a Spectrum of Congenital Deficiencies: A Treatment Algorithm Based on Clinical Examination *Plast Reconstr Surg*. 2006 May;117(6):1897–905.
3. Hostin R, James MA. Reconstruction of the hypoplastic thumb. *JHS(Am)*. 2004 Nov;4(4):275–90.
4. Kozin SH. Syndactyly. *JHS(Am)*. 2001 Feb;1(1):1–13.
5. Terzis JK, Kokkalis ZT. Outcomes of Hand Reconstruction in Obstetric Brachial Plexus Palsy *Plast Reconstr Surg*. 2008 Aug;122(2):516–26.

Syndactyly

It is a congenital hand condition due to failure of differentiation and resulting in a variable fusion of the soft tissues and/or skeletal elements of the adjacent digits.

EPIDEMIOLOGY
1:2k,
50% bilateral,
<40% FHx, +/- associated with other hand anomalies

FREQUENCY
Isolated: 3rd web > 4th > 2nd > 1st
Syndromic: 1st web > 2nd > others

TERMINOLOGY OF SYNDACTYLY
- Complete: where web space extends to include the fingertip
- Incomplete: where webspace occurs anywhere between the normal site and fingertip

("Normal site" is approximately the level halfway up the proximal phalanx, with 3rd web slightly distant than others)

- Simple: where syndactyly only involves skin and soft tissue connection
- Complex: above plus skeletal elements
- Complex-complicated: where accessory phalanges are interposed

Acrosyndactyly, is syndactyly with fenestrations in the web with a distal fusion. 50% are bilateral, 50% end with an amputation.

Management depends on i) severity of distant deformity, ii) position and size of sinus.

HISTORY AND EXAMINATION
As above

Principles of management
Operate at one year of age
Webspace reconstruction
Resurface digits
Staged separation, if multiple digits with border digit first

The management would take into account

- one/multiple webs involved
- extent of involvement of a (particular) web space, i.e. complete/ incomplete
- presence of bony fusion i.e. simple/complex

INVESTIGATIONS

- None for simple syndactyly
- X-rays, if their is concern about complicated syndactyly
- CT Angio, if syndromic and having a CT head for that indication

TREATMENT

1. Commissure/webspace reconstruction:
   - Minor incomplete syndactyly: simple Z / 4-flap / 5 flap Z-plasty
   - Most common method: Proximal dorsal rectangular skin flap +/- lateral wings

2. Separation of digits (needs careful planning)
   - Commonest method: Palmar and dorsal triangular flaps [Ref: Cronin's technique, PRS 1956]. Ref: Figure
   - Identify neurovascular bundles.
   - If bifurcation is found distal to webspace, i) give one proper digital vessel each digit ii) Interfascicular dissection of nerve proximally to the desired level

3. Resurfacing of the digit with local palmar/dorsal flaps +/- FTSG

4. Paronychial fold. Buck-Gramcko's "stilleto" flaps. (Ref Figure)

Figure: Steps of drawing a syndactyly release. [There are as many variations described as there are surgeons.]

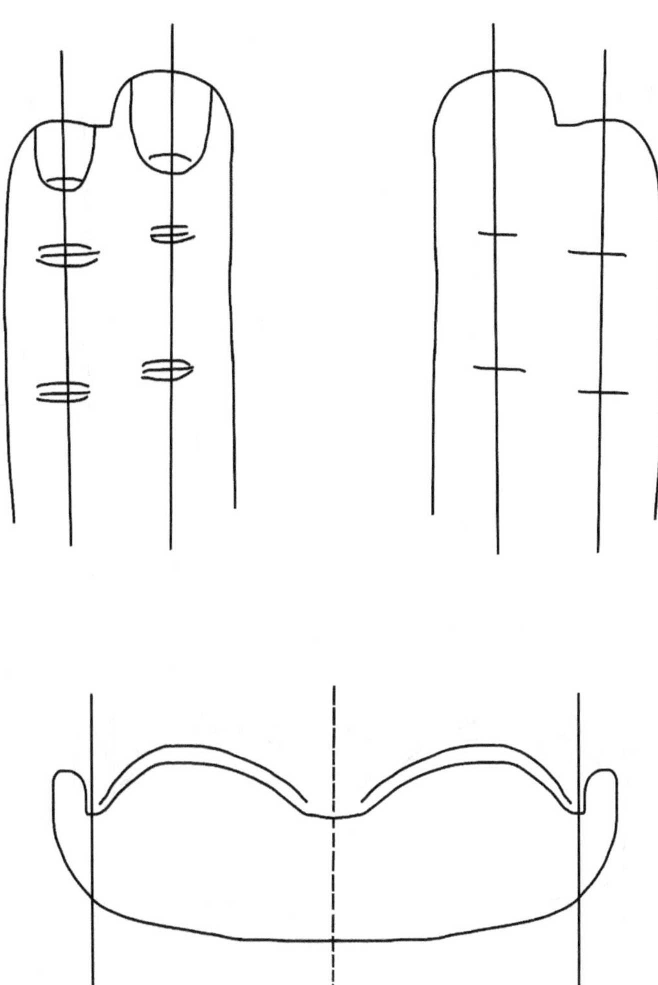

Figure (*contd.*): Steps of drawing a syndactyly release

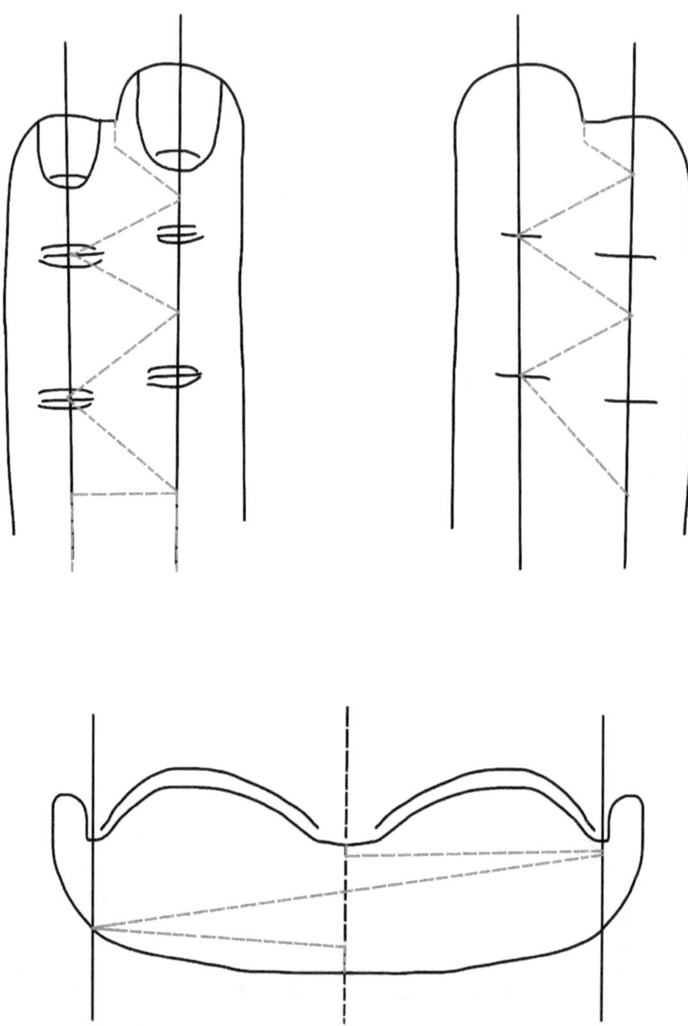

Apert hand

It is a complex hand deformity with possible shoulder and elbow anomalies. (Shoulder stiffness and anomalies at radio-capitellar joint, but rarely need operative intervention).

Table: Classification of Apert hand

	1st web	Central mass	4th web
Spade (=obstetrician's) hand	Incomplete simple	Flat digital mass in palmar plane Good MCPj	Incomplete simple
Spoon (= mitten)	Complete simple	Digital mass forms palmar concavity MC splayed but fingertips tightly fused	Complete simple
Rosebud	Complete complex	Thumb completely incorporated	Simple +/- 4th-5th MC synostosis

Principles of management

Management goal is complete separation of digits by two years of age to allow for growth and development of function.

1) Release of first web

Minor: local flaps for example 4/5 flap Z-plasty

Severe contracture: Free tissue transfer (groin / lateral arm flap)

Intermediate: Rotation advancement flap from dorsum

2) Release of centre digits
- This needs to be a staged reconstruction. Neurovascular anomalies are common therefore investigate with CT Angio (at time of head CT)
- Release distal bony union with a fishmouth incision (to convert a tightly bunched hand to "spade" configuration) and stabilise with a transverse K-wire
- Later use standard syndactyly releases

3) Release of small finger

Release synostosis plus fascia/fat interposition

Complications of syndactyly release

A) Early

       Wound dehiscence

       Infection

       Graft loss

       Vascular compromise

B) Late

       Web creep

       Joint conjecture, from scars contracting across PIPJ

       Beaked nail, (after complete syndactyly release) from loss of soft tissue bulk & scarring

       Joint instability, especially in complex-complicated ones

Symbrachydactyly = short stiff fingers combined with syndactyly. It is associated with Poland's, usually unilateral and of variable severity. Operate if digits are well formed and release MC ligament to increase mobility of fingers and appealing length.

Toe-to-thumb transfer

Ref: Green's Operative Hand Surgery

TIMING

1yr+ of age and acute injury has healed

PROS

Good mobility, sensibility and strength
Similar in appearance to a thumb
Preserved growth potential

CONS

Sacrifices a toe
Size mismatch (usually the great toe is slightly bigger, and 2nd toe is slightly smaller than the thumb)

Ideal amputation level, for which toe-to-thumb transfer is considered ideal, is mid to distal 1st MC

Pre-requisites = Normal CMCj + good thenar muscles (which will give the eventual range of motion and strength)

CHOICE OF TOE

Only between 1st vs 2nd. ipsilateral vs contra-lateral
Ipsilateral preferred because,
  - Favourable location of pedicle for anastomosis
  - 10-15degrees angulation at MTP & IPj allows for opposition
Skin from 1st webspace of toe used to reconstruct 1st web of hand

Ist toe:

Gait can potentially be affected

2nd toe:

- Less problem with gait, but
- Smaller in size
- Needs better planning of skin cover

POSTOP MANAGEMENT

Like a replant
Well hydrated, warm room, frequent observations

SUGGESTED REHAB

Gentle ROM at 1/52

Foot NWB for 2/52

Tendon repair protocol at 3/52

COURSE AND COMPLICATIONS

Postop thombosis (10-15%) needs re-exploration

95% overall survival

sensations return 4-6/12 to 2 years

SECONDARY PROCEDURES

Flexor tenolysis

Bone graft

Osteotomies

Nerve graft

1st web deepening

Tendon transfer e.g. opponensplasty

Aesthetics - except breast

Brow lift

CORE KNOWLEDGE
Brow-levator continuum
Compensated brow ptosis

APPROACH TO PATIENT - HISTORY
Basic information
- Age, occupation, hobbies, smoking

Extended information
- Past medical history. Hypertension, bleeding disorders, other medical conditions, psychiatric history.
- Medication. Anticoagulants, anti-inflammatory Vitamin E, herbals
- Allergies
- Smoking, alcohol, recreational drugs

Motives (BDD screen)
- Why? Why now? Who is paying? Partner/GP aware? Previous plastic surgery? Satisfied?

Problem area
- Vision, dry eyes, diplopia/glaucoma

Don't forget
- Clinical photographs

APPROACH TO PATIENT - EXAMINATION
Brow and orbit symmetry
Position of anterior hairline
Thickness of scalp hair
Transverse forehead lines
Glabellar frown lines

Excess skin/hollowness of upper lids
Lid margin (position)
Thickness of the eyebrow hair
Eyebrow. Height, axis, shape, mobility, old scars
Compensated brow ptosis
Consider various vectors of mobilisation

Figure: Aging forehead and peri-orbita

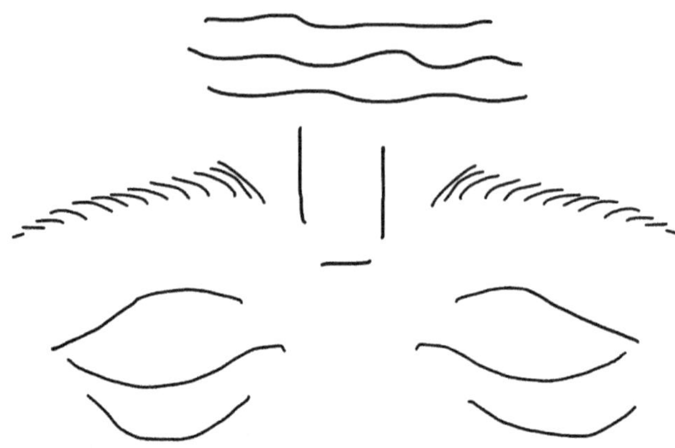

APPROACH TO PATIENT - TREATMENT

Endoscopic / Open approach

Open approaches.

1. coronal,
2. anterior hairline,
3. temporal lift by galeapexy (Fogli),
4. direct excision, (in transverse crease),
5. melon slice,
6. trans-blepharoplasty.

EXPECTED CLINICAL QUESTIONS

Normal eyebrow shape (Ellenbogen)

Compensated brow ptosis

Complications. Haematoma, alopecia, injury to sensory nerves causing forehead numbness, numbness posterior to skin incisions(expected), weakness of frontalis (for up to a year), separation of eyebrows, quizzical look

RECOMMENDED PAPERS

1. Flowers RS, Ceydeli A. The Open Coronal Approach to Forehead Rejuvenation. *Clin Plast Surg.* 2008 Jul;35(3):331–51.
2. Fogli AL. Temporal Lift by Galeapexy: A Review of 270 Cases. *Aesthetic Plast Surg.* 2003 Jun 1;27(3):159–65.

COMPENSATED BROW PTOSIS

It is a condition where eyebrow descent is masked by constant contraction of the frontalis muscle. This gives rise to deep forehead wrinkles and frontal headaches at the end of the day.

Describe a technique you are familiar with

It will be helpful to organise your thoughts under the following headings.

APPROACH

1. Open.
   - Bicoronal, largely historic
   - Temporal,
   - Anterior hair line
2. Endoscopic

EXTENT OF DISSECTION

Subgaleal to a variable degree
Shift to subcutaneous plane

METHOD OF FIXATION

Sutures
Bone anchors

Blephroplasty

CORE KNOWLEDGE
Brow-bleph continuum
Compensated brow ptosis

APPROACH TO PATIENT - HISTORY
Basic information
- Age, occupation, hobbies, smoking

Extended information
- Past medical history. Hypertension, bleeding disorders, other medical conditions, psychiatric history
- Medication. Anticoagulants, anti-inflammatory Vitamin E, herbals
- Allergies
- Smoking, alcohol, recreational drugs

Motives / BDD screen
- Why? Why now? Who is paying? Partner/GP are we? Previous plastic surgery? Satisfied?

Problem area
- Form. What exactly is the pt unhappy about
- Function. Vision, contact lens use, dry eyes
- Specific PMHx. Diplopia, glaucoma

Dont forget
- Clinical photographs (with eyes open and closed)

APPROACH TO PATIENT - EXAMINATION
Inspection
Position of eyebrows
Obvious eyelid pathology
Amount of excess eyelid tissue
Any excess of fat pads
Lagophthalmos
Enophthalmos
MRD
CV VII

Test

- Compensated brow ptosis. Explain the procedure to the patient. Ask them to keep the head upright and look down/close their eyes. Gently press the brows with both thumbs. Then ask them to open their eyes. Once eyes are in primary gaze, note any excess hooding of the upper lids. Then let go of the brow and note if they elevate. If they do, pt has a compensated brow ptosis and an upper bleph *alone* will *not* help them.
- Lower lid snap test - if lax, needs horizontal tightening.
- Location and size of fat pads - by gentle pressure on globe (warn the patient!!) to assess any herniation [Do not confuse fullness with herniation]
- Bell's phenomenon
- Offer visual acuity and fields

There is no need for Schirmer's test in every case (see below for Morphologically prone eye)

APPROACH TO PATIENT - TREATMENT
(see below)

PRINCIPLES
Proper brow positioning

Restoration of position of lateral canthus

Restoration of tone and posture of lower lids

Removal of only the tissue which is truly excessive (skin / muscle / fat) [see below]

EXPECTED CLINICAL QUESTIONS
- Characteristics of youthful eyes
- Markings for upper / lower bleph
- What would you tell the patient
- Describe the procedure (upper bleph, lower pleph, canthopexy), complications
- Retrobulbar hemorrhage scenario
- Rx of dry eyes
- Draw X-section of eyelid (upper / lower) Ref:Figure

Figure: Cross section of eyelids

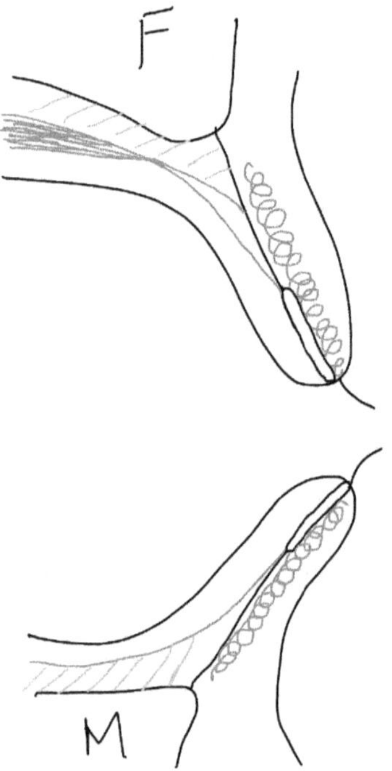

RECOMMENDED PAPERS

1. Friedland JA, Lalonde DH, Rohrich RJ. An Evidence-Based Approach to Blepharoplasty *Plast Reconstr Surg*. 2010 Dec;126(6):2222–9.
2. Trussler AP, Rohrich RJ. MOC-PSSM CME Article: Blepharoplasty *Plast Reconstr Surg*. 2008 Jan;121(MOC-PS CME Coll):1–10.

DEFINITION OF CONFUSING TERMS

- Dermatochalasis = involutional loosening of the lower lid skin
- Blephrochalasis = rare eyelid disorder with repetitive h/o eyelid edema eventually causing levator dehiscence
- Blephroptosis = drooping of eyelid
- Steatoblephron = prominence of fat (either due to true excess of fat, or from a lax septum)

Negative orbital vector / Mophologically prone eye (MPE)

In lateral view, a line drawn from the most prominent points on cornea, on lower lid and the inferior bony orbit is said to define the orbital vector. A "negative orbital vector" means that this vector points posteriorly i.e. cornea is projecting more than the lower lid which is projecting more than the bony orbit.

It is important to note this relationship as a lower lid tightening procedure *alone* (in presence of a -ve orbital vector) will cause the now-shortened lower lid to slide under the prominent globe. That will expose the lower conjuctiva and increase risk of dryness and exposure keratitis / conjunctivitis.

There is no such term as the "+ve orbital vector". One only refers to a patient having, or not having, a -ve orbital vector. The original description of negative orbital vector was by Jelks and Jelks, the condition is increasingly referred to as the "morphologically prone eye".

Schirmer's test is only usually recommended in a morphologically prone eye or in a patient with pre-existing dryness of eyes. [Do think of Sjogren's syndrome and related rheumatologic conditions and refer as appropriate].

WHAT WOULD YOU TELL YOUR PATIENT
[This is not an exhaustive list]

- Expect to be in hospital for half a day.
- You will be awake during the operation.
- You will have a slightly curved scar on the eyelid and a blue stitch coming out of it. This stitch will stay there for five days and will be removed in clinic.
- You can go home the same day, but someone will need to pick you up.
- You may need to go home with eye pads on - don't be alarmed.
- Your eye may be swollen and bruised for a few days (so adjust your social schedule accordingly).
- Avoid straining, heavy lifting, leaning over, ibuprofen/diclofenac.
- Do apply damp pads on eyes at night.
- We will see you in five days to take the stitches out.
- The scars will start out as pink after removal of stitches - you can camouflage them with makeup.
- Expect some dryness of eyes and tightness when you blink, which will settle over several weeks to a few months.

COMPLICATIONS
Intra-operative
- Ptosis, from levator injury
- Diplopia, from inferior oblique injury

Early
- Infection

Late
- Inadequate correction
- Lagophthalmos
- Excessive scleral show

Rare
- Retrobulbar hematoma (approx 1:40k) and return to theatre

Describe upper bleph procedure

MARKING
Lower: Stay cephalad to the tarsal plate. This determines where your scar is set. A higher incision gives a feminising look.

Upper: Depends on the amount of excess skin. Don't make it too high, or the upper lid will be too short. Leave at least 1cm intact below the brow.

Medial: Don't go medial to medial canthus. If there is excess skin, consider a fish tail incision.

Lateral: Go as far lateral as needed to remove the excess skin. If you need to come lateral to the lateral canthus, slant the incision supero-lateral, past the lateral end of brow. [Slanting it inferiorly will interfere with a lower bleph incision].

PROCEDURE
- Head up & reclining
- LA - precise amount
- Skin excision - always. Do double and triple check that you will be able to close the resulting wound e.g. using a pair of non-toothed forceps and with patient's eyes closed.
- Orbicularis and retro-septal fat. The indications are few and far between. [Unnecessary removal of fat gives a hollowed eye look that you may notice in some celebrities. It may be a different look but not a natural, rejuvinated look].

Please refer to Peter Neligan's book, or some of the excellent articles in PRS for discussion.

- Closure is with non-absorbable sutures of your choice

[Note that the adult globe is approx. 23mm in diametre giving an approx circumference of 72mm or a quadrant of 18mm. If you leave intact 7-8mm from ciliary margin and 10mm from the brow, that gives you 18mm to cover the upper lid *in primary gaze* - of course you need more for proper upper lid function]

Retrobulbar haemorrhage

CLINICAL FEATURES

- Pain
- Proptosis
- Ophthalmoplegia
- Decreasing vision (late sign !!)

If concerned, check for extra-ocular muscle ROM, RAPD and formal vision assessment *regularly.* Most haemorrhages evolve over a period of a few hours.

GOALS

1. Patient safety
2. Protection of vision

MANAGEMENT

1. Prevention
    - Short procedure with minimum trauma and good hemostasis.
    - Good analgesia
    - Heads up position and avoid valsalva

If you are not on-site
1. Confirm patient's vitals, pain score and symptoms progression
2. Who is available on site. Can a colleague assess and manage.
3. If no one is available.
    - Do attend asap.
    - In that interval, ensure pt is positioned head up, has good analgesia (and any antihypertension medication they forgot to take today).
    - Cool pads on the side of the face (but not on the globe directly)
    - Consider acetazolamide / mannitol if available and someone able to administer them.

If you are on site, decide whether it is or isn't a vision threatening condition.
1. Confirm patient's vitals, pain score and symptoms progression

2. Ensure positioning, analgesia, patient's regular antihypertensives, cool pads on side of face
3. If concerned, immediately decompress, preferably in theatre by releasing sutures and securing hemostasis. However, if vision is threatened be prepared to remove sutures by the bedside (and cover with sterile dressing) +/- do a bedside lateral cantholysis.

Do review regularly.

Management of lateral canthus

CANTHOPEXY

involves hitching the lateral canthus to the periosteum of the bony orbit.

CANTHOPLASTY

is securing the lateral canthus with a non-absorbable suture in to a hole made in the bony orbit. [Yes, the globe is very near]

Concepts around eyelid ptosis

[As a general plastic surgeon, you'll need to refer these cases to an ophthalmology colleague]

Classification

1. Congenital
2. Acquired
   - Neurogenic
   - Myogenic
   - Traumatic
   - Mechanical

MRD-1 is the distance in millimetres, between pupillary light reflex and the upper lid margin. Increased distance implies upper lid retraction.

MRD-2 is the distance in millimetres between pupillary light reflex and lower lid margin. Increased distance implies lower lid retraction.

MRD 1& 2 are measured with patient looking straight ahead and head upright. Light reflex refers to the reflection of the pen torch on the cornea when the pen torch is held in midline at horizontal level of the eye at an arms length.

Levator function is the distance in millimetres travelled by the upper eyelid margin between down gaze and up gaze, while the brow is held static by the examiner.

Explain the steps to the patient. Ask them to look down. Gently press one brow with your thumb and place a transparent ruler with the other hand in that eye's pupillary midline - away from the lashes. "Zero" the ruler on the lid margin. Ask the patient to look all the way up, as you use your thumb to prevent the brow from rising. Note the distance travelled in mm.

Table: Options for correction of upper eyelid ptosis

Ptosis	Levator function		
	Good (= 8-10mm)	Fair (=5-7mm)	Poor (4mm or less)
Mild (= 1-2mm)	Fasanella-Servat		
Moderate (=3-4mm)	Aponeurosis sling	Levator resection	
Severe (>4mm)			Brow/frontalis suspension

Myasthenia gravis is an autoimmune neuromuscular disorder caused by postsynaptic acetylcholine receptor block at the neuromuscular junction. It causes painless muscle weakness that worsens with activity. Typically it tends to be worse in upper lids (i.e. small muscles which are used a lot) and at the end of the day.

Edrophonium ("Tensilon") is a (reversible) cholinesterase inhibitor i.e. prevents breakdown of acetylcholine so that it lasts longer at the neuromuscular junction.

PTOSIS PROCEDURES

1. Fasanella-Servat = mullerectomy = conjunctiva, tarsal and Muller's muscle resection via a trans-conjunctical approach
2. Aponeurosis surgery = either repair of levator dehiscence, or levator aponeurosis advancement/plication
3. Levator resection = rarely needed
4. Brow suspension = slings suspend lids to brow, to substitute for poor levator function

Rhinoplasty

CORE KNOWLEDGE

Terminology
Anatomical landmarks
Instruments in a rhinoplasty set
Blood supply to nasal tip
Basic manoeuvres e.g. hump reduction

APPROACH TO PATIENT - HISTORY

Basic information

- Age, occupation, smoking, hobbies (do the job/hobbies depend on pt's sense of smell e.g. chef, wine taster)

Extended info

- Past medical history. Hypertension, bleeding disorders, other medical conditions, psychiatric history
- Medication. Anticoagulants, anti-inflammatories, Vitamin E, herbals
- Allergies
- Smoking, alcohol, recreational drugs (esp. cocaine use)

Motives

- Why? Why now? Who is paying? Partner/GP are we? Previous plastic surgery? Satisfied?

Problem area

- Form: What exactly about the nose is the problem?
- Function: Obstruction? Sense of smell?
- Specific PMHx: Allergic disorders/ hay fever / asthma. Trauma / surgeries to nose or sinuses

Don't forget

- Clinical photographs (frontal, both sides lateral, bird's eye view, worm's eye view)

APPROACH TO PATIENT - EXAMINATION

Know your landmarks *well* and how to describe them fluently. [This is a common clinical station in FRCS(Plast)]. Remember to look at it as a whole - deconstruct, and then reconstruct the shape. Adapted from Rohrich PRS 2011. See references for details.

FRONTAL VIEW

Facial proportions	"attractive" / well-balanced etc.
Skin type / quality	thin / good / sebaceous
Symmetry and nasal deviation	it tends to be the lobule only that is deviated
Dorsal esthetic lines	well formed / not formed
Upper 1/3rd (Bony vault)	wide / narrow
Middle 1/3rd	wide / narrow / collapsed, any ULC asymmetry
Lower 1/3rd	symmetrical / asymmetrical
Nasal tip	bulbous / boxy / narrow
Alar rims	flaring
Alar base	same/different level, wide/narrow
Upper lip	short / long

LATERAL VIEW

The most prominent feature is … (usually a dorsal hump / collapse)

Nasofrontal angle	deep / shallow*
Nasal length	appropriate for the face / apears long or short
Dorsum	straight / hump / collapsed
Supratip	break or not
Tip projection	appropriate, over- / under- projected
Tip rotation	over- / under- rotated
Alar-columellar relationship	normal / abnormal, and whether the cause is in the ala or the columella

Nasolabial angle	acute / obtuse*
Lip-chin relationship	normal / abnormal (with chin protrusion/retrusion)

* Don't claim to measure any angle by eyeballing it alone (nasofrontal, nasolabial or even Dupuytren's). That is what your clinical photographs are for, so that you can make a pre- and post-op comparison.

BASAL VIEW

Nasal projectiom	well projected or not
Nostril	symmetrical (if not, what is the asymmetry)
Columella	central / deviated
Alar base	narrow / wide
Alar flaring	

INTERNAL NASAL EXAM

External valve	
Mucosa	congested or not
Inferior turbinate	hypertrophy or not
Septum	deviation and its direction
Masses	if any
Cottle's test (for internal valve)	

APPROACH TO PATIENT - TREATMENT
(This is best described in Rohrich's paper or his chapter in Neligan. Use that as a minimum guide, before reading any particular surgeon's technique)

EXPECTED QUESTIONS
- Nasofacial analysis of a patient
- Cottel's test
- Steps of a hump reduction
- Counselling
- Choice of incision and why

RECOMMENDED PAPERS

1. Cochran CS, Landecker A. Prevention and Management of Rhinoplasty Complications *Plast Reconstr Surg.* 2008 Aug;122(2):60e – 67e.
2. Rohrich RJ, Ahmad J. Rhinoplasty *Plast Reconstr Surg.* 2011 Aug;128(2): 49e – 73e.

[For the FRCS exam you shouldn't need anything a lot more. Janis' book gives a good summary of techniques but it assumes that you know the principles.]

Facelift

CORE KNOWLEDGE
Anatomical planes
Danger zones for facial nerve
Principles of commonly used techniques
At least one technique in some depth

APPROACH TO PATIENT - HISTORY
Basic information
- Age, occupation, smoking, hobbies (do the job/hobbies depend on pt's sense of smell e.g. chef, wine taster)

Extended info
- Past medical history. Hypertension, bleeding disorders, other medical conditions, psychiatric history
- Medication. Anticoagulants, anti-inflammatories, Vitamin E, herbals
- Allergies
- Smoking, alcohol, recreational drugs (esp. cocaine use)

Motives
- Why? Why now? Who is paying? Partner/GP are we? Previous plastic surgery? Satisfied?

Problem area
- What specifically is the problem (forehead, jowls, nasolabial folds, eyelids, wrinkles, depression)?
- What does the patient not like?
- How is it causing problem?
- Can you see the same problem?
- Is facelift the only solution for it? Does it needmore/less?

Don't forget
Clinical photographs (frontal, both sides lateral, bird's eye and worm's eye views)

APPROACH TO PATIENT - EXAMINATION

Figure: Examination of an aged face

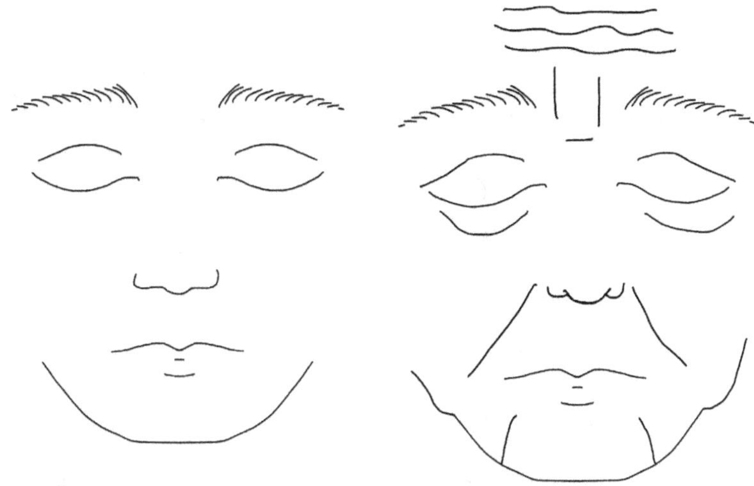

Transverse forehead creases
Temporal wasting
Lateral brow ptosis
Hollowing of upper lid sulcus
Inferior displacement of lateral canthus
Crow's feet

Tear trough
Midface flattenening
Cheek descent
Prominent nasolabial folds

Elongation of upper lip
Peri-oral wrinkles
Thin upper lip
Jowls
Marionette lines

Transverse neck folds
Platysmal bands

APPROACH TO PATIENT - TREATMENT

Operations can be classified by
1.   Plane of dissection
2.   Method of fixation

Plane of dissection	Procedure		Method of fixation
Subcutaneous	sub-cut		skin sutures
Subcutaneous	SMAS Plication		SMAS sutures
	Lateral SMAS-ectomy	Baker 1997	SMAS sutures
	Extended SMAS-ectomy	Stuzin	SMAS sutures
	High SMAS		SMAS sutures
	SMAS-Platysma plication	Berry & Davies	SMAS & Platysma
Subcutaneous	MACS	Tonnard & Varpeale	Sutures (only) at jowl, NLF +/- malar fat
	Deep plane	Hamra 1992	
Subperiosteal	Subperiosteal	Tessier 1979	

EXPECTED CLINICAL QUESTIONS
• Describe the age related changes on a face
• Describe a facelift operation that you know/have seen
• Anatomical planes
• "Lift and fill"

RECOMMENDED PAPERS
1.   Rohrich RJ, Pessa JE. The Fat Compartments of the Face: Anatomy and Clinical Implications for Cosmetic Surgery. *Plast Reconstr Surg.* 2007 Jun; 119(7):2219–27.
2.   Rohrich RJ, Ghavami A, Constantine FC, Unger J, Mojallal A. Lift-and-Fill Face Lift: Integrating the Fat Compartments. *Plast Reconstr Surg.* 2014 Jun; 133(6):756e – 767e.

3. Richard J. Warren, Peter C. Neligan. *Plastic Surgery: Volume 2: Aesthetic Surgery* (Expert Consult - Online and Print), 3rd edition. London ; New York: Saunders; 2012. 924 p.

Opinion:

Peter Neligan's book ("Plastic Surgery", volume 2: aesthetic surgery) very accurately describes the anatomical planes of facelift. It also aims to standardise what has been a very confusing amount of literature and nomenclature (especially about tissue layers in the temporal region). I strongly recommend reading that, however, the following points helped my understanding considerably.

1. There are five layers (not only) in the scalp, (but in) face as well as temporal region.

2. In each region, the corresponding layers and the structures passing through them are broadly similar.

3. Face can be divided into an anterior mimetic, mobile and superficial layer. (which is supplied by the facial nerve and is embryologically from the second branchial arch) and a more posterior and relatively less mobile set of muscles (related to mastication, embryologically derived from the first branchial arch and supplied by the trigeminal nerve). Most of the age related changes occur in the anterior face. Most methods of fixation anchor this more mobile part to the posterior less mobile part.

Abdominoplasty

CORE KNOWLEDGE
Huger's zones
Classification of excess abdominal tissue
Difference between male and female trunk
Types of abdominoplasty and their indications
Principle of high lateral tension

APPROACH TO PATIENT - HISTORY
Basic information
- Age, occupation, smoking, hobbies (e.g. yoga, cycling, running, fitness training), who is at home

Extended info
- Past medical history. Hypertension, bleeding disorders, other medical conditions, psychiatric history
- Medication. Anticoagulants, anti-inflammatories, Vitamin E, herbals
- Allergies
- Smoking, alcohol, recreational drugs

Motives
- Why? Why now? Who is paying? Partner/GP are we? Previous plastic surgery? Satisfied?

Problem area
- Form: What exactly about is the problem? Since when?
- Function: Family completed/more children planned?
- Specific PMHx: cholecystectomy, appendicectomy, thoracotomy

Don't forget
- Clinical photographs

APPROACH TO PATIENT - EXAMINATION
Consider a chaperone

Standing

> Appropriate exposure
> Striae
> Scars e.g. subcostal, upper midline, right iliac fossa, Pfennensteil
> Skin excess: supra-umbilical, infra-umbilical, posterior. Look for eczema or excoriation under the skin excess
> "Diver's test" = worsening of abdominal fullness suggesting myofascial laxity
> Ptosis of the umbilicus
> Ask to cough and look for hernias (epigastric, para-umbilical, inguinal, femoral)

Supine

> Cough and feel for hernias
> Resist forehead elevation and look for diverication

APPROACH TO PATIENT - TREATMENT
see below

EXPECTED VIVA QUESTIONS
- Huger's zones
- Classification of anterior abdominal skin excess
- Anterior rectus sheath anatomy
- Zones of adherence
- High lateral tension abdominoplasty
- Describe your technique

RECOMMENDED PAPERS

1. Bozola AR, Psillakis JM. Abdominoplasty: a new concept and classification for treatment. *Plast Reconstr Surg.* 1988 Dec;82(6):983–93.
2. Nahas FX, Ferreira LM. Concepts on Correction of the Musculoaponeurotic Layer in Abdominoplasty. *Clin Plast Surg.* 2010 Jul;37(3):527–38.
3. Friedland JA, Maffi TR. MOC-PS(SM) CME Article: Abdominoplasty: *Plast Reconstr Surg.* 2008 Apr;121(Supplement):1–11.
4. Matarasso A. Traditional Abdominoplasty. *Clin Plast Surg.* 2010 Jul;37(3): 415–37.
5. Lockwood TE. Maximizing aesthetics in lateral-tension abdominoplasty and body lifts. *Clin Plast Surg.* 2004 Oct;31(4):523–37.

Classification of abdominal excess tissue

[Matarasso classification (A-D), which most books describe, does not help your management at all - as the amount of tissue excess is quite subjective]

ABDOMINAL CONTOUR DEFORMITY

Bozola & Psillakis, 1988 (modified by Pitman, 1997).

Category	Skin excess	Fat excess	Musculo-aponeurotic laxity	Management
0	No	No	No	No surgery
1	No	+	No	SAL
2	+	+/-	No	mini-abdoplasty +/- SAL
3	+ (infra-umblical)	+/-	+/-	mini-abdoplasty +/- SAL +/- infra umbilical plication
4	+ (infra +/- supra umblical)	+/-	+/-	mini-abdoplasty + umbo relocation/ transection, plication supra & infra umbilical
5	+ (infra- & supra-umblical)	+/-	+/-	classic abdoplasty
6	++ (circumf-erential post MWL)	+/-	+/-	belt lipectomy

MUSCULO-APONEUROTIC DEFORMITY

Nahas (Clinics, 2010)

Type	Defect	Management
A	Post partum RD*	plication
B	RD + lateral and infraumblical laxity	plication + L-shaped plication of ext oblique
C	congenital lateral insertion of recti	Repositioning
D	RD + poor waistline	plication + advancement of ext obliques

* RD, rectus diastasis

"Standard" Abdominoplasty operation

PREOPERATIVE

Mark standing. Identify pubic bone and anterior superior iliac spine

Mark inferior incision first, at just above pubic symphysis in the midline at least 5 to 7 cm from vulvar commisure

Carried laterally to just under ASIS

Pinch test to assess how much tissue can be excised +/- mark the upper extent as a dotted line. Final decision would be made peroperatively

IN THEATRE

GA

Position. Supine, arms abducted and secured on a table that can be flexed intraoperatively.

"Specialing". Flowtrons, catheter

WHO checklist, IV antibiotics, prep, and drape

PROCEDURE

- Stand on patient's right side and check your markings & landmarks.
- Infiltrate LA
- Make the inferior incision & carry it down to Scarpa's fascia
- Control superficial circumflex iliac vessels [If you were doing a DIEAP, save these as a lifeboat]
- Elevate skin flap at level of Scarpa's until halfway to umbilicus
- Then switch the plane on to anterior rectus sheath/external oblique fascia
- Anticipate finding the umbilical stalk
- Incise skin around umbilcus
- Dissect the umbilicus free without skeletonizing it
- Rest of the dissection is only over the anterior rectus sheet up to the xiphisternum
- If there is divarication, zero-looped nylon as a running horizontal mattress and embedding it in the fat in the lower part of the wound
- Judge skin to be excised
- Split the excess down the midline to give 2 hemi-flaps
- Excise them
- Break table
- Check hemostasis
- Progressive tension sutures
- Re-site the umblicus (5/0 rapide)
- Place two drains
- 3 layer closure, 3/0 & 4/0 monocryl
- Histoacryl glue

POST-OPERATIVE

Nurse in hip flexed position

Ensure antibiotics and anticoagulation

Keep drains until <30ml in 24 hours or at seven days [or as you prefer]

Discharge plan when drains out [or home with drains, as you prefer]

Shower after three days.

Dressing clinic one week. No driving or exercise for six weeks. Outpatient one month for scar management advice. Outpatients three months for clinical photos.

COMPLICATIONS / CONSENT ISSUES

(not an exhaustive list)

Scars (location, length)

Wound healing complications (15% non-smokers, 50% smoker)

Infection <10%

VTE

Seromas

Malposition of umbo / loss of umbo

Numbness of lower skin flap

Revision surgery (has been quoted up to 40%)

Wont be able to walk fully erect for 1/52

Approximately 2-3/52 off work

No strenuous exercise/heavy lifting for 6/52

Massive weight loss (MWL)

CORE KNOWLEDGE
- Knowledge of MWL MDT
- BAPRAS guidelines, Soldin et al. August 2014
- What is MWL
- Types of bariatric procedures

APPROACH TO PATIENT - HISTORY
General
Age, Occupation, Hobbies, Who is at home, Smoking

Medical issues = PMHx, Meds (including "blood thinners" *)

PSHx - esp any chest wall / abdominal ops

DVT / PE

DM, HTN, High chol, sleep apneoa

Breast history

Pregnancy history

Psychiatric history

Substance misuse

Specific
Any bariatric surgical operations - when and what?

BMI - max, lowest, current, target

Weight changes in the last one year

Seeing a general surgeon

Seeing nutritionist / dietitian

Regular blood tests

B12/folate supplements? others (eg Fe, vitamins, trace elements)?

Ideas
How much do you know so far (internet search / family or friend had a similar experience)? What is bothering you?

Concerns
Anything you are especially worried about

Expectations
How can I help you?

Then go in to appropriate detail

APPROACH TO PATIENT - EXAMINATION
* Keep thinking of scar placement *

Start with standing

Look
> Scars of previous operations
> Skin excess
> Distribution of fat
> Number and location of "rolls"

Feel
> Skin quality and quantity
> Pinch thickness
> Tethering from previous surgical scars

Standing & lying
> Hernias of anterior abdominal wall
> Rectus diastasis
> +/- offer breast examination (if pt. is for breast surgery)

INVESTIGATIONS:
In liaison with all the specialties involved in pt care - general surgeon, physician, anaesthetist, clinical psychologist. The following are a suggested minimum,
- CXR, ECG
- FBC, U&E, Clotting
- Liver function
- Recent nutritional markers

PER-OP CONSIDERATIONS
Bariatric table
Positioning and padding, including position change during the procedure
Operative steps
Prevention of hypothermia
VTE prophylaxis - consider Flowtrons, TEDS & LMWH
Antibiotics
Fluids = maintenance + 10ml/kg/hr

APPROACH TO PATIENT - TREATMENT
Areas that *can* be addressed

Abdomen
1. Apronectomy. This is used for patients with a large overhanging pannus, especially if they have multiple comorbidities. There is no undermining of skin and the excess tissue is effectively amputated at the level of the lower abdominal scar.
2. Traditional abdominoplasty
3. Fleur-de-Lys abdoplasty

Lower body lift
This addresses lower trunk and thigh as a single unit as lateral zones of adherence are destroyed. The scar lies approximately one third of the way down the buttocks.

Belt lipectomy
The excision is more superior with respect to lower body lift and zones of adherence are preserved

EXPECTED VIVA QUESTIONS
Role of liposuction
- If @same operation = 1 op but more edema and risk to flap vascularity
- If @diff op => lipo 1st, excision 2nd. = 2 ops but adequate debulking and less edema

UK guidelines. Soldin et al 2014
High lateral tension abdoplasty
Superficial fascial suspension
Zones of adherence

RECOMMENDED PAPERS
1. Bossert RP, Rubin JP. Evaluation of the Weight Loss Patient Presenting for Plastic Surgery Consultation. *Plast Reconstr Surg.* 2012 Dec;130(6):1361–9.
2. Lockwood T. High-lateral-tension abdominoplasty with superficial fascial system suspension. *Plast Reconstr Surg.* 1995 Sep;96(3):603–15.
3. Lockwood TE. Superficial fascial system (SFS) of the trunk and extremities: a new concept. *Plast Reconstr Surg.* 1991 Jun;87(6):1009–18.
4. Matarasso A, Aly A, Hurwitz DJ, Lockwood TE. Body contouring after massive weight loss. *Aesthetic Surgery J.* 2004 Oct;24(5):452–63.
5. Sarwer DB, Thompson JK, Mitchell JE, Rubin JP. Psychological Considerations of the Bariatric Surgery Patient Undergoing Body Contouring Surgery. *Plast Reconstr Surg.* 2008 Jun;121(6):423e – 434e.

6. Soldin M, Mughal M, Al-Hadithy N. National Commissioning Guidelines: Body contouring surgery after massive weight loss. *J Plast Reconstr & Aesthetic Surg.* 2014 Aug;67(8):1076–81.

Consent

Some of the issues that may be addressed in the consent include:

1. What does the procedure involve. General anaesthetic, duration, stages, scars
2. Aims. What do we hope to be the final outcome
3. Alternatives, including the option of not having an operation
4. Complications and risks

A. Scar placement, infection, breakdown, migration, contracture, keloid, asymmetry
B. Bleeding, bruising, haematoma, Seroma, (lymphoedema in limbs)
C. Altered sensations, ethnic grocers, our creation with age and weight, DVT/ PE, allergic reaction, problem with intimate relations, patient dissatisfaction.

In UK 65% of the over 16 years age population is overweight. Between 2 to 3% are morbidly obese.

The purposed guidelines suggest that patients see their GP and if they meet the criteria they have clinical psychologist's opinion before having a specialist referral.

The general criteria include,
- age more than 16 years
- starting BMI, either more than 40, or more than 35 with comorbidities
- current BMI, less than 28
- wait stable for 12 months
- significant functional disturbance, which may be physical or psychological

If the patient does not meet the general criteria they may still be eligible for an operation in certain exceptional situations. These include
- starting BMI criteria are met
- final BMI is more than 28
- rest of criteria are met
- patient has lost more than 75% of excess body weight
- in this situation the patient be eligible for an apronectomy

Situations which exclude someone to be considered for massive weight loss operations include

- smoker adverse psych logical history
- deliberate self harm in the last two years
- previous diagnosis of body dysmorphic syndrome
- disproportionate view of problem
- drug or alcohol misuse.

Methods of weight loss

1. Diet and exercise
2. Pharmacological
3. Bariatric surgery
   A. Restrictive. By far the most popular procedure, this results in a smaller gastric pouch. The stomach is narrowed by encircling it with either a fixed size, or an adjustable band.
   B. Malabsorptive. Which divert nutrients e.g. biliopancreatic diversion, roux-en-Y gastric bypass
   C. combination

Potential medical improvements and benefits of MWL surgery

Hypertension
Diabetes
Hyper lipidaemia
Sleep apnoea
Life expectancy
Asthma, CCF, osteoarthritis, gastro-oesophageal reflux.

Breast - aesthetics / recon.

Breast augmentation

CORE KNOWLEDGE
Silicone controversy!
Polyurethane controversy!
PIP Implant controversy! [sounds ominous]
Saline vs Silicone
Capsular contracture
ALCL

APPROACH TO PATIENT - HISTORY
General
Age, occupation, hobbies, who is at home
Number of children, whether breastfed, more planned?
HTN, DM, smoking
Pills, hormone replacement therapy, herbal medicine
Height, Weight, BMI

Specific
Current cup size
Small/asymmetrical/odd shaped?
Issues with self confidence / intimate relations / dressing at beach (consider psychological support)
Personal/family history of CA breast, CA ovary, BRCA 1/2

Motives
Why? Why now
Who is paying? Partner/family/GP aware? What do they think
Previous plastic surgery procedures? Whether satisfied

Ideas & expectations
What can I do for you? i.e. wt is the exact problem patient wants addressed
What size are you aiming for? Are you satisfied with the other side?
Checked Internet for information or support groups
Spoken to family, friends and significant other ? what is their opinion?
Is any of them with the patient for this consultation?

APPROACH TO PATIENT - EXAMINATION

Ask for chaperone

Stand straight

Shoulders level, arms for Poland

Kyphosis/scars on back

Hands on hips

There is/is not CW deformity from front

Are there any scars (e.g. from previous aesthetic/diagnostic procedure)

Comment if the two sides are symmetrical

Ask to lift the breast to see position of IMF [only if it is a pendulous breast, else it would be obvious]

Comment on

- footplate (if height & width are symmetrical),
- breast volume (if one side is less/more),
- grade of ptosis (Regnault),
- skin envelope (whether it conforms to the underlying parenchyma i.e. hanging loose or not),
- NAC position (symmetrical or not - both in horizontal and vertical placement) [Remember, asymmetry is the "norm"]

Ask about NAC discharge

Are there any scars (again)

Hands above head

Look for tethering

Hands on hips again and press down

Feel for pect contraction (i.e. ant. axillary fold) on both sides

Consider oncological examination of breast and axillae ["Offer" in an exam scenario. In clinic always do it]

Measure

SN:N, N:IMF

BW, N:midline

Pinch thickness

APPROACH TO PATIENT - TREATMENT
see below

EXPECTED CLINICAL / VIVA QUESTIONS
Implant controversies

Types of implants

Types of augmentation

How to choose an implant & dissection plane

Dual planing

Consent

Complications

Capsule formation

Implant failure/rupture

RECOMMENDED PAPERS
1. Berry MG, Cucchiara V, Davies DM. Breast augmentation: Part II – adverse capsular contracture. *J Plast Reconstr & Aesthetic Surg*. 2010 Dec;63(12): 2098–107.
2. Berry MG, Cucchiara V, Davies DM. Breast augmentation: Part III– preoperative considerations and planning. *J Plast Reconstr & Aesthetic Surg*. 2011 Nov;64(11):1401–9.
3. Berry MG, Davies DM. Breast augmentation: Part I – a review of the silicone prosthesis. *J Plast Reconstr & Aesthetic Surg*. 2010 Nov;63(11): 1761–8.

4. Blondeel PN, Hijjawi J, Depypere H, Roche N, Van Landuyt K. Shaping the Breast in Aesthetic and Reconstructive Breast Surgery: An Easy Three-Step Principle. *Plast Reconstr Surg*. 2009 Feb;123(2):455–62.
5. Blondeel PN, Hijjawi J, Depypere H, Roche N, Van Landuyt K. Shaping the Breast in Aesthetic and Reconstructive Breast Surgery: An Easy Three-Step Principle. Part II—Breast Reconstruction after Total Mastectomy. *Plast Reconstr Surg*. 2009 Mar;123(3):794–805.

6. Adams & Mallucci. CME: Breast augmentation. *Plast Reconstr Surg*. 2012
7. Tebbetts JB. Dual Plane Breast Augmentation: Optimizing Implant–Soft- Tissue Relationships in a Wide Range of Breast Types. *Plast Reconstr Surg*. 2001;107(5):1255-72
8. Hedén P, Montemurro P, Adams WP, Germann G, Scheflan M, Maxwell GP. Anatomical and Round Breast Implants: How to Select and Indications for Use. *Plast Reconstr Surg*. 2015 Aug;136(2):263–72.

9. Hammond DC, Migliori MM, Caplin DA, Garcia ME, Phillips CA. Mentor Contour Profile Gel Implants: Clinical Outcomes at 6 Years. *Plast Reconstr Surg.* 2012 Jun;129(6):1381–91.

10. Maxwell GP, Van Natta BW, Bengtson BP, Murphy DK. Ten-Year Results From the Natrelle 410 Anatomical Form-Stable Silicone Breast Implant Core Study. *Aesthetic Surgery J.* 2015 Feb 1;35(2):145–55.

11. Maxwell GP, Van Natta BW, Murphy DK, Slicton A, Bengtson BP. Natrelle Style 410 Form-Stable Silicone Breast Implants: Core Study Results at 6 Years. *Aesthetic Surgery J.* 2012 Aug 1;32(6):709–17.

12. Spear SL, Murphy DK, Slicton A, Walker PS. Inamed Silicone Breast Implant Core Study Results at 6 Years. *Plast Reconstr Surg.* 2007 Dec; 120(Supplement 1):8S – 16S.

13. Spear SL, Murphy DK. Natrelle Round Silicone Breast Implants: Core Study Results at 10 Years. *Plast Reconstr Surg.* 2014 Jun;133(6):1354–61.

14. Stevens WG, Harrington J, Alizadeh K, Broadway D, Zeidler K, Godinez TB. Eight-Year Follow-Up Data from the U.S. Clinical Trial for Sientra's FDA-Approved Round and Shaped Implants with High-Strength Cohesive Silicone Gel. *Aesthetic Surgery J.* 2015 May 1;35(suppl 1):S3–10.

15. Stevens WG, Harrington J, Alizadeh K, Berger L, Broadway D, Hester TR, et al. Five-Year Follow-Up Data from the U.S. Clinical Trial for Sientra's U.S. Food and Drug Administration–Approved Silimed® Brand Round and Shaped Implants with High-Strength Silicone Gel. *Plast Reconstr Surg.* 2012 Nov;130(5):973–81.

16. Hedén P, Boné B, Murphy DK, Slicton A, Walker PS. Style 410 cohesive silicone breast implants: safety and effectiveness at 5 to 9 years after implantation. *Plast Reconstr Surg.* 2006 Nov;118(6):1281–7.

Silicone controversy

WHAT WAS THE CLAIMED PROBLEM

Silicone filled implants were claimed to cause connective tissue disorders. (Implant shell, though made of a silicone elastomer, was never in question).

WHAT STARTED IT

Some patients in USA claimed to develop rheumatic symptoms after implantation with silicone filled implants. In 1991 a US court awarded damages to a claimant based on what is now believed to be limited medical evidence. [Even though new medical devices need to get FDA approval, breast implants pre-dated the FDA and so were "grand fathered" in to the relevant legislation].

ESCALATION

In 1992, FDA placed a "voluntary moratorium" on the use of silicone filled implants for aesthetic purpose until further information became available. A media hype developed followed by a class action law suit against the manufacturer, Dow Corning that was upheld by court. Dow Corning faced a several billion dollar bill and filed for bankruptcy. [Dow Corning have since diversified and now manufacture the gorilla glass used as a cover on all iPhones & iPads].

EVIDENCE & POSITION STATEMENTS

- American College of rheumatology statement, 1995
- Sanchez-Guerrero et al. 1995, NEJM
- Independent review group (IRG) report August 1998 (from UK)
- Nyren et al. BMJ 1998, and many more

No evidence found linking silicone gel with autoimmune disease

WHAT HAS HAPPENED SINCE

USA almost exclusively used saline filled implants while the rest of the world continued with silicone filled implants. In 2006 cohesive gel implants were allowed as part of long term clinical studies and in 2011 all restrictions were effectively removed by FDA.

PIP scandal

PROBLEM

Over a period of nearly 10 years, Poly Implant Prosthese company knowingly used non-medical grade silicone to manufacture breast (& other) implants and systematically evaded detection by fabricating quality control. These implants were noted to have a high rupture rate but the company was allowed to manufacture and sell them worldwide.

RESULT

The owner, Jean-Claude Mas, was jailed for four years and the company liquidated in 2010.

IS THERE A KNOWN HEALTH RISK

The implants have a very high rupture rate and figures range up to 35% (Ref: Quaba & Quaba). In many cases the silicone from a ruptured implant is taken up by the lymphatic system and found in the axillary lymph nodes as siliconomas. *At the time of this writing*, there is no known evidence of any other systemic disease or cancer.

UK GUIDELINES IN THE AFTERMATH (DOH / BAPRAS)

The patients should be contacted. They should be counselled that there is no known risk to life with these implants. They may be offered explantation on the NHS (irrespective of where the surgery was done). If the initial surgery was not in the NHS, only explantation may be offered. Consider USS / MRI

Old polyurethane implant controversy

ISSUE

Implants were thought to be carcinogenic.

EVIDENCE

No evidence in humans. The only concern raised was from studies in mice and when using supra-physiologic doses of polyurethane.

Newer polyurethane (Silimed) controversy

ISSUE

Revocation of european CE mark due to concern about presence of "foreign materials" on the polyurethane shell made by a specific manufacturer in Brazil (Silimed).

EVENTS

EU regulator were inspecting the manufacturing facility as part of giving them a CE mark in 2015. The surface of implants were found to be covered with "nano particles" above the limit specified by EU. As a result, the CE mark was not extended for use in EU which was actioned by MHRA in UK and by BAPRAS.

EVIDENCE

At the time of this writing, evidence is being collected.

WHAT HAPPENS IN THE MEANTIME

BAPRAS has recommended its members, not to use Silimed implants and counsel the patients who have been implanted.

How to choose a breast implant?

Books can be written on this subject and we've all heard eminent figures hotly debating one implant or approach over another. As a day one consultant in the NHS (what you are being judged for in the FRCS exam) stay in the middle of the road! The following description is of a "simple" case i.e. young patient, primary breast augment, has no skeletal abnormality, no soft tissue asymmetry, good skin quality and no medical comorbidities.

AIM

Minimise complications (haematoma, implant exposure, adverse capsular contracture) and longevity of result by achieving a harmonious tissue-implant interaction ("tissue based planning").

This represents a scientific way to approach BAs instead of sticking in the largest volume possible.

1. SILICONE VS SALINE (VS POLYURETHANE!)

In the UK you will be most often using silicone implants. Unless you have extensive experience in using polyurethane implants, do not mention these as your first choice of implant in the exam scenario [especially since their CE marking has been revoked and use discontinued throughout EU, at the time of this writing]

Please refer to the excellent review by Dai Davies on implant generations and silicone controversy. Current generation of silicone implants are form stable ("gummy bear" implants).

Many junior colleagues, when asked how to choose an implant start with Tebbetts' High-5. Note that High-5 system has two components, i) a theoretical one which explains the 5 decisions that need to be made (e.g. if you are using silicone implants via inframammary incision), and ii) the implant template which lets you find the implant volume by the steps of addition and subtraction.

The theoretical component is vitally important to understanding the underlying concepts. But the numerical component, I think, is to breast surgery what MESS scoring is to limb trauma i.e. painstakingly detailed/accurate but cumbersome and rarely used in the real world. Even Tebbetts himself (reading from his papers) needs a written template to work out the final implant volume. Moreover, he does not say how he arrived at the numbers being added and subtracted at each stage.

The principle, you should know well, but implement it based on your training.

2. TEXTURE

Texturing is "producing an implant with an uneven surface". Texturing of implant surface has been shown to decrease the risk of capsular contracture. Most surgeons would choose textured implants for this reason.

Capsule contracture is likely due to parallel arrangement of fibroblast n myofibroblasts in the capsule which results in a synergistic pull. Texturing of the surface is considered to disrupt that parallel arrangement so the myofibroblasts have a different vector of contraction so these vectors effectively cancel each other out and there is no net vector of contraction.

The 2 main implant manufacturers each have a proprietary texturing method. Siltex™ (Mentor, formerly McGhan) is an imprinting method where a mould is pressed onto the surface of the implant to give it the required texture. The resolution of the texturing is related the amount of detail in the mould. Biocell™ (Allergan, formerly Inamed) use a "lost salt" technique which allows for relatively larger indentations ("macro-texturing"). The clinical data does not show any significant difference between rate of capsular contractures between either manufacturer (Ref: Core studies referenced above).

[Mathes' Plastic Surgery textbook (i.e. the version between those edited by McCarthy & by Neligan) gives a very detailed review of the process].

3. INCISION

With a silicone implant your only real choice is a sub-mammary incision. This is a 5 cm incision which sits across the breast meridian in a 2:3 ratio (medial:lateral).

The classic teaching is that IMF lowers itself by about a centimetre as the implant settles in its pocket over few months, so the incision scar appears to move up the lower pole of the breast. [However that is incorrect and the IMF can be reliably fixed].

4. POCKET - SUBGLANDULAR VS SUBMUSCULAR VS DUAL PLANE

The idea behind choosing a pocket is to cover the implant with soft tissue all over, or else it may be visible, palpable and at risk of extrusion.

A **subglandular** pocket is sufficient if the patient has enough native tissue to cover/support it. Since the upper pole is the thinnest part, >2cm pinch thickness on the upper pole is taken to mean that there will be sufficient soft tissue cover for the rest of the implant and it can go subglandular.

A **submuscular** plane is strictly only partially submuscular, as the lower part of the implant is still covered by breast parenchyma (see discussion about ADMs below).

A **total submuscular** plane has been used historically to avoid implant visibility/palpability. It involved raising the serratus as well as the pect major & if needed, the upper part of the rectus. The technique can be considered for patients with very little breast tissue in the lower pole. Currently, many surgeons will use an ADM in this situation.

Subfascial plane has recently been introduced which involves raising the fascia over the pect major and placing the implant under it. [Like any new technique people either swear by it, or roll their eyes].

Dual planing implies that there are two planes of dissection. The first plane is between the chest and and the pectoralis major muscle. The second plane is between the muscle and the chest wall (i.e. ribs). The implant always goes between the muscle and the chest wall. The dissection between the breast parenchyma and pectoralis major muscle helps to free the breast tissue and re-drape it over the lower pole of the implant. The types of dual planing depend upon how far the dissection between breast tissue and the muscle is carried. The pect major muscle attachment from the sternum is *never* disturbed, because this would lead to the window shade effect and the muscle will bunch cephalad to the implant giving you more problems than you bargained for. (Ref: Figure).

Type 1 dual planing = conventional submuscular augment i.e. you raise the *costal* attachments of pect major (which can be a bit variable), then dissect your pocket under the pect major and place your implant.

Type 2 dual planing = do sub*glandular* dissection up to the lower border of NAC, *then* dissect the submuscular plane as above

Type 3 dual planing = do sub*glandular* dissection up to the upper border of NAC, *then* dissect the submuscular plane (as above)

Opinion:

Some colleagues argue that a breast augment does 'lifts' the breast & so can address ptosis too. This is true with a proviso. Notice that the ptosis is a function of the direction of the nipple as much as its vertical location. Breast augmentation can certainly move the underlying "platform" so that the base of the nipple is slightly superior. But it does not affect the direction of the nipple significantly. Dual planing can improve this situation by redraping the lower pole (but it does not work for extreme ptosis which requires augmentation-mastopexy).

Why & when should you dual plane?

Dual planing is for slightly ptotic breasts (predominantly Regnault 2 ptosis).

A pert breast (Regnault 1) will take any implant [please excuse the blanket statement] and will stay pert- in fact will be more pert due to the extra projection added by the implant (Ref: Figure).

But a ptotic breast (Regnault 2 or 3) after implant, will be a *more projected ptotic* breast. This is because the breast tissue is held in lobules separated by ligaments of Astley Cooper which extend from pectoral fascia to the NAC. Ptosis of breast comes from relaxation of these ligaments while the IMF remains relatively fixed. This causes the nipple to point downwards and the breast tissue to "sag". No matter how much volume you place behind it, this anatomical relationship will not change until you specifically address it.

Figure: Submuscular augmentation in a *non*-ptotic breast

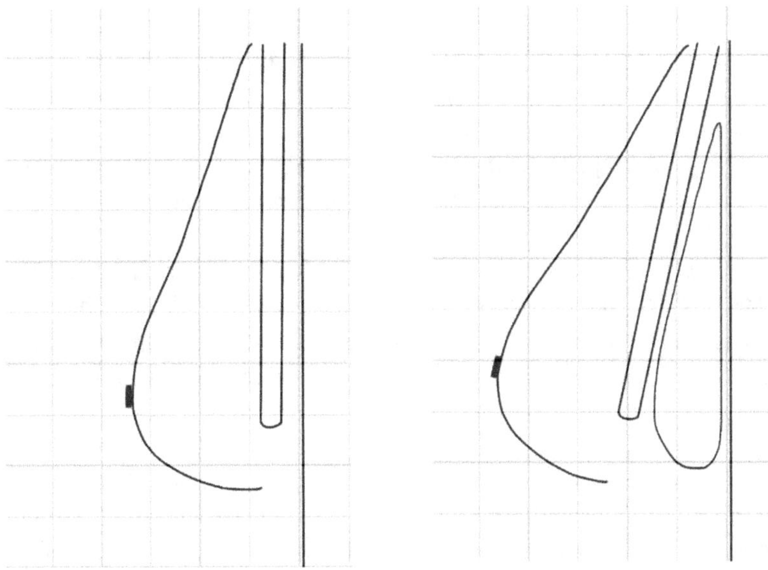

Figure: Submuscular augmentation in a ptotic breast

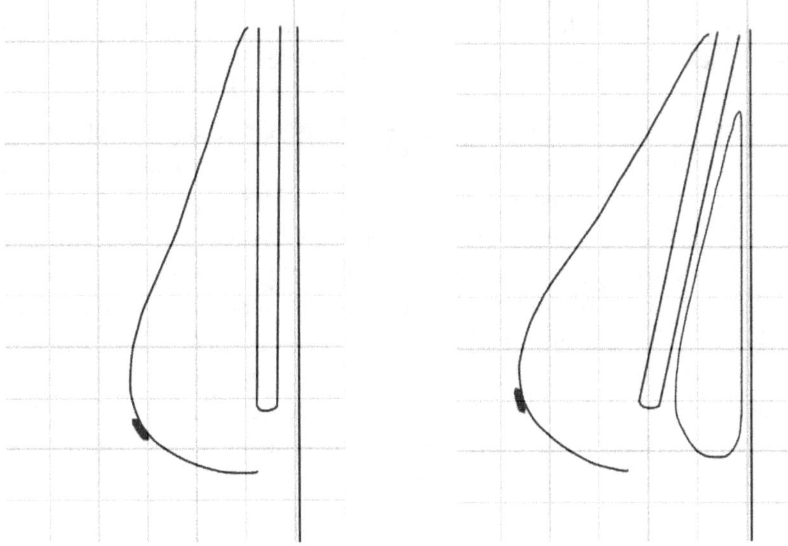

Dual planing addresses this problem by detaching the ligaments of Cooper holding the inferior pole (where majority of breast volume now exists) and allowing the lower pole tissue to redrape.

As you may suspect, this only works for up to a certain degree of ptosis, after which an augmentation mastopexy is the most appropriate solution.

5. IMPLANT SHAPE - ROUND VS ANATOMICAL

Round implants (especially subglandular) give a steep upper pole "take off" while anatomical ones result in a more subtle change. Anatomical shape is also more suitable in tall patients who have a narrow chest. The implant pocket needs to be fairly snug to prevent rotation of the anatomical implant.

A recent study where observers blinded to the plane of dissection were asked to rate the aesthetic appearance of post-op BA patients, failed to showed any significant difference in the aesthetic appearance. It may mean either that the choice of implant shape is irrelevant, or that the patient selection was appropriate for each implant type.

Although anatomical implants are chastised for a 2% rotation risk, the *total* risk of complications is much higher with the round implants (mainly due to higher capsular contracture). Anatomical implants do require a tighter pocket to prevent rotation.

6. IMPLANT VOLUME

This is another sticking point. Consider the end result that the implant needs to stay in vivo for a long time and hence need to stay harmoniously within the available pocket (or as harmonious as a foreign body can).

The volume of any implant is determined by its dimensions (which in turn depend on patient's body habitus). The width of the implant has to be constrained by the patient's existing breast width (approximately from parasternal to anterior axillary line). The height is constrained by the upper pole (at level of a horizontal line drawn between the 2 anterior axillary folds) and the IMF. There may be a 1cm leeway in deciding these dimensions to account for pinch thickness (=soft tissue cover) all around.

The manufacturers make implants in certain specific dimensions only. That means that once height and width are decided, the only variable left that can influence implant volume is its projection.

In general, surgeons decide an implant volume pre-operatively after measurement of and discussion with the patient.

VARIATIONS ON THE THEME

The upper pole may not be immediately obvious. But it is never above the line joining the anterior axillary folds.

Most (possibly all) breasts are asymmetrical. This may be in
- vertical dimension (upper pole, IMF position),
- horizontal dimension (axillary tail, axillary roll, asymmetric medial end of IMF) or
- volume (e.g. infro-medial vs infro-lateral quadrant).

Add to that horizontal & vertical asymmetry of the position of NAC, as well as variation in size of nipple and areola, the surgeon can only have a limited control of these variations. Of course we try to improve these as much as possible, but it is vitally important to point these to the patient pre-operatively and explain that these asymmetries will become more prominent once these are placed on a more projected base.

Many patients for BA have very little breast tissue and a small N:IMF distance. Use the arc length of the implant to guide you to the placement o the scar and the lower level of the implant. Note that cleavage is achieved only in a bra.

ADJUNCTS

An acellular dermal matrix covers the newly created space in the infero-lateral quadrant of the breast. It mechanically supports the lateral and inferior part of the implant. Because of these functions, the surgeon can use larger volume implants without risking implant exposure. (Of course ADMs have their own risks).

Implant failure / "rupture"

[Note "rupture" is a rather alarming term for the patients, esp. now that the 5th generation implants are form stable]

The commonest presentation is due to asymmetry, or a fairly rapid change in shape. Sometimes, a capsular contracture masks an implant rupture or it may be an incidental intra-operative finding.

There may be history of trauma or it may be insidious event. The diagnosis rests on clinical suspicion and an imaging modality. Both USS and MRI can make the diagnosis (but with different accuracy). USS may be cheaper and more easily available than MRI in many places, but MRI is considered the gold standard. In a study on 2nd generation implant ruptures, Chung et al. (1998) gave a good summary of the then available evidence (Ref: Table).

Category	Pre test probability	USS	MRI
Asymptomatic	6.5%	37.8% if +ve 2.2% if -ve	86%
Symptomatic, with implant <10years	31%	79.7% if +ve 16% if -ve	97.5%
Symptomatic, with implant >10years	64%	94% if +ve	not needed

Heden et al. (2006) showed 0.3% rate of silent implant rupture (Style 410, on MRI) in *asymptomatic* patients. The MRI was indeterminate in 0.7% cases. A meta-analysis by Chung et al. (2011) showed 87% sensitivity & 89.9% specificity of MRI in picking up an implant rupture in *symptomatic* patients.

[Of course one limiting factor with most imaging studies is that they look at a spectrum of implants usually of different generations of manufacturing].

Capsular contracture

"Capsule" around a breast implant is a foreign body reaction causing fibrosis and walling off of the perceived foreign body.

All breast implants have a capsule around them to a variable degree (Ref: Table) which appears soon after implantation and continues to evolve over time at a variable rate. Due to its fibroblast & myofibroblast content, the capsule may contract over time resulting in a palpable or visible deformity and be painful for the patient.

Table: Baker's classification (adapted)

Type	Explanation
I	Breast appear "normal"
II	Capsule palpable
III	Capsule visible as well
IV	Painful capsule

Breast implant capsule that is symptomatic for the patient (visible or painful) is referred to as an adverse capsular contracture (ACC).

IMPLICATED CAUSES / SUSPECTED ASSOCIATIONS

- Reactive e.g. secondary to haematoma
- Foreign body e.g. powder latex gloves
- Subclinical infection

MANAGEMENT

1. Avoid. Meticulous haemostasis, change gloves &/or re-prep for insertion of implant.
2. Treat.
   - Capsul*otomy* only scores the capsule and allows the implant to sit in a larger cavity. It possibly only delays the inevitable.
   - Capsul*ectomy* removes all capsule except that stuck to the chest wall. Often combined with change of implant (e.g. to a textured one) & a change of pocket. Optionally the capsule left behind on the chest wall may be scored.

Breast reduction

CORE KNOWLEDGE
Pedicles
Eponymous names
Markings
Describe your technique (at least one)

APPROACH TO PATIENT - HISTORY
General
Age, occupation, hobbies, who is at home
Number of children,? Breastfed,? More planned
HTN, DM, smoking
Pills, hormone replacement therapy, herbal medicine
Height, Weight, BMI

Specific
Current cup size
Personal/family history of CA breast, CA ovary, BRCA 1/2

Symptoms
Backache, intertrigo, shoulder straps digging, unwanted comments

Motives
Why? Why now
Who is paying? Partner/family/GP aware? What do they think
Previous plastic surgery procedures? Whether satisfied

Ideas & expectations
What can I do for you? i.e. what is the exact problem patient wants addressed
What size are you aiming for?
Checked internet/social media for information or support groups
Spoken to family, friends and significant other & what do they think

APPROACH TO PATIENT - EXAMINATION
Ask for chaperone
Stand straight
Shoulders level, arms for Poland
Kyphosis/scars on back

Hands on hips

> There is/is not CW deformity from front
> Are there any scars (e.g. from previous aesthetic/diagnostic procedure)
>
> Comment if the two sides are symmetrical
> Ask patient to lift the breast to see position of IMF
>
> Comment on
> - footplate (if height & width are symmetrical),
> - breast volume (if one side is less/more),
> - grade of ptosis (Regnault),
> - skin envelope (whether it conforms to the underlying parenchyma i.e. hanging loose or not),
> - NAC position (symmetrical or not - both in horizontal and vertical placement) [Remember, asymmetry is the "norm"]
>
> Ask about NAC discharge
> Are there any scars (again)

Hands above head

> Look for tethering

Hands on hips again and press down

> Feel for pect contraction (i.e. ant. axillary fold) on both sides

Consider oncological examination of breast and axillae ["Offer" in an exam scenario. In clinic, always do it]

Measure
SN:N, N:IMF
BW, N:midline
Skin quality / elasticity

APPROACH TO PATIENT - TREATMENT

Any operation offered on NHS has to be justified on the local CCG guidelines, so know them well for your area. Broadly, these are related to problems with form (excessive size which may in turn cause unwanted attention & anxiety) and function (backache*, intertrigo, sweating).

* Although removal of excessive breast tissue can improve the posture, it does not always improve the backache - something that the patient should know specifically during the consent process.

EXPECTED CLINICAL QUESTIONS
- Blood supply of breast tissue
- Who described various pedicles (Strombeck, McKissock, Asplund)
- Blood supply for each pedicle named above
- Specific techniques (Lejour, Marchac, Hall-Findley, SPAIR)
- How will *you* mark a breast reduction

RECOMMENDED PAPERS

1. Hammond DC, Loffredo M. Breast Reduction. *Plast Reconstr Surg.* 2012 May;129(5):829e – 839e.
2. Nahai FR, Nahai F. MOC-PSSM CME Article: Breast Reduction. *Plast Reconstr Surg.* 2008 Jan;121(MOC-PS CME Coll):1–13.
3. Noone RB. An Evidence-Based Approach to Reduction Mammaplasty. *Plast Reconstr Surg.* 2010 Dec;126(6):2171–6.
4. Fahmy FS, Hemington-Gorse SJ. The Sitting, Oblique, and Supine Marking Technique for Reduction Mammaplasty and Mastopexy. *Plast Reconstr Surg.* 2006 Jun;117(7):2145–51.
5. Asplund OA, Davies DM. Vertical scar breast reduction with medial flap or glandular transposition of the nipple-areol. *Br J Plast Surg.* 1996;49:507-5

see references for mastopexy as well

Marking for a breast reduction

Consent, chaperone, ensure privacy

Point out all asymmetries to pt while marking & document them

Measure SN:N, N:IMF

Measure N:midline

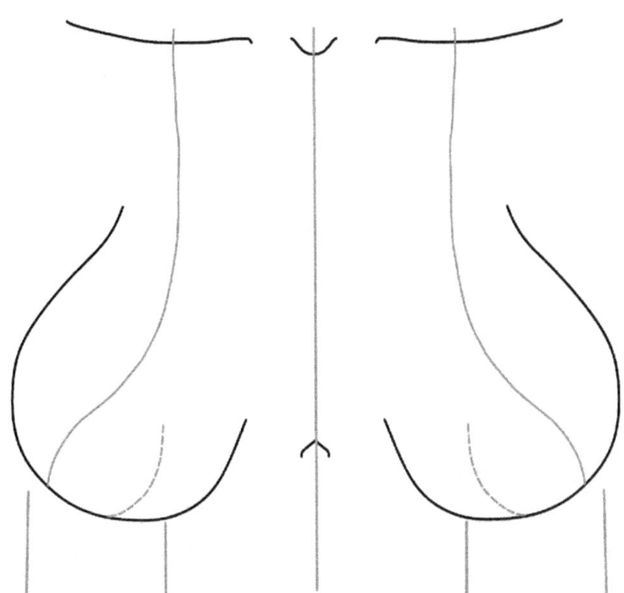

VERTICAL LINES

Midline. From supra-sternal notch to the xiphisternum and towards umbilicus

Meridian. Let the measuring tape fall as a plumb line from the patient's neck on either side. Eyeball it to make sure it lies in the central vertical meridian of each upper hemi-thorax (i.e.vertically down from mid-clavicular point*) and of the breast conus (ignoring the position of NAC, which may or may not be in the centre of the breast conus).

Follow this meridian in the inferior pole of the breast up to infra-mammary fold (IMF) and then onto lower chest/abdominal wall. The distance between the inferior most part of this line, and the vertical midline should be the same on both sides.

*Many colleagues measure 5-7cm from sternal notch for mid-clavicular point.

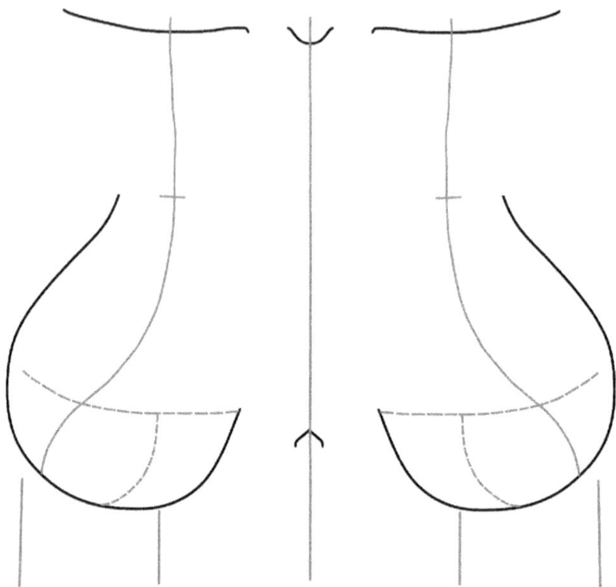

HORIZONTAL LINES

Upper pole. You may want to mark the position of the upper pole as a short horizontal line to serve as a visual reference. In cases where the upper pole is empty, mark its ideal position which is at a level just below that of the anterior axillary fold.

IMF. Ask pt to hold up both sides. Draw a horizontal line from the lowest point on IMF (this should be where the breast meridian drawn earlier meets the IMF) to the vertical midline. This would give you a visual reference that (usually) IMF are not at the same horizontal level.

Also mark the medial and lateral extent of IMF. If you are doing a Wise pattern excision, keep the scar inside these markings else it would be visible and painful in a bra postop. The medial ends are usually asymmetrical, so use the one which is lower as your guide. The lateral extent can be difficult to find especially if the patient has a fat roll. This shouldn't extend beyond anterior axillary line and any residual fat there can be liposuctioned instead.

All the previous markings are about the landmarks of the existing breast. From here onwards we are marking for the future breast.

New nipple position / Pitanguay's point. Pitanguay's point is the projection of the centre of IMF on to the breast meridian anteriorly, *with the breast weight taken off* (or else the NAC position would end up too high). This is the key point so be absolutely certain of it before you move further. There are three ways to locate it.

1. Direct palpation between the fingers of two hands (Pitanguay's original description).
2. By measuring distance from the supra-sternal notch (as pt takes the weight of both breasts)
3. Mid humeral point. Everyone talks about it but no one actually measures it!

It is best to step back and judge the position by eyeballing it. Experience helps! so does asking the patient to flex her elbow at 90° and rest it across the torso, which makes the judgement easier.

All of the above will likely give slightly different level - go for the lowest one. Eyeball it and measure again from sternal notch to ensure the distance is symmetrical.

OBLIQUE LINES / SKIN EXCISION PATTERN

Pendulum test. Swing the breast laterally. Judge the volume (and contour) to be left behind on the medial half. Then draw a vertical from Pitanguay's point to the previously marked meridian on the lower hemi-torso. Make this line approximately 8-10cm long. Then swing the breast medially and repeat. These will make an inverted-V shape, with apex at Pitanguay's point.

If the NAC was central on the breast mound, then these lines should be equidistant from the NAC. If NAC was not central, then u have the chance to adjust its position by moving the inverted-V shape design towards where you want the NAC to move (usually NAC is slightly too lateral). Any such adjustment needs to be carefully planned and executed as overcorrection will leave very little tissue medially and distort the final shape.

Figure: "Pendulum" manoeuvre (shown here on both side simultaneously)

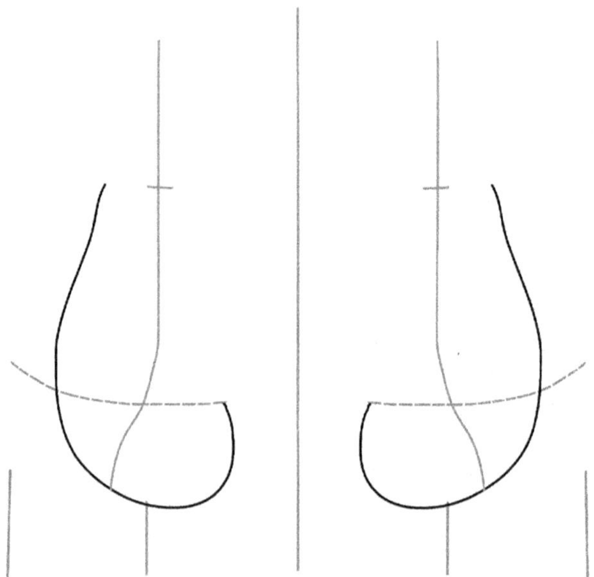

Aside:

Markings for a vertical scar differ at this stage. Once the new NAC position is determined (as above), most surgeons will draw a free hand marking of the NAC ("mosque dome" pattern) and the judge vertical limbs based on the pendulum test. The vertical limbs are parallel (as opposed to diverging) and are joined by a tapered "U" shape at there inferior extent. All these markings stay on the breast.

Figure: Vertical limbs (for a Wise pattern)

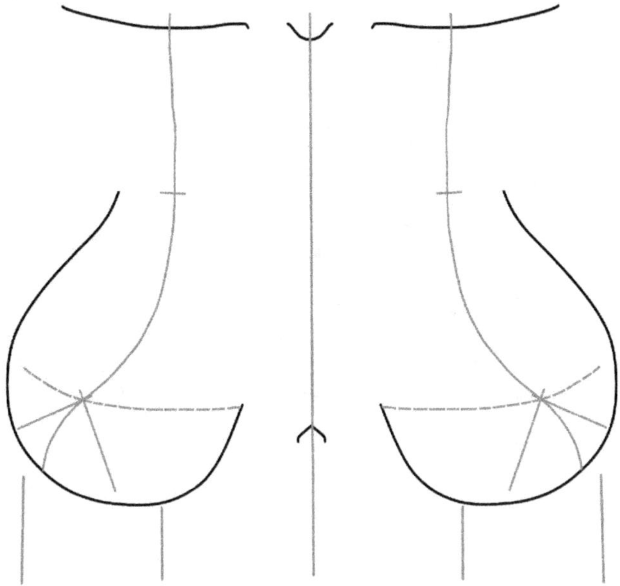

Figure: (above) Horizontal limbs, for a Wise pattern

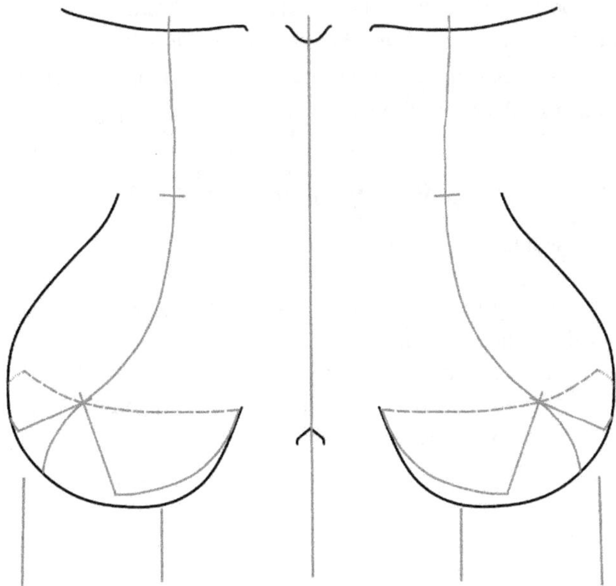

Figure: Marking the pedicle

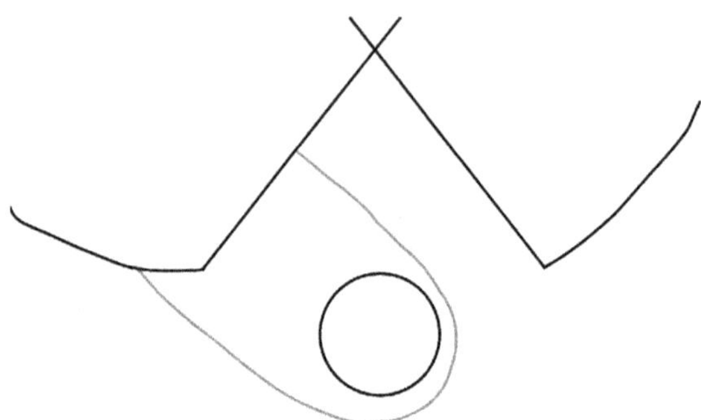

The pedicle is marked with 7cm width, with ideally 2/3rd of the pedicle within the vertical limbs and 1/3rd outside it. This provides a good configuration for the NAC to rotate during inset.

For a robust blood supply, keep the pedicle width similar to its length. Pedicle thickness should be at least 1 cm. Avoid raising a too long / too thin pedicle. Limit undermining it and rotate only as needed. [It is a circle- there is no need to twist it by 90 degrees! That will only congest its blood supply].

Opinion: When to lift and when to rotate the NAC

Do whichever is simplest.

The size of the existing breast, the amount of reduction and the dimensions of the pedicle will dictate the best option. The only paper that refers to a measurement is by Asplund & Powell (BJPS 1996) stating that lifting alone is suitable in reductions less than 500gm and when NAC moves less than 5cm.

Mastopexy

CORE KNOWLEDGE
Types & who described them
Spear's rules for concentric mastopexy
Lejour principle
Augmentation-mastopexy

APPROACH TO PATIENT - HISTORY & EXAMINATION
As above for BBR, plus be sure of:
- Is the patient concerned about shape or volume, or both
- Is she concerned about both side
- Degree of ptosis
- Quality of skin
- Do both sides have the same problem

Do go through the BDD screen. Remember it is an aesthetic procedure

APPROACH TO PATIENT - TREATMENT
Know precisely what is concerning the patient and address that

Per-op, plan to correct the more challenging side first and then match the "easier" side.

Always "tailor tack" the tissue & double check excision markings before any excision.

EXPECTED CLINICAL QUESTIONS
- Expect to see a picture and decide what type of mastopexy may be suitable
- What do you think is the patient's main problem
- How can it be solved [Know your 3-step principle]
- Markings, pedicles
- Eponymous techniques (name and definitions)
- Augmentation mastopexy, 1 vs 2 stage, reasons and steps

RECOMMENDED PAPERS
1. Goes JCS. Periareolar mammaplasty: double-skin technique with application of mesh support. *Clin Plast Surg.* 2002;29:349-64
2. Hall Findley EJ. Pedicles in vertical breast reduction and mastopexy. *Clin Plast Surg.* 2002;29:379-91

3. Hall-Findlay EJ. Discussion: A Matched Cohort Study of Superomedial Pedicle Vertical Scar Breast Reduction (100 Breasts) and Traditional Inferior Pedicle Wise-Pattern Reduction (100 Breasts). *Plast Reconstr Surg.* 2013 Nov;132(5):1077–9.

4. Lejour M. Pedicle Modification Of The Lejour Vertical Scar Reduction Mammaplasty. *Plast Reconstr Surg.* 1998;101(4):1149-50

5. Hofmann AK, Wuestner-Hofmann MC, Bassetto F, et al. Breast Reduction: Modified "Lejour Technique" in 500 Large Breasts. *Plast Reconstr Surg.* 2007 Oct;120(5):1095–104.

6. Spear SL, Giese SY, Ducic I. Concentric mastopexy revisited. *Plast Reconstr Surg.* 2001;107(5):1294-99

7. Spear S. Augmentation/Mastopexy:Surgeon, Beware. *Plast Reconstr Surg..* 2003 Sep;112(3):905–6.

Spear's rules for concentric mastopexy

Mark *eccentric* ovals,

- One centred on current nipple & diameter=the preferred final nipple diameter
- Other centred on the ideal (=new) nipple location & diameter detemined by the "rules" below
- Don't try to lift nipple >4cm (preferably 2cm only)

Rule 1	Excise more areola, less skin
Rule 2	Don't make outer circle, 3x the inner's dia. (keep it less than 3x in proportion & <10cm in measurement, i.e. keep inner circle <3.3cm dia)
Rule 3	The final scar is mid way between the inner and out incisions Keep the final scar closer to the nipple margin

Hall-Findley

"Vertical scar supero-medial pedicle with an inferior parenchymal excision similar to a Wise pattern. No skin puckering of the vertical limb. IMF is usually moved superiorly and part of vertical scar ends up on the chest wall"

Note that the NAC position is determined by superior border of the foot plate (8-11cm).

INDICATIONS
Small to medium reductions

CONTRA-INDICATIONS
Very large breasts
Inelastic skin (unlikely to redrape)
Very long pedicle

MAJOR MARKINGS
Upper border
Breast meridian (ignoring NAC) + CW meridian
New nipple position (err low, not high)

SKIN RESECTION MARKINGS
Draw areola (mosque dome)
Rotate medial and lateral to draw vertical limbs (stay 2-3cm above the IMF).
Join with a "U" at the bottom
Mark wings of the wise pattern (for conus excision) keeping 5-7cm pillars

PEDICLE MARKING
"Medial pedicle", where half of its base is in the mosque dome and the other half in the vertical limb
OR, "superomedial" for longer pedicles

Note that in contrast to Lejour's technique, Hall-Findley's technique gives immediate on-table results.

Lassus

"Vertical scar, thin (7-8mm) dermoglandular superior pedicle with stepwise parenchymal excision in a semi-recumbent position, and minimal undermining."

MARKING
1. NAC position, at 2cm below mid-humeral level
2. Lower extent of skin excision, marked as (3), 6 or 9 cm IMF-to-NAC distance. These two points are joined by rotating the breast medially and laterally.

Draw pedicle

STEPS
Semi-sitting
De-epithelise pedicle
Isolate pedicle as a thin flap

Pyramidal resection of parenchyma (base superficial and apex deep ??) under centre of NAC

Tacking sutures to vertical limbs (and assess the inferior dog ear)

Another layer of tacking sutures and excise a vertical melon slice

Repeat tacking and melon slice if needed

Dermal & skin closure

Lejour

"Vertical scar, superior pedicle technique with wide retroglandular undermining"

The vertical scar is crimped, making it shorter. The resulting skin wrinkles disappear over time and the breast conus "settles down" in approximately 3 months.

Tubular breast

CORE KNOWLEDGE
Elements of a tubular breast
Classification
Reconstruction techniques

APPROACH TO PATIENT - HISTORY
(as above)

APPROACH TO PATIENT - EXAMINATION
(as above)

APPROACH TO PATIENT - TREATMENT
(see below)

EXPECTED CLINICAL QUESTIONS
[You are more likely to see the patient in clinical section and be expected to pick up the deformity]

- What is it
- What classification
- What would you do
- Why two stage
- What else
- What implant, where, when

RECOMMENDED PAPERS
1. Persichetti P, Cagli B, Tenna S, et al. Decision Making in the Treatment of Tuberous and Tubular Breasts: Volume Adjustment as a Crucial Stage in the Surgical Strategy. *Aesthetic Plast Surg*. 2005 Dec;29(6):482–8.
2. von Heimburg D, Exner K, Kruft S, Lemperle G. The tuberous breast deformity: classification and treatment. *Br J Plast Surg*. 1996 Sep;49(6): 339–45.
3. von Heimburg D. Refined version of the tuberous breast classification. *Plast Reconstr Surg*. 2000 May;105(6):2269–70.
4. Blondeel's 3 step principle

Tubular breast deformity

Narrow base

High IMF

Hypoplasia of one or more quadrants

+/- herniation if breast tissue through a constricting ring

Tuberous = decreased BW & BH, mega-areola

Tubular = decreased BH, normal areola

Classification

Von Heimburg BJPS, 1996

I.   hypoplasia of lower medial quadrant
II. both lower quadrants, adequate sub-areolar skin
III. Inadequate sub-areolar skin
IV. severe breast constriction

[Opinion: This classification is pretty much irrelevant if you stick to the 3 step principle].

Management options

1 stage if adequate skin envelope

2 stage if inadequate skin envelope

If there is volume deficit *alone*, that will needs addressing. Usually this difference is too large to be addressed by fat grafting alone and an implant is needed.

Know what you need to do and when you need to do it e.g. in a very young patient (early teens) since the breast development is not completed, a definitive procedure will have to be deferred. However if the volume difference is becoming very noticeable (and pt is not keen on using external prostheses/ padded bras anymore) it is appropriate to place a tissue expander that is expanded at the same rate as the contralateral breast development.

The commonest cohort of patients seen are younger patients who don't want donor site scars and a 2 stage expander-implant with release of constricting fascia is a good option.

ALTERNATIVES

1. 1 stage anatomical implant
2. Northwood index. Ref: Pacifico MD, Kang NV. The tuberous breast revisited. *J Plast Reconstr & Aesthetic Surg.* 2007 May;60(5):455–64.
3. Ribiero technique of auto-augmentation. Useful if there is adequate volume but abnormal shape. Uses inferior quadrant tissue to augment volume behind the NAC and redrapes the remaining tissues around it. Ref: Ribeiro L, Canzi W, Buss A, Accorsi A. Tuberous breast: a new approach. *Plast Reconstr Surg.* 1998 Jan;101(1):42–50; discussion 51–2.

Poland's

CORE KNOWLEDGE
Definition
Cause
Epidemiology
Who described it
What do patients present with
Management principles

APPROACH TO PATIENT - HISTORY
(as for breast patient)

APPROACH TO PATIENT - EXAMINATION
[Consider a chaperone]
Pt standing, hands by side
> Point out obvious asymmetry of chest wall.
> Absence of anterior axillary fold

Hands on hips
> Ask to press down 7 look for anterior ax fold again and feel for contraction of pect major
> Look at back & check for LD presence (symmetry of posterior axillary fold & feel for contraction).

Ask to see both hands
> Compare size & comment if the affected side is smaller (usu not operated on as little functional deficit)

If the pt is postop, there may be an implant there already.

APPROACH TO PATIENT - TREATMENT
(see below)

EXPECTED CLINICAL QUESTIONS
Make a spot diagnosis
Describe the condition
Incidence
Age of presentation

RECOMMENDED PAPERS
1. Pryor LS, Lehman JA, Workman MC. Disorders of the Female Breast in the Pediatric Age Group. *Plast Reconstr Surg.* 2009 Jul;124(Supplement):50e – 60e.
2. van Aalst JA, Phillips JD, Sadove AM. Pediatric Chest Wall and Breast Deformities. *Plast Reconstr Surg.* 2009 Jul;124(Supplement):38e – 49e.

Poland's deformity

Poland's is a congenital condition affecting upper limb development due to an insult to the subclavian artery in the fetal period. Characteristically the pt lacks the sternal head of pectoralis major (on ipsilateral side) with variable hypoplasia of soft tissue and bony components of the upper limb and chest wall (including hypoplasia of serratus anterior, LD, absent ribs).

Described in 1841 by Alfred Poland, then a medical student at Guy's Hospital.

The true incidence is unknown but is thought to be more common in males. However females present more commonly to plastic surgery service due to associated effect on breast development. There is an association with brachysyndactyly.

Most patients go unnoticed through childhood, unless there is a stark limb discrepancy.

Male patients present due to concerns about flat chest on one side and being unable to build muscle. They may report feeling embarrassment in swimming costume. The pt is missing volume. If you decide to operate, the volume can be built incrementally with autologous fat grafting, or using custom made implants. A CT helps the prosthetist plan the implant, and rules out any bony anomalies (which should be dealt by thoracic surgeons).

Female patients present in their teens with asymmetry of breast development. Both the pt and the parent may be quite worried & keen to start a surgical plan. A common way is to insert a tissue expander in the affected side (remember there is no pect major!) which is inflated in keeping with contralateral breast development. Once the breast development comes to a halt, the TE is exchanged for an implant.

Breast - reconstruction

CORE KNOWLEDGE
Patient journey
Principles of management

APPROACH TO PATIENT - HISTORY
General
Age, occupation, hobbies
Who is at home, Is the significant other here today?
Number of children,? Breastfed,? More planned
HTN, DM, smoking
Pills, hormone replacement therapy, herbal medicine
Surgical History, esp. Abdomen/back operations

Oncological history
CA breast (type), CA ovary, BRCA 1/2
Tumour size, one/more tumours
Mastectomy/Lumpectomy and when, by whom
ANC
Chemotherapy (neo-adjuvant/ adjuvant), RT
Last mammo

Morphologic info
Current cup size
?satisfied with the opposite side
Height, Weight, BMI

Ideas & expectations
Specifically be sure of the following:
What can I do for you? i.e. wt is the exact problem patient wants addressed
What size are you aiming for? Are you satisfied with the other side?
Checked Internet for information or support groups?
Spoken to family, friends and significant other
Seen breast care nurses (given any DVD or leaflets)

APPROACH TO PATIENT - EXAMINATION
(assuming unilateral mastectomy and an uninvolved contralateral breast)

Ask for chaperone

Stand straight
>Shoulders level, arms for Poland
>Kyphosis/scars on back

Hands on hips
>There is/is not CW deformity from front
>Are there any scars (eg from mastectomy, WLE, axillary procedure)
>If the patient has had a mastectomy
>- Mention which side
>- Look for telengiectasias, radiation
>
>Contralateral side
>- Comment if the two sides are symmetrical
>- Ask to lift the breast to see position of IMF [only if it is a pendulous breast, else it would be obvious]
>- Comment on footplate (if height & width are symmetrical), Breast volume (if one side is less/more), grade of ptosis (Regnault), skin envelope (whether it conforms to the underlying parenchyma i.e. hanging loose or not), NAC position (symmetrical or not - both in horizontal and vertical placement)
>
>Ask about NAC discharge
>Are there any scars (again)

Hands above head
Look for tethering

Hands on hips again and press down
Feel for pects contraction (i.e. ant. axillary fold) on both sides

Consider oncological examination of breast and axillae ["Offer" in an exam scenario. In clinic always do it]

Measure
SN:N, N:IMF
BW, N:midline
Skin quality & tissue thickness

Examine donor sites:

Abdomen (DIEAP/TRAM): Scars, volume of tissue, hernias, divarication of recti

Back (LD): Scars, volume of tissue, test presence of LD

APPROACH TO PATIENT - TREATMENT
(see below)

EXPECTED CLINICAL QUESTIONS
- What does the patient have
- What does she want
- What can you offer
- Risks, complications

RECOMMENDED PAPERS

1. Blondeel PN, Hijjawi J, Depypere H, Roche N, Van Landuyt K. Shaping the Breast in Aesthetic and Reconstructive Breast Surgery: An Easy Three-Step Principle. *Plast Reconstr Surg.* 2009 Feb;123(2):455–62.
2. Blondeel PN, Hijjawi J, Depypere H, Roche N, Van Landuyt K. Shaping the Breast in Aesthetic and Reconstructive Breast Surgery: An Easy Three-Step Principle. Part II—Breast Reconstruction after Total Mastectomy. *Plast Reconstr Surg.* 2009 Mar;123(3):794–805.
3. Blondeel PN, Hijjawi J, Depypere H, Roche N, Van Landuyt K. Shaping the Breast in Aesthetic and Reconstructive Breast Surgery: An Easy Three-Step Principle. Part III—Reconstruction following Breast Conservative Treatment. *Plast Reconstr Surg.* 2009 Jul;124(1):28–38.
4. Munhoz AM, Montag E, Arruda E, Pellarin L, Filassi JR, Piato JR, et al. Assessment of immediate conservative breast surgery reconstruction: a classification system of defects revisited and an algorithm for selecting the appropriate technique. *Plast Reconstr Surg.* 2008 Mar;121(3):716–27.
5. McCulley SJ, Macmillan RD. Planning and use of therapeutic mammoplasty—Nottingham approach. *Br J Plast Surg.* 2005 Oct;58(7):889–901.
6. McCulley SJ, Macmillan RD. Therapeutic mammaplasty—analysis of 50 consecutive cases. *Br J Plast Surg.* 2005 Oct;58(7):902–7.
7. Clough KB, Lewis JS, Couturaud B, Fitoussi A, Nos C, Falcou M-C. Oncoplastic techniques allow extensive resections for breast-conserving therapy of breast carcinomas. *Annals of Surgery.* 2003;237(1):26–34.
8. Kronowitz SJ. Delayed-Immediate Breast Reconstruction: Technical and Timing Considerations. *Plast Reconstr Surg.* 2010 Feb;125(2):463–74.

9. Nahabedian MY. Breast Reconstruction: A Review and Rationale for Patient Selection. *Plast Reconstr Surg.* 2009 Jul;124(1):55–62.

REVIEWS:

1. Sigurdson L, Lalonde DH. MOC-PSSM CME Article: Breast Reconstruction. *Plast Reconstr Surg.* 2008 Jan;121(MOC-PS CME Coll):1–12.
2. Berry MG, Fitoussi AD, Curnier A, Couturaud B, Salmon RJ. Oncoplastic breast surgery: A review and systematic approach. *J Plast Reconstr & Aesthetic Surg.* 2010 Aug;63(8):1233–43.

RADIOTHERAPY:

1. Nava MB, Pennati AE, Lozza L, Spano A, Zambetti M, Catanuto G. Outcome of Different Timings of Radiotherapy in Implant-Based Breast Reconstructions. *Plast Reconstr Surg.* 2011 Aug;128(2):353–9.
2. Schaverien MV, Macmillan RD, McCulley SJ. Is immediate autologous breast reconstruction with postoperative radiotherapy good practice?: A systematic review of the literature. *J Plast Reconstr & Aesthetic Surg.* 2013 Dec;66(12):1637–51.
3. Spear SL, Boehmler JH, Bogue DP, Mafi AA. Options in Reconstructing the Irradiated Breast. *Plast Reconstr Surg.* 2008 Aug;122(2):379–88.

Oncological considerations for breast reconstruction

Patient journey (Ref: Figure) starts by either finding the breast cancer by self examination (and attendance at GP) or detection by a breast screening program (NHSBSP). NHSBSP invites all females age 50 to 70 for regular mammography. (Ref: Asides on NHSBSP & Controversy in breast screening, Canadian study).

Figure: Journey of a breast cancer patient

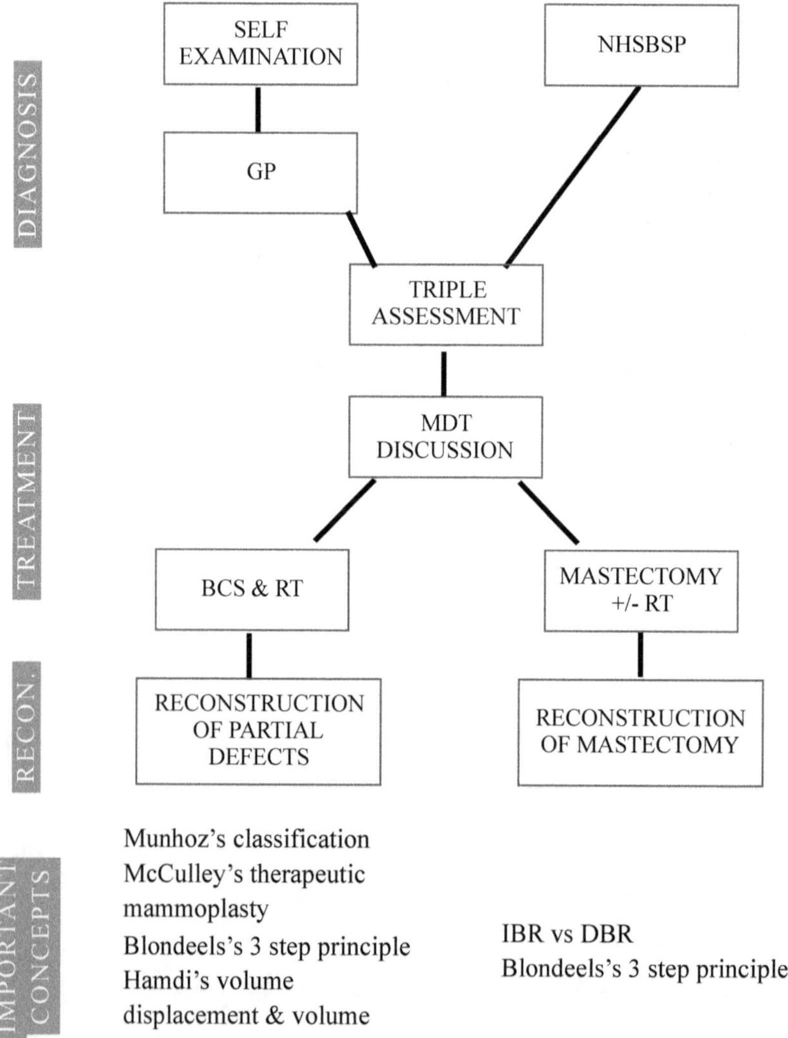

In UK this would be referred to the breast MDT as a two weeks referral for
triple assessment. Triple assessment involves
1. physical examination,
2. radiological localisation (ultrasound/mammography) and
3. tissue diagnosis (i.e. FNAC or biopsy Ref: Tables x2).

Table: FNAC reporting

FNAC report	Meaning
C1	Inadequate sample
C2	Benign
C3	Atypia, probably benign
C4	Atypia suspicious of CA
C5	CA

Table: Biopsy reporting

Biopsy report	Meaning
B1	Normal
B2	Benign
B3	Uncertain malignant potential
B4	Suspicious
B5	Malignant

If the breast CA is confirmed, the options are either
1) Breast conserving surgery with radiotherapy, or
2) Mastectomy (Ref: Table)

Table: Indications for Mx

Tumour factors	Large tumours in small breast Multifocal CA Diffuse micro-calcifications on mammo. Inflammatory CA Failed BCT
Patient choice	Patient choice, including BRCA

Sometimes radiotherapy is given after mastectomy as well (Ref: Aside). Note that if the patient undergoes breast conservation surgery, it will by definition involve radiotherapy afterwards (Ref: Veronesi U, Zucali R, Luini A. Local control and survival in early breast cancer: the Milan trial. *Int J Radiat Oncol Biol Phys*. 1986 May;12(5):717–20).

Aside: Indications for RT after Mx

- Involved margins
- 4+ nodes

The total number of options for mastectomy are:
1. (Radical mastectomy) which has been confined to history
2. Modified radical mastectomy, i.e. Mastectomy + axillary dissection, has been the standard technique (before SSM & IBR) and is still used for patients who are not candidates for IBR.
3. Skin sparing mastectomy (SSM), is the standard procedure for IBR
4. Nipple sparing mastectomy

Note all axillae are staged with a pre-op USS +/- FNAC. Those which are FNA-negative have a per-op nodal sampling, while those that are FNA +ve undergo a (level 2) axillary dissection.

After mastectomy options of reconstructions are either immediate or delayed breast reconstruction, as decided by the breast MDT. Immediate breast reconstruction is appropriate for early-stage breast cancer patients and not expected to need radiotherapy. Delayed breast reconstruction is chosen for patient who will certainly need radiotherapy after mastectomy (as adequate treatment of cancer takes priority over reconstruction). Delayed reconstruction is the only option for patients who had a mastectomy in the past when immediate breast reconstruction was not available. (Ref: Exceptions - IBR needing RT).

Aside: Delayed-Immediate reconstruction

More recently the concept of Delayed-Immediate recon has been described by Kronowitz which involves temporising the mastectomy wound for several days until histology results are available.

The options for both IBR or DBR can be either autologous, implant-based or both. An implant based reconstruction is chosen only if patient is not likely to need radiotherapy (in an IBR scenario), or has not had radiotherapy (DBR scenario). Autologous-only reconstruction can be used irrespective of radiotherapy use. (Ref: Exception RT needed after IBR with implant, or TE+RT+Implant)

Aside: Exceptions where RT may be needed after an implant

1. IBR needing RT
2. Delayed-Immediate recon (Kronowitz)

The concern with RT arises from evidence on higher rates of capsular contracture and implant exposure. The irradiated dermis is thin and is less likely to be able to support a prosthesis (Ref: core studies).

Aesthetic considerations for breast reconstruction

Think in terms of footplate, conus, envelope. This is valid for defects after mastectomy as well as those after lumpectomy (Figure: Defects after BCS).

1. The size of this defects *relative to the breast size* is more important than its numerical value. This forms the basis of Munhoz's classification.
2. For smaller defects (in relation to breast size), local breast tissue flaps may be used. The location of these defects form the basis of Scenarios A & B in McCulley's therapeutic mammoplasty.

Aside: Clough's classification of post-mastectomy defects

Ref: Clough et al. Annals of plastic surgery 1998

The first major classification was by Clough who described 3 situations, depending on whether their is no apparent defect of the treated breast (so no treatment), there is some defect (needing partial reconstruction) or their is major defect (needing mastectomy & total reconstruction). [I feel that it has been superseded by the other systems of classifications mentioned].

Table: Defects after BCS (Summarised from Munhoz PRS 2008). I-III are increasing breast sizes. Defect types A-C have little, moderate or a large defect *relative* to the breast size. LTDF=Lateral thoracodorsal flap

	A	B	C
I		*Lateral defect*, LTDF *Central/medial defect*, LD	Mx & total reconstruction
II	Breast tissue advancement flaps	Bilateral Mx	*Favourable location**, manage as I-B
III		bilateral red. mastopexy	*Favourable location**, bilateral red. mastopexy

* If unfavourable location, needs mastectomy and total reconstruction

McCulley's therapeutic mammaplasty is more relevant for the Type A defects in Munhoz' classification i.e. those which require breast tissue advancement flaps. in this situation, McCulley described two scenarios:

A. Scenario A, when the defect lies at a location that is normally removed during breast reduction. The solution is easy - just do a breast reduction (with an appropriate choice of pedicle).
B. Scenario B, when the defect does *not* lie in an area excised during breast reduction. The recommendation, in this situation is to,
    1. Decide skin pattern,
    2. Decide NAC position,
    3. Decide how to fill the defect, either by extending the NAC pedicle, or by creating a secondary pedicle from tissue that would otherwise be excised in a breast reduction.

It is well worth reading both his original papers.

Post-mastectomy reconstruction planning

	IBR	DBR
Has...	Footplate intact (including the IMF) Skin envelope intact	Footplate absent Volume absent Skin envelope absent
Needs...	Needs volume	Needs all 3
How to...?	Volume can be from an implant, or from autologous tissue	**Footplate** can be copied from the opposite side, or recreated do novo - no problem! **Volume** can be from an implant, or from autologous tissue **Skin envelope** recon varies depending whether an implant or autologous tissue is chosen for recon
What if ... implant?	Implant is one stage	Definitive **implant** can provide volume but not skin envelope, so a TE is needed initially to build skin envelope. A **tissue expander** can provide skin, but pt needs one op to insert the TE and another to exchange TE to a definitive implant (i.e. 2 stage recon) To avoid 2 operations, an **expander-implant** (i.e. Becker 35) can be used for 1-stage recon. But prediction of final volume and shape can be difficult
What if... autologous?	Autologous tissue can be taken based on availability, patient choice and size of breast desired	Autologous tissue can provide both volume as well as skin. Hence a one stage reconstruction is possible
	LD is always available, but by itself can only provide small to moderate volumes	same
	Abdominal tissue (pedicled/ free/muscle sparing TRAM, DIEAP**) is increasingly synonymous with DIEAP flap	same
	Less commonly used autologous sources include SGAP, IGAP, TUG flaps	same
How to decide between implant and autologous?	Determined by expected need for XRT* and (if no XRT is needed) patient choice	h/o RT is CI to implant recon

* XRT need can only be anticipated based on info available to the MDT preop. Theoretically, need for XRT may become apparent *after* IBR (e.g. if the mastectomy specimen shows a multicentric tumour), in which case XRT has to go ahead irrespective of its effect on implants (as CA treatment takes priority over everything else). If there is a small risk of needing postop RT and pt wants IBR, then a TE may be placed to keep the tissue planes open at the time of MX and final recon done after RT is completed- the final result may not be ideal in this case.

** For choice of abdominal tissue (see below)

Table: Choice of abdominal tissue. Note, MS-TRAM classification was described by Nahabedian (PRS 2002)

Types of TRAM		Description
Pedicle TRAM		Uses the non-dominant pedicle (superior epigastric)
Free TRAM		Uses the dominant pedicle (deep inferior epigastric) and hence is more reliable
Muscle sparing TRAM		Both of the above options use the complete width of the muscle and hence weaken the anterior abdominal wall, so muscle sparing flap may have an advantage
	MS-0	It is a backronym for a free TRAM i.e. no muscle is spared. Has 3-6 perforators
	MS-1	Muscle lateral to the perforator is saved
	MS-2	Both lateral & medial saved. A small strip around perforator is taken with the flap
	MS-3	All of the rectus muscle is spared = DIEAP flap

Size and shape of the desired breast is either copied from the opposite side (unilateral cases), or created de novo (in bilateral cases, or in unilateral cases where pt wants the opposite side adjusted).

"TRAM" zones

Skin paddle on the anterior lower abdominal wall are numbered in order of decreasing reliability of vascular supply.

WHAT EVERYONE AGREES ON
Zone 1 = Ipsilateral medial part of skin island, w.r.t. donor vessel

Zone 4 = Contralateral lateral, to the donor vessel

Zones 2 & 3 - Ref: Table

Table: Zone 2 vs Zone 3:

Author	What they mean
Hartrampf, 1982	Thought there is better blood supply across the midline Zone 2 = Contralateral medial Zone 3 = Ipsilateral lateral
Holm, Ninkovic et al., 2006	Intra-operative indocyanine green showed better perfusion in "ipsilateral lateral" Zone 2 = Ipsilateral lateral Zone 3 = Contralateral medial
Rohrich, 2010	3D CT angio Zones depend on whether a medial or a lateral row perforator is taken
Losken, 2012	ICG at 12 standardised data points No difference between Zones 2 & 3

Opinion:

Hartrampf's zone (or any variation) are not clinically relevant anymore as the flap perfusion is dependent on the choice of perforator and on the arborisation of microvasculature from that perforator. You are best off seeing how flap perfusion looks on table, either using dermal bleeding as your guide [do check pt's systolic BP on the monitor] or one of the commercial systems utilising indocyanine green or equivalent.

Hand surgery

Hand surgery principles

"Function, Function and Function"! For each injury/pathology, consider how this affects the patient's function. For every management option, consider how this will improve the patient's function.

Functions of hand

Functions		Description	Example
3 pinches	**1. Fine pinch**	between the distal most tip of the thumb & IF (next to the hyponychium)	picking up a needle, or a thread
	2. Pulp to pulp pinch	between the pulps of thumb and IF	holding a newspaper, or turning a page
	3. Lateral / key pinch	between thumb pulp & radial border of IF	holding a key and turning it in the lock
3 grips	**1. Chuck / tripod grip**	between thumb, IF & MF pulps	twisting open a water bottle or salt dispenser
	2. Hook grip	between the gutter formed by extension of MCPj2-5 and flexion of respective IPjs. (Thumb not involved).	lifting a shopping bag
	3. Power grip	all fingers and thumb rolled around a narrow cylindrical object	turning a door handle, lifting a kettle, striking a hammer
Grasp		fingers and thumb rolled part way around a wide cylindrical object	holding a pint
Open hand		thumb adducted and in the plane of a flat palm	pushing a door open

At the end of your history, you should always know how these are affected in your patient, especially in elective cases. Your management should restore lost function, without worsening any existing function. Note that every single one of the above mentioned functions are affected in an ulnar nerve lesion.

Dupuytren's

CORE KNOWLEDGE
Palmar fascia layers and pathology they cause

APPROACH TO PATIENT - HISTORY
General
Age, occupation, hand dominance, hobbies, who is at home
PMHx, Meds, Allergies

Specific
Disease course
When did it start
One hand, or both
Rx so far
Have you had any operations so far (When, who, where, what improvement, any complications postop., specifically ask for sensations in all sides of all digits and cold intolerance)

Functional issues
What is the current problem
What difficulties in ADLs. (Typically it pokes the face while washing, or catches the digit in trouser pockets)
Functional status. (Pinches and grips" - see above)

"How can I help you?"
[This may seem like an obvious question but do not assume its answer].

APPROACH TO PATIENT - EXAMINATION
[Show as you go. The swiftest way to examine is to show the patient with both your hands]

Look
Both hands exposed to elbow [don't be caught out by an ulnar n. injury]. Palms up

Move (AROM)
Flex the involved finger
Extend fully. Note cascade & any restrictions. "Looks like DD"

Palm down

Look for Garrod's pads (+ exclude hyperextension at ulnar MCPjs)

Palm up again

Feel

"Dz it hurt anywhere?"

Palpate the normal hand first and quickly feel for fascia in palm as well as in fingers and thumb. [In exam, say that you are going to feel the normal side first. Examiner may just move you along].

Go to the side that you are examining

Start at palm and feel along each ray. Describe disease as bands, cords, nodules and their location [the examiner may ask you to point them out]

Assess passive extension of digit (gently!).

- If you can't extend fully at PIPj try passively flexing MCPj (which slackens the diseased fascia) to see if it helps open PIPj (i.e. if it extends).
  - If yes, you are likely to get PIPj straight(er) with an operation
  - If not, PIPj may have fixed flexion deformity that will persist even after disease excision. [It is important to warn the patient of this! Also consider if you will attempt arthrolysis of PIPj. The decision depends on patient's functional demands & expected compliance. Ask your patient's view]

If there is obvious skin involvement: look for donor sites in antecubital fossa or medial upper arm. (Explain the patient that a skin graft will be needed).If skin involvement is doubtful, let the patient know of that and that you may make an intra-operative decision to use a skin graft.

APPROACH TO PATIENT - TREATMENT

Management can be nonoperative or operative.

Non-operative management may be suitable for early onset and slowly progressive disease which is not affecting the activities of daily living. In past, splints have been used but they have not shown to be effective, are cumbersome for the patient and can result in poor patient compliance (defeating the purpose to have them in the first place).

When to operate

Some colleagues quote various angles at which to offer an operation. This notion originated with McFarlane who described the threshold for operating on DD at

- 30° MCPj flexion, or
- any PIPj contraction.

Opinion:

Problem with using an angle to base your decision is that you lose track of how the condition affects your patient and you fail to individualise your management. Monitoring the angle is an objective way to track the progress / recurrence of the disease but is less than an ideal way to decide upon an operation. For example, what if the patient comes to you in clinic 2° short of your threshold but struggling with ADLs. Will you bring them back once the joint is over your "threshold for operation" - I hope not.

McGrouther & Bayat (2006) suggested that decision to operate should be based upon how well the patient is coping with their activities of daily living.

Options for operation

Keep your options simple and limited to the techniques that you have seen. A simple classification is:

Operative*
- Segmental fasciectomy, which removes a segment of the diseased fascia
- Dermo-fasciectomy, which removes the diseased fascia alongside involved skin (usually over proximal phalanx)

Non-operative/minimally invasive
- Needle fasciotomy
- Enzymatic fasciotomy (using collagenase injection)

*These are the most common techniques used. If you start with eponymous names (like Meurman & McFarlane), expect a higher level of scrutiny.

Strictly speaking the above are all approaches to the fascia. When you describe your technique, qualify your description with your approach to the skin, to the fascia and to the joint.

SKIN
1. Straight line incision with Z-plasties at the end, if needed. The commonest place for these Z-plasties is over distal palmar crease and the proximal digital crease (Skoog's approach). You can be asked to draw these Z-plasties. (Ref: Figure)
2. Zig-Zag incisions ('Brunner')
3. Combination

Figure: Z-plasties with Skoog's incisions. a) Make sure to keep the final scar in an existing crease, keep the length of Z-plasty limbs equal, round off the tip slightly, make one limb then transpose it before incising the 2nd limb, hold the flaps with a skin hook and not your forceps. b) Make a second Z-plasty if needed.

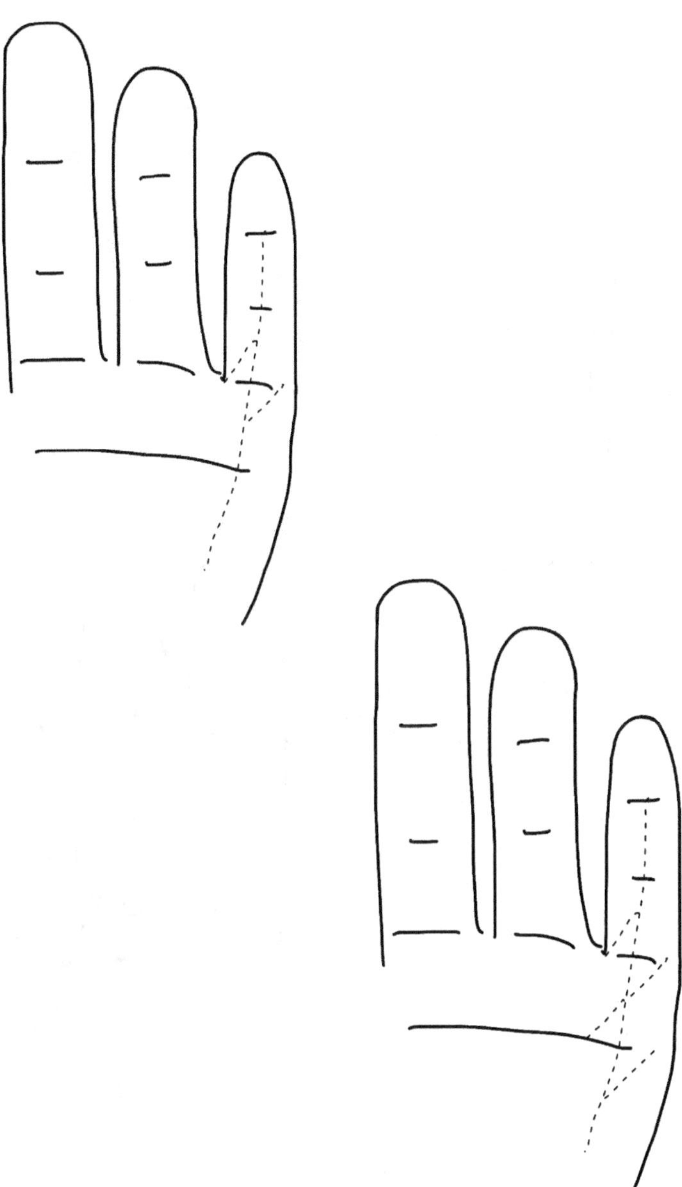

Figure: Z-plasties with Skoog's incisions (*contd.*) c) Know how *you* make a Z-plasty if operating on an adjacent digit. If the adjacent digit needs a single Z-plasty, its direction does not matter much. d) However if the adjacent digit needs a second Z-plasty, the direction of scars becomes very relevant. The volar skin of the webspace is more likely to be at risk. The opposing Z shapes in the figure are more likely to preserve the inter-metacarpal perforator (shown) and preserve viability of the island of skin.

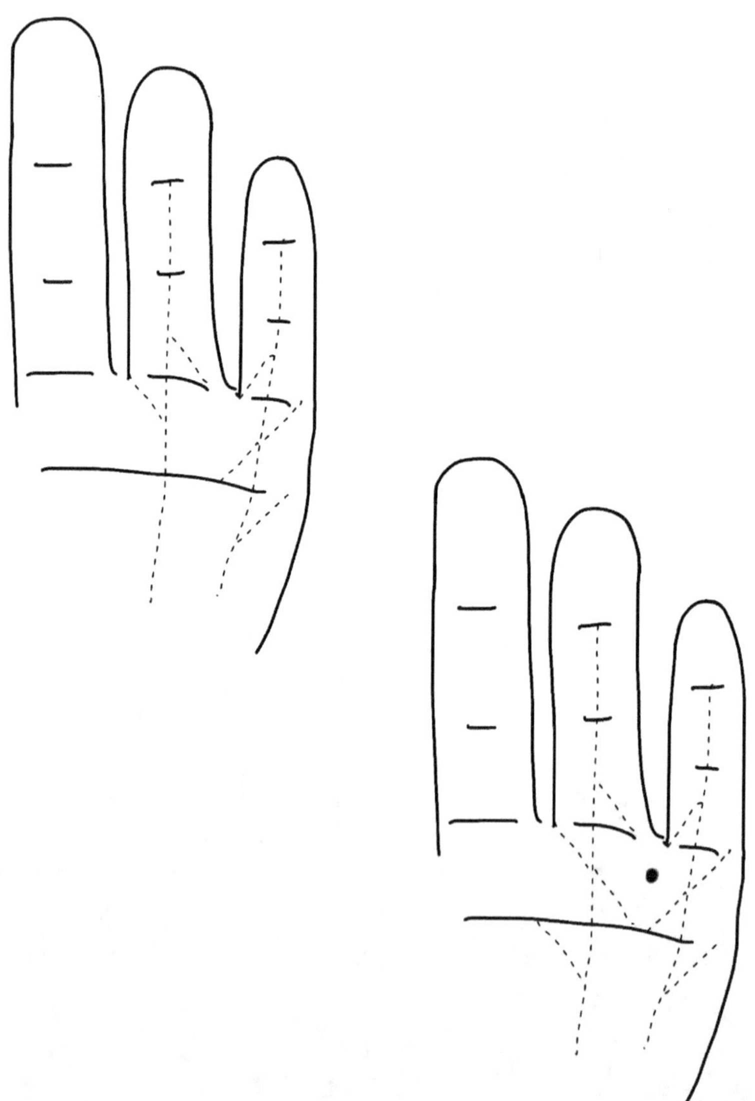

With any of the skin incision types, be clear how will you adjust your incisions when operating on adjacent digits, or when re-operating next to a previous scar (which may not match your technique). If your dissection is careful, there may be a helpful perforator coming in between metacarpal heads to perfuse that tricky area.

Do check your skin flaps and their tips at the end. These skin flaps are very thin and so may well take as full thickness skin grafts. In worst case, they breakdown and heal, but that takes longer and your counselling and rehab regimen will need to take account of that.

Most surgeon make the incision in stages, i.e. palm first, and then distally in an incremental fashion as space becomes available under what may be a very flexed PIPj.

If you are doing a dermo-fasciectomy, know whether you'll make your incision in midline on the digit [because you like a challenge] or mid-lateral [which is usually not involved, so you can see normal anatomy before digging in to DD].

FASCIA

Segmental fasciectomy removes a length of diseased fascia. Some surgeons like to remove the adjacent (i.e. within the same scar) un-involved fascia as well. Know your preference and the reason for it.

Needle fasciotomy has a high (up to 80%) recurrence rate. It is suitable only for a select group of patients with
i.   an isolated cord in the palm,
ii. a slowly progressive disease,
iii. a low functional demand, especially if they don't have the support to take the 3 months needed to rehab fully after an operation
[Remember the question, Who is at home with you and can take care of you]. You need to explain to the patient that the problem is likely to recur within the coming years.

Enzymatic fasciotomy (using collgenase injections) may be popular but it still considered an experimental procedure and is not widely used in the NHS. So most people have little experience in it, certainly not as much as they have in operative management of Dupuytren's. Know collagenase for your exam [and you will be expected to know it] but don't offer it as a first solution for every case. Knowing its theory and evidence is important.

ARTHROLYSIS

1.   Passive gentle manipulation.
2.   If needs be, release the volar plate. Access the volar plate by incising the pulley [identify the "swallow tail" and the transverse branch of the digital artery running through it], move both flexors out of the way and make a transverse incision into the volar plate.
3.   If the joint does not open, *consider* releasing the accessory collateral ligaments (on either side). If PIPj still does not open, *consider* incising proper collateral ligaments. Note that the joint will be grossly unstable after releasing the proper collateral ligaments, so you'll need to stabilise it in the short term (e.g. with K-wire across PIPj). Only once that fixation is removed can the joint be mobilised unhindered [so needs aggressive mobilisation and a compliant patient].

McCash

McCash is a loaded word in the world of Dupuytren's correction! Even though McCash described the "open palm technique", you'll find hand surgeons will squirm if you (and I've seen many) describe a failed graft as "leave it to heal by McCash's technique".

Open palm technique is only a small part of "McCash's technique". When you describe a technique by a named surgeon, make sure to know its details.

McCash's technique is *all* of the following:
1.   Multiple transverse stab incisions in the palm and digit
2.   Extensive undermining of skin in-between
3.   Traction on that skin to move it distally to allow preferential closure of skin on the digit, and
4.   Leaving the palm wounds open to heal by second intent

Collagenase

Collagenase is an enzyme that lyses collagen and the product used for Dupuytren's disease is from the bacterium clostridium histolyticum. The treatment can be done in clinic under aseptic conditions. The enzyme comes in a vial that needs to be reconstituted with sterile saline before injection into the diseased cord without anaesthesia [much like BoTNA]. The patient returns next day and the diseased joint is manipulated to attempt cord rupture. Complications include bruising and minor skin tears that heal easily.

Important trials are

Study	n	Design	Results
CORD 1	308 joints in 308 pts. (collagenase to 204, placebo to 104)	RCT	77% MPj & 40% PIPj improved to <5° contracture (vs 7% & 6% with placebo). Increase in ROM, 37° vs 4°
CORD 2	66 joints in 66 pts. (collagenase to 20 MPj & 25 PIPj, placebo to 11 MPj & 10 PIPj)	RCT Up to 3 injections	Improvement in contracture, 75 +/- 29% (vs 13 +/- 26%) Increase in ROM, 35° +/- 17°
CORDLESS (3 year results)	1080 joints (648 MPj & 432 PIPj)	Pooled pts. from 5 previous trials for longer f/u. Recurrence is >20° worsening of joint	27% MPj & 56% PIPj recurrence (mean= 35%)
CORDLESS (5 year results)	1081 joints in 644 patients (648 MPj & 432 PIPj)	Pooled pts. from 5 previous trials for longer f/u. Recurrence is >20° worsening of joint	27% MPj & 56% PIPj recurrence (mean= 35%)
JOINT 1 & 2	879 joints in 587 patients (531 MPj & 348 PIPj)	Open label studies. Up to 3 injections per cord (5 per pt.)	Full correction in 70% of MPj & 37% PIPj. 73% pts had at least 50% improvement Mean improvement 55° in MPj & 25° in PIPj

EXPECTED CLINICAL QUESTIONS

- Identify pits, nodules, cords, bands
- How are various pathologic structures formed (i.e. parts of diseased fascia)
- When would you operate
- Would you operate on this patient
- What operation
- Differences between various techniques. How do *you* do it

RECOMMENDED PAPERS

CORD I:

1. Badalamente MA, Hurst LC, Benhaim P, Cohen BM. Efficacy and safety of collagenase clostridium histolyticum in the treatment of proximal interphalangeal joints in dupuytren contracture: combined analysis of 4 phase 3 clinical trials. *J Hand Surg Am*. 2015 May;40(5):975–83.

2. Hurst LC, Badalamente MA, Hentz VR, Hotchkiss RN, Kaplan FTD, Meals RA, et al. Injectable collagenase clostridium histolyticum for Dupuytren's contracture. *N Engl J Med*. 2009 Sep 3;361(10):968–79.

CORD II:

3. Gilpin D, Coleman S, Hall S, Houston A, Karrasch J, Jones N. Injectable collagenase Clostridium histolyticum: a new nonsurgical treatment for Dupuytren's disease. *J Hand Surg Am*. 2010 Dec;35(12):2027–38.e1.

CORDLESS:

4. Peimer CA, Blazar P, Coleman S, Kaplan FTD, Smith T, Lindau T. Dupuytren Contracture Recurrence Following Treatment With Collagenase Clostridium histolyticum (CORDLESS [Collagenase Option for Reduction of Dupuytren Long-Term Evaluation of Safety Study]): 5-Year Data. *J Hand Surg Am*. 2015 Aug;40(8):1597–605.

5. Peimer CA, Blazar P, Coleman S, Kaplan FTD, Smith T, Tursi JP, et al. Dupuytren contracture recurrence following treatment with collagenase clostridium histolyticum (CORDLESS study): 3-year data. *J Hand Surg Am*. 2013 Jan;38(1):12–22.

JOINT I & JOINT II:

6. Witthaut J, Jones G, Skrepnik N, Kushner H, Houston A, Lindau TR. Efficacy and safety of collagenase clostridium histolyticum injection for Dupuytren contracture: short-term results from 2 open-label studies. J Hand Surg Am. 2013 Jan;38(1):2-11

Rheumatoid arthritis

Rheumatoid arthritis is a systemic disease that manifests as a symmetrical polyarthritis of small joints of hand and feet that spreads to involve the larger joints. The diagnosis is usually pretty obvious by the time patient reaches the surgeon. In clinical practice, the American College of rheumatology criteria are only used in difficult or atypical cases.

CORE KNOWLEDGE

- Pathophysiology
- Diagnostic criteria (ARA criteria)
- General info about DMRDs
- Progression of hand pathology
- Principles of management

It is one of the commonest inflammatory arthritis affecting 0.5-1% adult population. It is three times more likely in women. Its features include:

- Early arthritis. Early-morning stiffness for at least half an hour
- Joints are painful, swollen and symmetrical
- 80% are positive for RA factor, or ACPA (anti citrullinated protein antibodies)
- evidence of systemic infection inflammation for example raised ESR and CRP.
- If untreated extrapulmonary manifestations can occur

The current management for rheumatoid arthritis is primarily medical. Any surgical management needs to take place as a combined team approach with the patient's rheumatologist.

60-70% patients respond to disease modifying agents (DMARDs e.g. Methotrexate, sulphasalazine, leflunamide, low dose prednisolone). The current NICE guidelines recommend that these be used in combination.

Biological agents have a further 20-30% remission rate. However these can cause infections including TB, and potential problems with later joint replacement. Among the cytokines implicated in RA TNF-α and IL-1β are pro-inflammatory, while IL-1Ra and sTNF-R (soluble TNF receptor) are anti-inflammatory. TNFα is targeted by infliximab, adalimumab and etanercept. IL-1β is targeted by anabrine.

APPROACH TO PATIENT - HISTORY

General
Age, Occupation, Hand dominance, Hobbies, Who is at home
Other PMHx, Meds, Allergies

Specific
When did RA start (i.e. adult onset, or juvenile)
Who is the rheumatologist and what medications has the patient been on for RA
What surgery has been done so far, when and by whom
Any general anaesthetic in the past
Any neck Xrays, Any neck symptoms

Functional issues
What are the functional problems & how are they affecting patient's daily life (washing, clothing, shopping, driving)
Specifically ask about the hand grips
What specific function/issue that the patient will like to be addressed

APPROACH TO PATIENT - EXAMINATION

Rest both hands in a position that is comfortable for the patient. This may necessitate a cushion or a pillow on the patient's lap over which she rests her hands.

Look for swelling and deformities: (both sides, systematically)
Wrist
- Prominent ulnar head (Please do NOT try the 'Piano Key' sign- it is very painful and adds no information)
- Pronation / subluxation of the carpus w.r.t. radial head

MCPj
- Ulnar deviation (of digits)
- Volar subluxation

Fingers
- Dropped fingers
- Ulnar drift
- Swan neck
- Boutonniere

Thumb
- Z-deformity

See below for their pathophysiology

Feel:
Synovial swelling on the dorsum of wrist, hand and fingers.

Move:
- Differentiate between sagittal band lesion, extensor tendon rupture & PIN palsy. Relocate the dropped fingers into anatomical position (of full extension at MCPj & IPj) and ask the patient to keep them there. If the patient can maintain active finger extension, the problem is with laxity/ rupture of sagittal bands. Inability to keep that position implies tendon rupture or PIN palsy. PIN palsy is suggested by the radial deviation of wrist on attempted dorsiflexion (due to preservation of ECRL supplied by the radial nerve proper).
- Assess the ROM of joints

APPROACH TO PATIENT - TREATMENT

Aims of management:
1. Reduce pain and inflammation
2. Slow disease progression
3. Minimise loss of function
4. Prevent complications

Remember to treat the patient and not the Xray. The radiographs can show advanced destruction but may not have much associated pain/functional deficit for the patient.

Treatment options:
1. Non-operative
   - Optimise medical management. Talk to patient's rheumatologist!
   - Analgesics
   - Activity modification
   - Splints. Talk to your hand therapist
2. Operative
   - Excise, e.g. synovectomy, ulnar head resection (Darrach's procedure)
   - Fuse e.g. ulnar head (Sauve-Kapandji procedure), wrist fusion
   - Replace eg. MCPj, PIPj

Indication for surgery:
- Pain, not controlled by medication
- Progressive deformity

- Functional loss
- (Cosmetic). Deformity alone is not an indication for surgery. Never compromise function for cosmesis, or expose patient to risk of unnecessary complications.

PRIORITIES OF SURGICAL TREATMENT
- Address pain and function
- Tendon ruptures
- Significant nerve compression e.g. carpal tunnel compression
- Stability takes priority over mobility
- Proximal joints take priority over distal
- Do predictable/low-cost operations. "Bet on a winner"

DECISION MAKING PRIOR TO ANY SURGERY
1. Fitness for surgery and anaesthesia. Consult an anaesthetist, consider neck X-rays
2. Surgical plan. Know your priorities and operative sequence. "Bet on a winner"
3. Rehab plan
4. Patient compliance, and how can you help to improve it
5. Know your options for "next" surgery, if things don't improve

EXPECTED CLINICAL QUESTIONS
- Progression of hand pathology
- Principles of management

(Operative details are not expected to be asked except in a hand surgery exam)

RECOMMENDED PAPERS
1. Chung KC, Pushman AG. Current Concepts in the Management of the Rheumatoid Hand. *The Journal of Hand Surgery*. 2011 Apr;36(4):736–47.
2. Rehim SA, Chung KC. Applying Evidence in the Care of Patients with Rheumatoid Hand and Wrist Deformities. *Plast Reconstr Surg*. 2013 Oct; 132(4):885–97.

Pathophysiology of common lesions

PANNUS

This is overgrown synovium with fibroblast, chondrocyte & synovial cell proliferation as well as presence of collagenase and elastase enzymes.

WRIST

The pannus destroys the DRUJ and relaxes the ligaments around it
→ Radius subluxes volarly with the carpus,
→ making the ulna relatively more prominent
→ the prominent ulnar head causes attrition rupture of the extensor tendons (classically from ulnar to radial)

There is associated synovitis around tendons too.

MCPJ

There is a combination of
- ulnar drift,
- ulnar shift (of P1 base over MCP head) and
- volar subluxation of P1 w.r.t. MC head

Extensors to IF are positioned slightly on ulnar side of MCPj centre + Lateral pinch motion initially drives the digits ulnarly (starting from IF)
→ ulnar deviation + synovitis of the extensor tendons cause stretch of radial sagittal bands
→ the extensor tendons sublux in web spaces ulnar to their anatomical location
→ subluxed extensors increase the force of ulnar drift

Pannus stretches the MCPj capsule → volar subluxation of the proximal phalanges

IPJ

These joints are a very finely balanced system and problem at one joint readily affects the next. Boutonniere deformity is usually caused by a local problem at PIPj and has little functional consequence. Swan neck, however, can be caused by problems at PIPj or the joint below or above. Swan-necking is functionally a lot more significant since the patient cannot flex the digits to grip an object.

Boutonniere deformity

Synovitis at PIPj → relaxes the ligaments → relative lengthening of central slip → weakening of its extension force on PIPj + continued pull from the FDP → Flexed PIPj + Extended IPj (i.e. Boutonniere).

Swan neck

@MCPj:	Intrinsic tightness → increased extension force at PIPj
@PIPj:	Volar plate stretch +/- FDS rupture (due to synovitis)
@DIPj:	Mallet deformity (from any cause)

TYPES OF TENDON RUPTURES IN RA

1. Vaughan-Jackson lesions, Attrition rupture of extensor tendons due to friction over a prominent ulnar head (classically from ulnar to radial direction).
2. EPL rupture
3. Mannerfelt lesion, FPL rupture

Management options

1. Good medical management alongside a rheumatologist
2. Activity modification, or modification of home/work environment. Talk to your occupational therapist
3. Analgesia
4. Splints. Talk to your physiotherapist
5. Surgical options

- Always know why are you operating on a patient.
- What functional problems is the patient having in their ADLs,
- How any procedure that you would do with improve patient's functional condition.
- Ask the patient which specific activities are they having problem with.
- Is there any activity of daily life that can be modified or any splints that can be used.
- Give a trial of several weeks to a few months before deciding on surgery,
- Function, function, function!

Many a times a rheumatologist will refer a patient to your clinic who wants to explore any surgical options. It doesn't mean the patient wants or needs surgery. The consultation can be used to assess patient's current functional status and for a discussion of potential options in future. Do not talk yourself (and the patient) into offering an operation that the patient does not need. Never risk function for cosmesis.

> **Opinion:**
> Management of RA hand is highly specialised. You need to know the management principles including the option of not operating on the patient. If you find yourself being asked operative details of specific procedures like FDS tenodesis or central slip reconstruction, either you are doing brilliantly or you have said something stupid about 30 seconds ago.

Surgical options

Operating on rheumatoid hands is a specialised field. With early diagnosis and good rheumatologist support, these procedures are becoming less frequent. The following is an overview of management strategies. Make sure to use your toolbox wisely, start with a winner, plan ahead as to what procedure the patient may need in future and keep a lifeboat.

It is useful to think of the surgical options as:
- soft tissue procedures, and
- bony procedures

1. Synovectomy

Almost always used in combination with another management strategy. Rarely it may be used alone for florid synovitis to prevent risk of tendon rupture.

2. Surgical options for tendon ruptures

- Address the underlying cause i.e. prominent ulnar head or Lister's tubercle
- Tendon transfer (and do not repair)

LIST OF TRANSFER OPTIONS

Ruptured extensors	Possible solution
Extensors to LF only ruptured	Buddy to RF
LF & RF ruptured	EIP transfer to both
LF, RF & MF ruptured	EIP to ring & little + MF extensor buddied to index EDC
Extensors to LF, RF, MF & IF ruptured	FDS ring & middle
EPL	EIP

3. Surgical options for wrist

	Procedure	Principle	Comments
Darrach	Excision of ulnar head	No ulnar head => no tendon attrition rupture	Risk of ulnar subluxation of carpus
Sauve-Kapandji	Distal ulnar osteotomy + fusion of DRUJ	Fuse the problem joint + allow supination-pronation at osteotomy site	Fusion unpredictable if poor bone stock
Chamay	Radio-lunate fusion	Only fuse the problem area	Only possible if midcarpal joint is stable
RSL fusion	radio-scapho-lunate fusion	Fuse the problem joint	
Total wrist arthrodesis	Wrist fusion plate across distal radius, carpus and base of 3rd MC + bone graft intervening joints	Fuse the small bones in their anatomical relationship	Excellent pain control Be wary of poor bone stock
Denervation	Excision of sensory branch of PIN to the wrist joint	Pt can't feel any pain	For intractable wrist pain (if wrist stable), or With another wrist procedure

Figure: Darrach's procedure (excision of ulnar head)

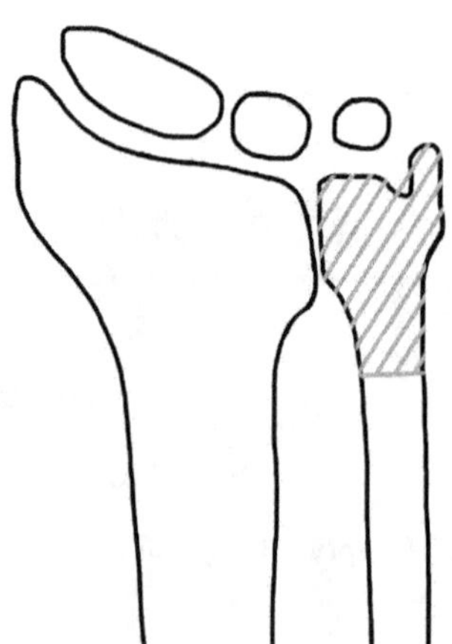

Figure: a) Sauve-Kapandji (DRUJ fusion & distal ulna osteotomy), b) Chamay (radio-lunate fusion), c) RSL fusion

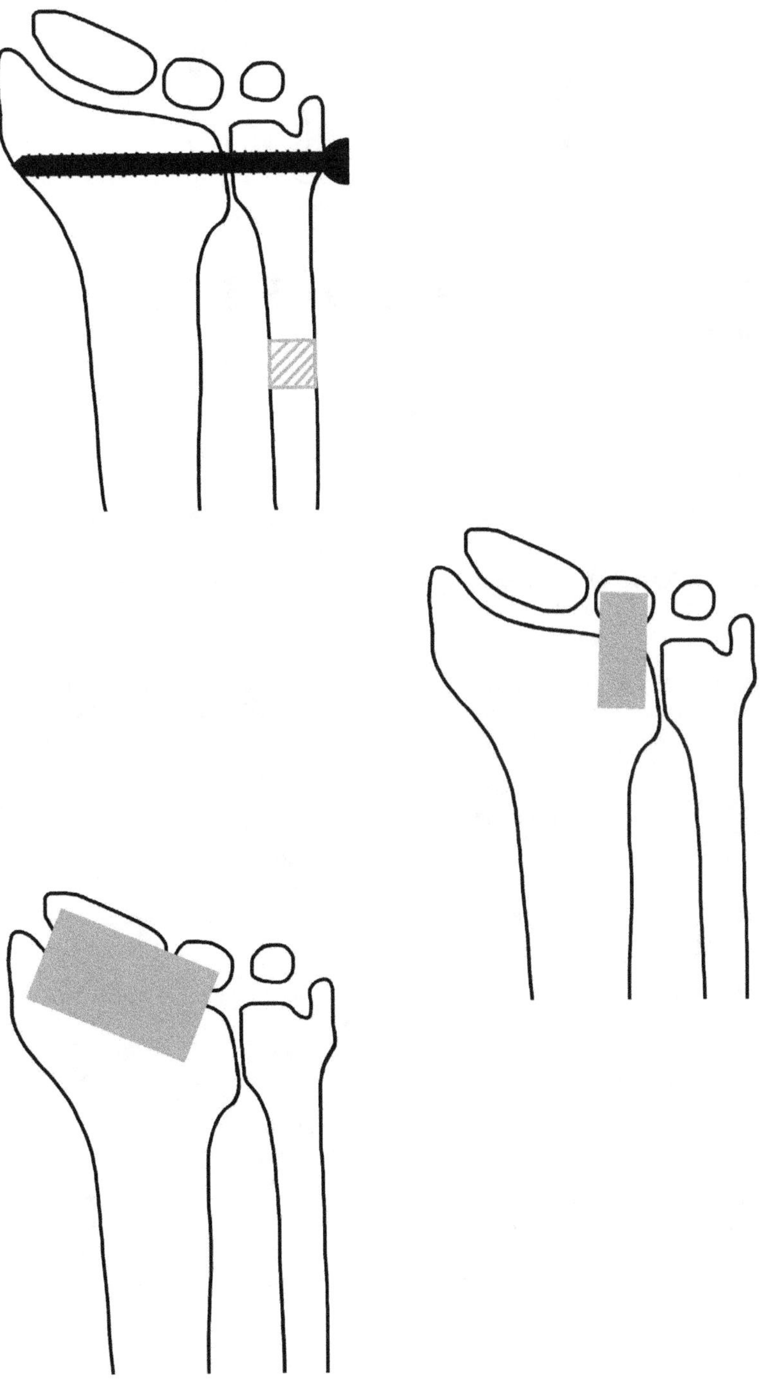

Figure: Total wrist arthrodesis (most surgeons bone graft around the intercarpal joints)

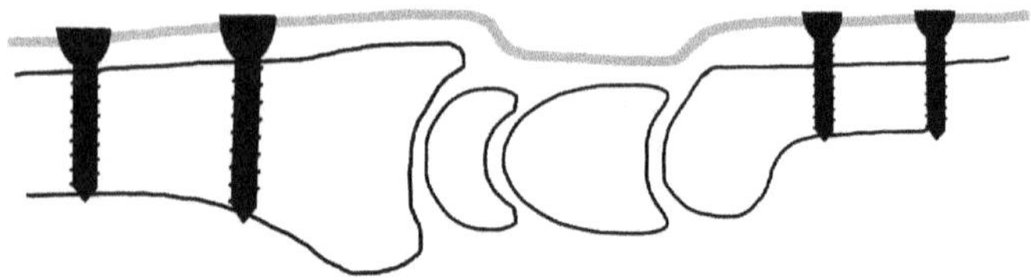

4. Surgical options for MCPjs

Problem:

Soft tissue component: Sagittal bands & extensor tendon

Joint / bony component: MCPj subluxation + ulnar drift of digits

Solution:

	Procedure*	Principle	Comments
Intrinsic release	Detach intrinsics and do not re-attach	Remove the deforming force behind ulnar deviation & sequalae	
Cross intrinsic transfer	Detach intrinsics attachment from ulnar side of P1 and re-attach to radial sides of adjacent digits	Rebalance the forces deviating the digits	Difficult in small finger (which may need division of AbdDM)
Repair of radial sagittal bands + tendon centralisation	Extensor tendon is relocated and sagittal bands repaired	Restoration of anatomical ralationship	Usually in combination with a procedure on intrinsics
Silicone arthroplasty	Replacement of MCPj with a silicone spacer	Get rid of diseased joint surface Move the arc of motion of the joint to more extension Decrease length to help intrinsics to relax	Usually in combination. ROM is not significantly changed
(Tupper arthroplasty)	Detach proximal part or volar plate and re-attach on dorsum of MC	Create a pseudoarthrosis	Historically, this preceeded silicone replacement. Infrequently used today, except as a salvage procedure

*These procedures can be combined with synovectomy (and each other).

5. Surgical options for digits

Check whether the deformity is flexible or fixed

- Flexiblilty implies good joint surface & lax ligaments, so soft tissue reconstruction can help.
- Fixed deformity means joint surface is compromised (in addition to any soft tissue component), so it needs either restoration of surface (joint replacement) or arthrodesis.

SWAN NECK

It is functionally limiting for the patient as she is unable to achieve fine pinch, pulp to pulp pinch or grasp an object (e.g. cup or mug). This is a difficult problem to treat as the original pathology may be in intrinsics, at PIPj or at DIPj.

Soft tissue: retinacular ligament recon, FDS tenodesis
Bony: Arthroplasty / arthrodesis

BOUTONNIERE

It is less of a functional problem (than swan neck) as patient can still grasp objects.

Soft tissue: Synovectomy + lateral band relocation +/- central slip recon
Bony: Silicone arthroplasty

PIPj arthrodesis is quite a limiting procedure for the patient's ROM. With good rheumatologist support, it is best that the patient doesn't have to reach this stage in the first place.

Opinion:

Note all these procedures for RA are quite extensive, need a prolonged period of rehabilitation, can be quite mutilating and take a long time to heal and rehabilitate. (Remember the steroids and MTX the patient is taking). I therefore cannot over-stress the importance of good medical management of rheumatoid in preventing surgery.

If and when surgery becomes necessary, know what functional problem is concerning the patient, start with a smaller procedure that carries little morbidity but has a high functional return for "that" patient. And don't forget "Function, function, function".

Nerve compression

CORE KNOWLEDGE
Tinel-Hoffman sign
Motor and cutaneous supply by median, ulnar and radial nerves
Reflex arc
Electrodiagnostic studies
Brachial plexus

APPROACH TO PATIENT - HISTORY
(as for any hand injury)

APPROACH TO PATIENT - EXAMINATION
Examination of median, ulnar and radial nerves

APPROACH TO PATIENT - TREATMENT
see below

EXPECTED CLINICAL QUESTIONS
- Draw brachial plexus
- Importance of reflex arc in interpretation of electrodiagnostic studies

RECOMMENDED PAPERS
1. Brauer CA, Graham B. The surgical treatment of cubital tunnel syndrome: a decision analysis. *J Hand Surg (Eur)*. 2007;32(6):654–62.
2. Hentz VR, Lalonde DH. MOC-PS(SM) CME Article: Self-Assessment and Performance in Practice: The Carpal Tunnel: *Plast Reconstr Surg*. 2008 Apr; 121(Supplement):1–10.
3. Shores JT, Lee WPA. An Evidence-Based Approach to Carpal Tunnel Syndrome: *Plast Reconstr Surg*. 2010 Dec;126(6):2196–204.

4. Mallik A. Nerve conduction studies: essentials and pitfalls in practice. *Journal of Neurology, Neurosurgery & Psychiatry*. 2005 Jun 1;76(suppl_2):ii23–31.
5. Whittaker RG. SNAPs, CMAPs and F-waves: nerve conduction studies for the uninitiated. *Practical Neurology*. 2012 Apr;12(2):108–15.
6. Terzis JK, Kostopoulos VK. The Surgical Treatment of Brachial Plexus Injuries in Adults. *Plast Reconstr Surg*. 2007 Apr;119(4):73e – 92e.
7. Terzis JK, Kokkalis ZT. Paediatric brachial plexus reconstruction. *Plast Reconstr Surg*. 2009;124(6):370e-385e

Examination of median nerve

Expose both sides

LOOK
Wasting of long flexor origin / thenar muscles
Trophic changes on index & middle fingers

FEEL
Sensations
Tinel along the course of the nerve from palm to axilla

MOVE
FDS to IF, MF, RF & LF
FDP to IF & MF
PT
FCR
PL
FPL
'O' sign

PROVOCATIVE TESTS
Phalen
Reverse phalen
Direct compression at wrist

Examination of ulnar nerve

Expose both sides [consider a chaperone]

LOOK
1. Wasting of medial forearm proximally
2. Claw deformity (hyperextension at MCPj and flexion at PIPj of small and ring fingers)
3. Wasting of hypothenar eminence, first dorsal interosseus (1st DIO)
4. Guttering of inter-metacarpal spaces (on dorsum)
5. Trophic changes on small finger

FEEL
1. Test light touch (show on an un-involved dermatome, then test over ulnar nerve distribution)
2. Tinel over the course of the nerve, up to the axilla
3. Provocative test for ulnar nerve by elbow flexion

MOVE

1. FCU, against resistance
2. FDP 4,5
3. Abd Dig Min (both sides together for comparison)
4. IF abduction (for 1st DIO)
5. Cross IF and MF (uses 1st PIO to IF, and 2nd DIO to MF)
6. Froment's sign

FURTHER SPECIAL TESTS

Unassisted angle. Ask pt to maintain lumbrical plus position (L+) & measure extensor deficit at PIPj

Assisted angle. Perform Bouvier's manoeuvre (i.e. ask pt to maintain a L+ position, the examiner passively flexes P1 to 90° and asks pt to extend PIPj). This is the single most important test to decide about surgery.

Result of Bouvier's manoeuvre	Nomenclature	Importance
Pt. can fully extend PIPj by themselves	Bouvier active positive	anti-claw procedure will be helpful
Pt. can't extend PIPj themselves, but the examiner can correct it fully	Bouvier passive positive	?? use anticlaw splint
If examiner can't correct it as well	Bouvier negative	joint contracture and tendon surgery will not help by itself
If PIPj can be corrected, but is hypermobile		risk of L+ position if anticlaw procedure is too tight

Ulnar paradox

Distal ulnar nerve lesions cause more pronounced clawing (than proximal lesions).

Aside: Mechanism of ulnar paradox
"Claw" deformity = ↑ extension @MPj + flexion @IPjs Normal intrinsic muscle action = MPj flexion + IPj ext ↓ Ulnar n. palsy → No intrinsics → extension @MPj + flexion @PIPj High ulnar n. palsy → additional loss of FDP to RF & LF → poor flexion @IPj → less clawing

Wartenberg sign

= spontaneous abduction of LF due to injury to the deep branch, due to unbalanced attachment of EDM & EDC to LF (which attach slightly ulnar).

The functional problem with ulnar nerve palsy is the claw as the patient can't grasp an object because PIPj flex (long flexors) before MCPs on any attempt to grasp.

Options = activity modif, physio, op when all joints supple, anticlaw splint, dynamic procedure

Examination of radial nerve

Expose both sides

LOOK
Wrist drop
Wasting of extensor origin, triceps

FEEL
Test light touch over superficial radial nerve territory
Tinel over the course of the nerve up to axilla

MOVE
The radial gives its branches a lot more proximal to the respective muscles (as compared to other nerves).

1. Triceps
2. ECRL, ECRB - feel for their contraction at their insertion on 2nd & 3rd MCs. (ECRB is first muscle supplied by the posterior interosseous nerve)
3. All EDCs - Hold the wrist, and ask to extend fingers against resistance
4. EIP & EDM - independent extension of index and small finger
5. EPL - retropulsion of thumb on a flat surface

Wartenberg syndrome:
(not to be confused with Wartenberg's sign in ulnar nerve lesions)
Pain & paraesthesia over the radial nerve distribution due to compression of the superficial branch of the radial nerve at the level of the wrist.

Examination if you don't know the exact nerve lesion

See examination for brachial plexus lesions. Tailor it if needs be.

Brachial plexus injury

APPROACH TO PATIENT - HISTORY
General
Is it an acute or chronic problem?
Age, occupation, handedness, hobbies, who is at home, medical issues.

Specific
Mechanism of injury
Time since injury
Treatment/Management carried out since then
Any associated injuries (& how have they been managed)

Functional issues
What is the patient's current problem and what can I do (as a surgeon) to help the patient

APPROACH TO PATIENT - EXAMINATION
ATLS (in acute situation)

Expose both upper limbs and the neck. [It will involve the patient tying a gown around their waist. Strongly consider having a chaperone].

Look:
Posture
Muscle bulk
Fasciculations
Horner's syndrome

Feel:
- Light touch over all sensory dermatomal distributions [judge if it is a dermatomal or peripheral nerve pattern]
- Sweating over the digits

[Alternatively, you can do motor examination first]

Aside: Motor examination in brachial plexus injury

In acute situation, be aware of other injuries and fractures which may be painful for the patient. In chronic cases, there may be joint contractures so don't forget the active and passive range of movements.

Move (& feel for contraction):

Joint	Movement	Explanation
Shoulder	Elevation	Trapezius (for CN XI transfer)
	Retrusion	Rhomboids
	Protrusion	Serratus anterior (for transfer)
	Abduction	Deltoid Supraspinatus
	External rotation	Teres major, minor
	Internal rotation	Subscapularis
Elbow	Flexion in supination	Biceps & brachialis
	Flexion in mid prone	Brachiradialis
	Extension	Triceps
	Supination in full extension	Supinator
	Pronation	Feel Pronator teres [Median n.*]
Wrist	Flexion	Feel FCR[median n.], FCU [ulnar n.]
	Extension	Feel ECRL, ECRB, ECU [Radial n.]
Fingers	Thumb retropulsion	[Radial n.]
	Digit extension	[Radial n.]
	Long flexors	FDS [Median n.]
		FDP to IF, MF [Median n.]
		FDP to LF, RF [Ulnar n.]
	LF abduction	[Ulnar n.]
	Interossei	[Ulnar n.]
	Froment	[Ulnar n.]

* Differentiation between individual branches of radial, median or ulnar nerves is less important in acute brachial plexus injuries than in peripheral nerve compression syndromes. In brachial plexus injuries, it is more important to assess the individual's proximal branches of the brachial plexus (e.g. nerves to serratus, rhomboids or supraspinatus) which cndicates the highest level of injury and helps rule out injury at the level of nerve roots ("root avulsion", which is the most challenging to manage).

Range of movement Active and Passive ROM of all joints, in chronic cases (Consider A/PROM as you do motor testing at each joint).

Tinel:

Test *at*,

1. Supra-clavicular, over plexus origin
2. Infra-clavicular, over coracoid
3. along the full course of ulnar, median and radial nerves

Test *for*,

- maximum Tinel
- most advanced point of Tinel

Investigations:

- Immediate = Chest Xray, to look for associated fracture of the clavicle, or position of the diaphragm (raised hemi-diaphragm in phrenic nerve palsy. Phrenic nerve is a potential donor)
- @3/52 = NCS and CT myelography (for possible root avulsion. see below for rationale)

APPROACH TO PATIENT - MANAGEMENT
see below

EXPECTED CLINICAL QUESTIONS
- Draw brachial plexus
- Importance of reflex arc in interpretation of electrodiagnostic studies
- Tinel-Hoffman sign and its clinical significance

RECOMMENDED PAPERS

1. Giuffre JL, Kakar S, Bishop AT, Spinner RJ, Shin AY. Current concepts of the treatment of adult brachial plexus injuries. *J Hand Surg Am.* 2010 Apr; 35(4):678-88
2. Giuffre JL, Bishop AT, Spinner RJ, Shin AY. The best of tendon and nerve transfers in the upper extremity. *Plast Reconstr Surg.* 2015 Mar;135(3): 617e-630e
3. Terzis JK, Kostopoulos VK. The surgical treatment of brachial plexus injuries in adults. *Plast Reconstr Surg.* 2007 Apr 1;119(4):73e-92e.
4. Terzis JK, Papakonstantinou KC. The surgical treatment of brachial plexus injuries in adults. *Plast Reconstr Surg.* 2000 Oct;106(5):1097-1122
5. Slutskey. Nerve conduction studies in hand surgery. J Hand Surg. 2003: 3(3); 152-169

Figure: Draw brachial plexus

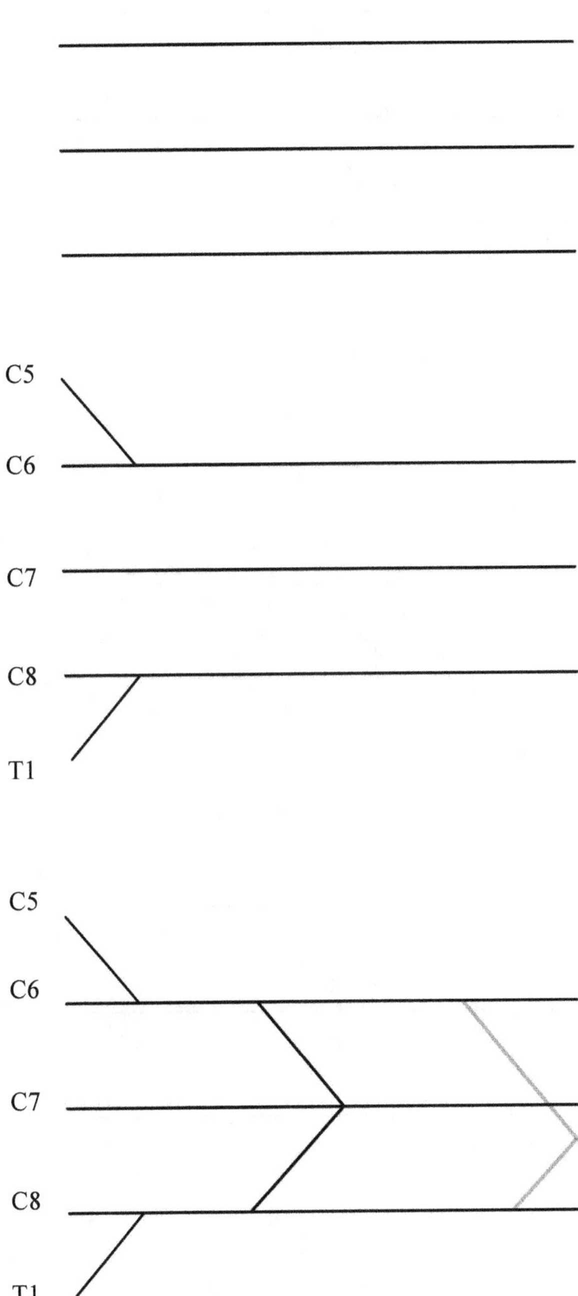

Figure: Draw brachial plexus (contd.)

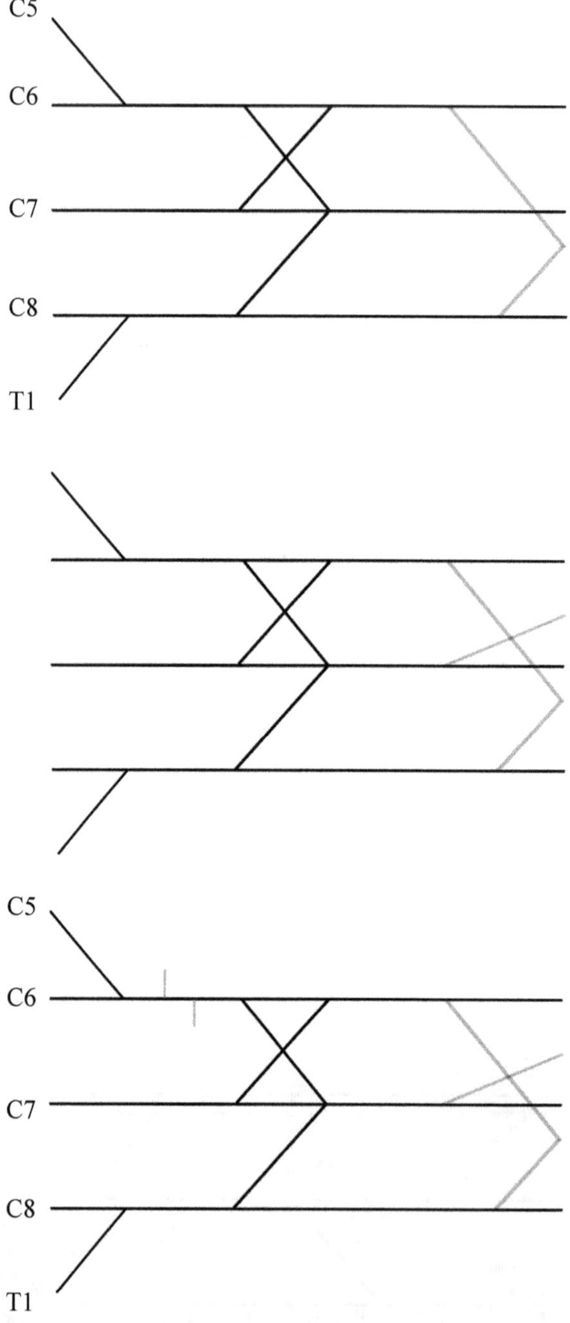

Figure: Draw brachial plexus (contd.)

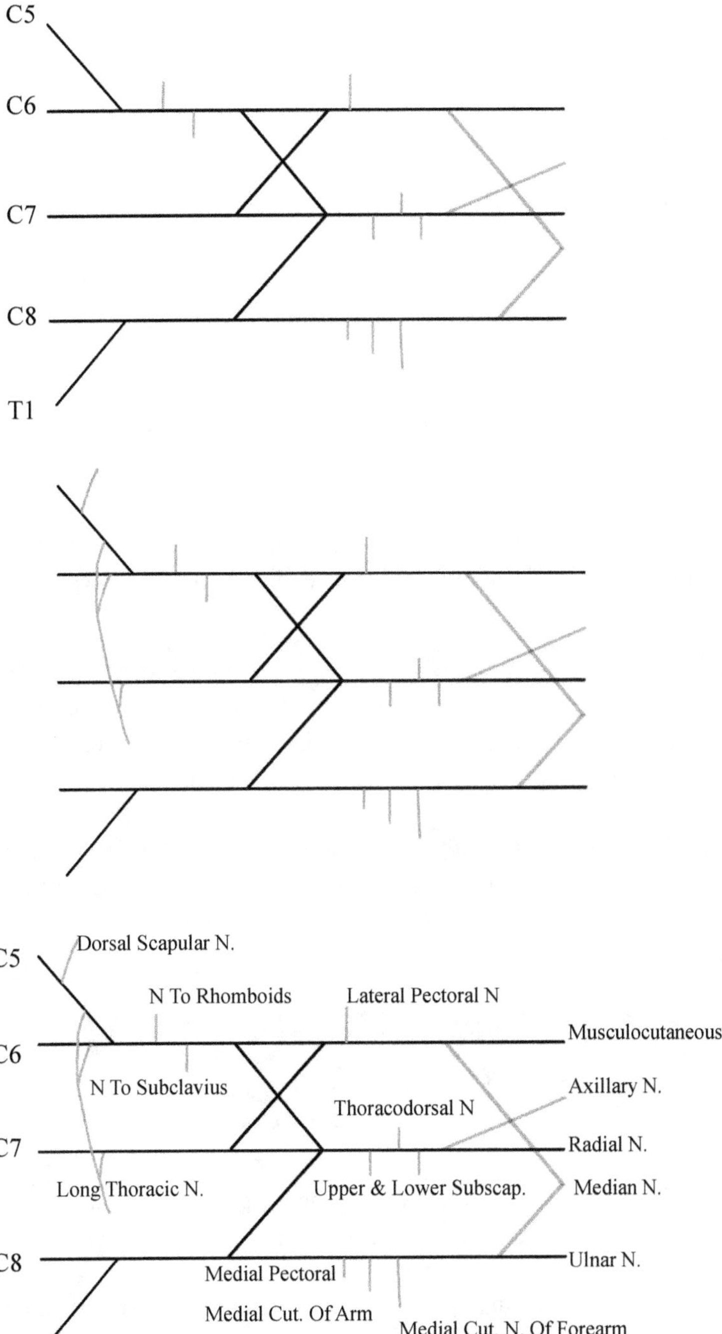

Classification of nerve injuries

Table: Seddon / Sunderland classifications of nerve injuries

Seddon (1943)	Sunderland (1951)
Neurapraxia	I = Neurapraxia
Axonotmesis	II = Pure axonotmesis, endoneurium is intact
	III = Axon + endoneurium gone
	IV = axon + endoneurium + perineurium gone
Neurotmesis	V = axon + endo. + peri + epinuerium gone (i.e complete disruption)
	VI = combination of any of above (added later in the classification by McKinnon)

How an injured nerve is improving, can be assessed clinically (by Tinel-Hoffman sign) or quantitatively (with neurophysiologic studies).

The Tinel-Hoffman sign

The Tinel-Hoffman sign is a clinical indicator of recovery of peripheral nerve injuries. A light tap on the nerve either produces localised discomfort or paraesthesia in the sensory distribution of that nerve.

This test is most commonly known for testing median nerve compression under the transverse carpal ligament, but can be used for assessing nerve compression or recovery from a nerve injury at any site. All further discussion in this chapter focuses on traumatic injuries.

Aside: Tinel and Hoffman

A frenchman Jules Tinel and a german physiologist Paul Hoffman described this useful clinical sign around the time of WW1.

The likely mechanism is that the regenerating axons have a lower threshold of excitation. This makes them susceptible to mechanical stimulation which can elicit an action potential. As the axons regenerate, this point of excitation can move distally, stay static, or both, i.e. positive at the site of injury as well a component that moves distally (Ref: Table).

Table: Significance of the Tinel-Hoffman sign

Advancing	Axonal regeneration (ideally at 1mm/day, or 1inch/month)
Static	Neuroma
Partly advancing and partly static	Some axons are regenerating but others are not. This may represent a physiologic delay or presence of scar tissue. If it does not improve (alongside corroborating clinical and electrophysiologic evidence) consider surgery to identify and rectify the problem.

Neurophysiologic studies

Sometimes called NCS, Nerve Conduction Studies assess the pattern of conduction in peripheral nerves and electrophysiologic activity in their respective muscles.

A typical study tests the nerve and the muscles, individually and together as a unit. The apparatus consists of a stimulating electrode and one (or more) pick up electrodes. Motor nerve conduction is tested in both orthodromic and retrodromic directions.

Motor fibres of a nerve are tested by application of a (proximal) stimulus and picking up a distal response. An applied stimulus results in an orthodromic action potential in a large number of axons (Combined Motor Action Potential, CMAP). Its amplitude is proportional to the number of fibres, while the conduction velocity is proportional to the diameter and myelination of the fibres.

Each peripheral nerve has a known velocity at which the applied signal travels. Knowing the distance between the electrodes (and the time between application and pickup of the signal) allows for calculation of conduction velocity in the nerve being tested. Varying the site of electrodes helps specify the location of any conduction block (e.g. across the carpal tunnel).

Sensory testing is done by applying a stimulus to the sensory distribution of the appropriate nerve and listening for an action potential more proximally (Sensory Nerve Action Potential, SNAP). The absolute value of the sensory action potential is much smaller than that of the motor one.

Now, an action potential needs an intact axon and an intact cell body connected to that axon. The cell bodies for motor neurons reside in the anterior horn of the spinal cord but those for sensory neurons live in the dorsal root ganglion (i.e. outside the spinal cord). Injuries to the distal parts of the brachial plexus preserve both these cell bodies which results in a positive action potential in both motor and sensory testing proximal to the injured level.

Presence of a sensory response from a dermatome with *absence of a corresponding motor* response implies that although the nerve is intact from the sensory cell body (in dorsal root ganglion) to the tested site, it is disrupted proximal to the dorsal root ganglion. Such an pattern is highly suggestive of a root avulsion injury (i.e. the rootlets exiting the spinal cord have been avulsed from the cord itself). These avulsed rootlets cannot regenerate their connections within the spinal cord. Hence the need for early exploration to confirm the diagnosis +/- to perform nerve transfers (vide infra for principles of management).

Lack of both sensory and motor responses beyond a certain level suggests an injury distal to the nerve roots (vide infra).

The reason for delaying NCS by 3 weeks after injury, is to give time for any Wallerian degeneration to occur (to avoid a false positive response) and for any neurapraxia to show signs of improvement.

Principles of management

[Obtain an accurate history and have a high index of suspicion. Identify and deal with life threatening injuries first]

OPEN INJURIES

Any open injuries should be explored immediately, to identify severed nerves and attempt primary repair, ideally before edema sets in.

CLOSED INJURIES

We need to determine:

- Firstly, if this deficit is due to neurapraxia (various grades, which improve spontaneously over time) or neurotmesis (Table: Seddon & Sunderland classifications)
- Secondly what is the exact level of injury (hopefully a single level injury!).

This distinction is made by regular detailed clinical examination + nerve conduction studies (NCS) +/- CT myelogram.

@3/52:

We wait for three weeks for any Wallerian degeneration to set in. At this stage Sunderland grade 1 or 2 injuries (Ref: Sunderland and Seddon grades) will have shown rapid clinical improvement. Sunderland 3 or 4 will not show much clinical recovery at this stage. (Sunderland 5 are usually open injuries that need early exploration).

Abnormal nerve conduction studies at three weeks may,

i.   show nothing. So watch & wait, and monitor clinically
ii. show improvement early on. So watch & wait, and monitor clinically
iii. suggest root avulsion from the spinal cord (Ref: nerve conduction studies, above). This will neither improve by itself nor can the avulsed roots be operated upon to anastomose them inside the spinal cord. The only option to recover function in such a situation, is to find new nerves which can be coapted onto the distal nerve stump and serve as donor axons.

A CT myelogram/MRI may also show corroborative evidence of root avulsion at 3 weeks.

@6/52:

If there is no sign of clinical recovery at 3 weeks, the surgeon hopes that this may still be Sunderland grade 3 or 4 injury. So the patient examination and nerve connection studies are at done at 6 weeks post injury and then at 6 weekly intervals, until either clinical improvement or decision to operate (see below).

Clinical monitoring:

Patients managed non-operatively are monitored at 6 weekly intervals to look for an advancing Tinel-Hoffman sign and with NCS.

Decision to operate:

1. In case of suspicion of nerve root avulsion, an early MRI can provide both corroborating evidence for root avulsion and identify associated injuries.
2. If there is no recovery at all, this may be a Sunderland grade 5 (i.e. neurotmesis) which needs exploration and a primary repair.
3. If the nerve function started to recover but has stalled ("Tinel's failure to progress") there may be a neuroma, which usually manifests as a strong localised Tinel but no progression.
4. If the recovery has been slow and incomplete, this may be a Sunderland 6 injury, which again needs operative exploration.

Figure: Outline of management algorithm of acute brachial plexus injury

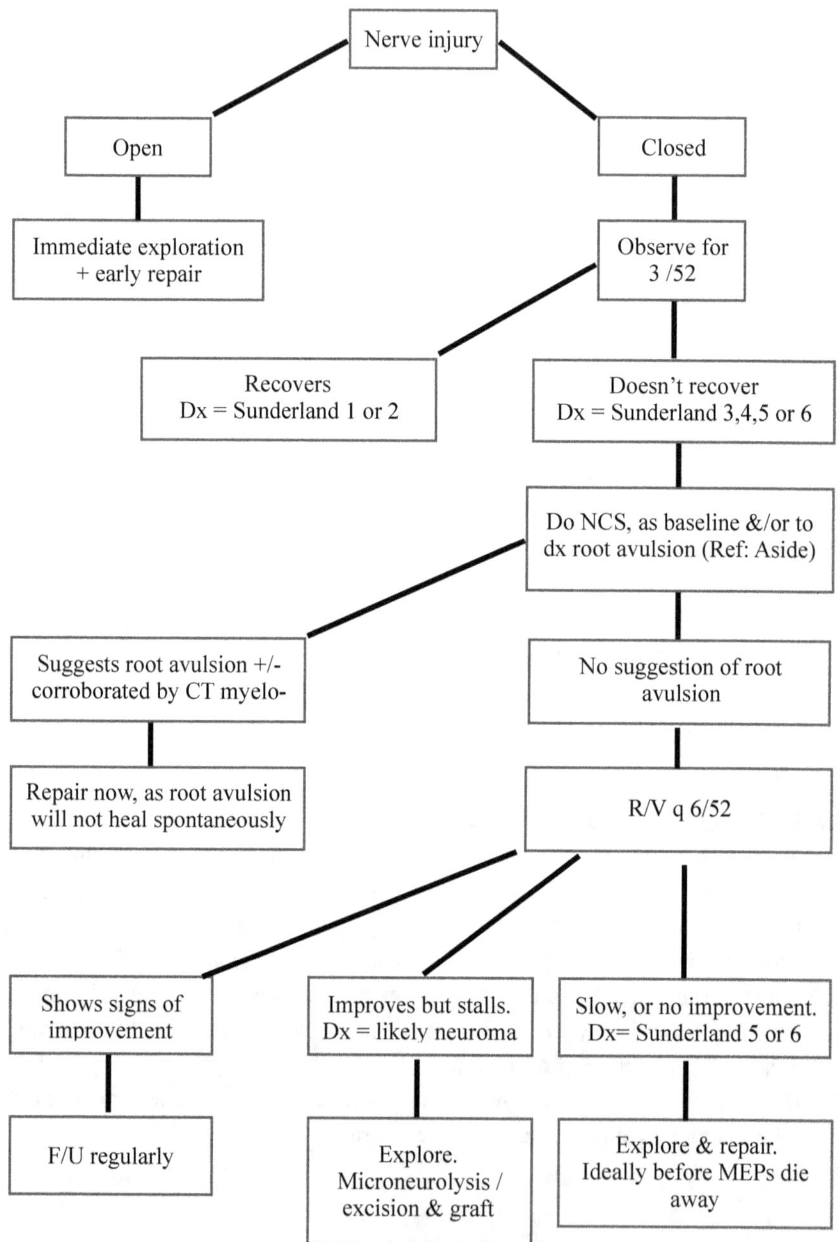

Timing of operation:

The endpoint of treatment is to restore patient's function to its premorbid state. If this happens spontaneously that's very good. But if not, then the upper limit for axonal recovery (from the site of injury on to the motor end plate on the muscle) is 12-15 months. At this point, the motor end plates (MEPs) degenerate and any (spontaneous or post-op) axons arriving at the MEP after that will not restore muscle function.

Note that the regenerating axons (after the initial period of Wallerian degeneration and in optimal conditions) grow at approximately 1 mm/day from the site of injury, or approx. one inch/month. This implies that the regeneration needs to happen at a certain pace, otherwise the muscles will lose MEPs before axons reach them ("neurotisation"). Practically that implies that any (proximal) lesion which has not shown signs of improvement by six months needs an operation (to bring in new axons) otherwise you miss the boat to neurotise the muscle in time. Of course, if you that the pt. is unlikely to improve spontaneously, there is no point in waiting for 6 weeks.

If the muscles has not been neurotised in time (e.g. late presentation) the only option to restore function is muscle transfer. (Ref: Priority in muscle transfer, see below).

Intra-operative decisions:

Nerves which have been transected need direct repair (if possible), or interposition nerve grafts (if some length is missing, or has to be debrided).

A proximal neuroma within brachial plexus is a good sign which suggests that there are good axons arriving at this site (i.e. there is no proximal injury). If this neuroma is dealt with, there are good chances of nerve growth. A distal neuroma, however, may have axons arriving from any branch of the brachial plexus, so it cannot be relied upon to rule out a more proximal injury.

A neuroma present in the continuity of the nerve either needs microneurolysis, or excision and nerve graft.

Options of reconstruction:

The tool box for a brachial plexus surgeon consists of:

1. Direct repair
2. Interposition nerve grafts. Classically sural or saphenous nerve grafts, more recently vascularised ulnar nerve graft
3. Motor nerve transfer
4. Muscle transfer
5. Tendon transfer
6. Arthrodesis

PRINCIPLES IN CHOOSING A DONOR

- If the MEPs are there - use a nerve
- If too late to neurotise MEPs - choose between stability and function i.e. either transfer muscle / tendons or arthrodese

1. Know what is missing and what function you want to restore (and how that will help in patient's daily life)
2. Know what is available (with acceptable morbidity). The donors can be un-injured nerves of the plexus, or from outside the plexus [intercostal nerves are your "Get out of Jail" card]
3. Set your priority list e.g. shoulder abduction > elbow flexion > wrist stabilisation > sensibility > arthrodesis
4. Find what is expendable
5. Donor should have similar action as the target

For the reasons cited above, early recon is with nerve transfers and later with muscle transfers (note the similarity in principles with facial nerve injury).

SHOULDER STABILISATION

1. CN XI to supra-scapular n.
2. Triceps branch of radial to axillary n. ('Somsak/Leechavengvongs transfer')
3. Intercostal to sub-scapular n.
4. Phrenic nerve. Only if no previous respiratory condition *and* a pre-op CXR has been checked (to rule out pre-existing phrenic nerve injury, by looking for an elevated hemi-diaphragm).
5. Glenohumeral arthrodesis. Which provides the patient with a stable post to help move the rest of the upper limb.

ELBOW FLEXION:

Elbow flexion takes priority so the patient can feed himself [vast majority are male patients].

Target = Biceps +/- brachioradialis

Donor options
- Intra-plexal. Ulnar nerve branch to biceps ('Oberlin transfer', JHS Am 1994)
- Intra-plexal. Median nerve fascicle to motor branch of brachialis (Oberlin II)
- Extra plexal. CN XI, or intercostals
- More recently, direct muscle neurotization with ulnar of median nerve fascicles

Late recon options
- Transfer of local muscles (if partial injury) e.g. pect major / minor, triceps, LD
- Proximal advancement of flexor pronator mass (Steindler's flexoroplasty)
- Free functioning muscle transfer e.g. Gracilis (powered by CN XI, or 2x intercostals), LD or rectus femoris.

ELBOW EXTENSION
Intercostals to branch of triceps

HAND FUNCTION
So far the results have been poor, which is not surprising considering that nerve transfers (assuming brachial plexus injury at / above axilla) cannot neurotise small muscles of hand in time to preserve MEPs and muscle transfers cannot be accomodated in the small spaces of the hand. Doi et al. described use of double gracilis transfer

SENSATIONS
Sensory part of intercostal nerve to lateral root of median nerve (C6/7 dermatome).

Summary:

Think,
1. Where is the problem?
2. What does the patient need?
3. Translate that need to a donor nerve or muscle
4. Know what is available
5. Think through your donors (intra- / extra-plexal nerves, synergistic muscles etc.)

Basic Science

Basic science

Structure of skin

Describe in terms of
- Epidermis
- Dermis
- Sub cut

as well as,
- Cells
- Organs
- Hair follicles & associated apparatus

Skin healing

Hemostasis (immediate)	Vessel wall contraction → denuding of epithelium
	+
	Platelet adherence to endothelium
	    - degranulation → TxA2
	    - ↑ platelet attraction
	    - platelet plug formation
	+
	Activation of coagulation cascade
	    - fibrinogen to fibrin
	    - platform for platelets to adhere

Inflammation (minutes to 3 days)	Neutrophil (within 24hr) infiltration
	    - phagocytose FB/necrotic material
	
	Macrophage (in 48hr) from monoctyes
	    - ↑ phagocytosis
	    - orchestrates wound healing
	        • re-epithelisation
	        • granulation tissue
	        • angiogenesis
	        • cytokines
	        • wound contraction

Proliferation (3d. - 3wk)	**EPIDERMIS:**
	Loss of contact inhibition → migration →mitosis→ differentiation
	
	DERMIS:
	Fibroblasts move in (esp. @day7) →↑rate of collagen synthesis
	GAG production (= HA), then
	     - chondroitin SO_4
	     - dermatan SO_4
	
	ANGIOGENESIS:
	= formation of new blood vessels from existing ones

Remodelling (3wk- 1yr+)	@3-5wks = equilibrium between collagen breakdown and synthesis
	
	Collagen
	     - ↑ organisation
	     - ↑ cross links
	     - Type III → Type !
	
	↓ GAGs / water content / vascularity

Factors affecting wound healing

LOCAL

Foreign bodies

Necrotic material

Infection

REGIONAL

Arterial disease

Venous disease

Oedema

SYSTEMIC
Congenital

Spectrum of rare collagen disorders (= Ehlers-Danlos, Progeria and Werner's, but NOT Pseudoxanthoma elasticum or Cutis laxa)

Acquired

Age

Medication, eg. steroids, cyclosporine

Medical conditions

- diabetes,
- peripheral vascular disease,
- chronic cardiopulmonary disease,
- renal failure

Environmental

- smoking,
- malnutrition (protein / vitamin / trace elements)
- radiation exposure

Fetal wound healing

= ability of the skin of early gestational fetuses to heal with regeneration (i.e. without a scar).

Characteristics of fetal wound healing

1. Site specific, i.e. where is the scar
2. Wound size specific, i.e. how large it is
3. Fetal age specific, i.e. at what fetal age did it occur

The following are the major differences:

A) Extracellular matrix

Collagen, Type III & rapid turnover

HA, Less inhibitors

Proteoglycan, ↑MMPs vs tissue-derived inhibitors

Adhesion proteins, allow ↑cell movement (*tensein*) & ↑cell anchoring (*fibronectin*)

B) Mediators:

Ref: Table (next page)

Table: Differences in mediators of fetal wound healing (as compared to adults)

Cellular	Platelets	↓degranulation ↓ aggregation ↓ TGF β1&2
	Neutrophils	↓ number
	Fibroblasts	Simultaneous proliferation & collagen production No myofibroblasts
Cytokines	TGF β	β1&2 unchanged β3 increased
	IL-1	↓IL6&8

RECOMMENDED READING:

Larson BJ et al. Scarless fetal wound healing: A basic science review. *Plast Recon Surg*. 2010; 126(4): 1172-1182

Assessment of adverse scar

CORE KNOWLEDGE
Scar assessment scales
Wound healing
Keloid vs HT scars
Management strategies and evidence

APPROACH TO PATIENT - HISTORY
General
Patient PMHx, medications, Allergies

Specific
Age of scar
Cause e.g. laceration, surgery, burns, chronic wound, acne
Healing process. Did it never heal (chronic wound), healed and broke down (what may be the cause), breaks down regularly (unstable scar, or e.g. ill fitting shoe)
What treatments have been done so far, including any steroids

Ideas & expectations
Whose idea was to refer
What happened now that the patient needed referring
What is the problem now - aesthetic, functional, psychological (Ref: Table) or a combination

Table: An adverse characteristic of a scar may be,

Aesthetic	Social issues, esp. if • discolored • persistent erythema • $\uparrow$ / $\downarrow$ pigmentation
Functional	Restrictive • contracture • tethered
Psychological	esp. if on face

APPROACH TO PATIENT - EXAMINATION

On examination try to place the scar in one of the categories

- Mature / Immature
- Linear / Wide spread

as well as,

- Linear / widespread hypertrophic
- Minor / Major keloid

Look:

(try to assess scar maturity)

Site	
Size	Approx. dimensions Straight / curved / streched
Colour	
Contour	Flat / raised / depressed
Pigmentation	↑ or ↓
Pliability	pliable vs non-pliable, or supple/firm/contracture
Texture	
Vascularity	
(Maturity)	Redness
	Contour

Feel:

Maturity	Tenderness Lumpiness Itching (ask!)
Functionality	Contracture bands

Move:

Check AROM

APPROACH TO PATIENT - TREATMENT

Do s:

1. Do consider a trial of non-operative management for several months or until scar maturation
2. Do consider a combination therapy approach
3. Do warn about patient dissatisfaction (irrespective of management option)

Non-surgical options:

Do nothing

Massage +/- camoflague

Silicone gel (for exposed ares) / sheet (for covered areas)

Pressure garments

Steroid injections

Laser, usually PDL (585nm), or CO_2 (10800nm)

Others (= rare / specialised)

- anti-mitotics, 5FU, Bleomycin
- RT (for keloids)
- IFN (also been described for keloids)

Surgical options:

Direct excision	If lies along an RSTL and linear, incl. ice pick scars of acne
Serial excision +/- TE	where scar is too large to close without tension
Re-orientation	If scar is at an acute angle to the RSTL, consider Z-plasty If scar is at right angle to local RSTL, consider W-plasty

Release	Superficial scar
	  • Graft
	  • Local flap, e.g. Y-V plasty to lengthen scar without undermining
	Deep scar
	  • Need tissue interposition e.g. trachy scars

Camouflage, by W-plasty	gives a broken line closure
Resurfacing	Autologous, SSG / FTSG Synthetic, ADM
Soft tissue augmentation	

Postop. care
- Massage
- Taping
- Silicone
- Pressure garments, usually in combination

EXPECTED CLINICAL QUESTIONS
- Ideal scar
- Scar assessment scales
- HT vs keloid
- Management of a specific scar

RECOMMENDED PAPERS
1. Mustoe TA, Cooter RD, Gold MH, et al. International Advisory Panel on Scar Management.. International clinical recommendations on scar management. *Plast Reconstr Surg.* 2002 Aug;110(2):560-71
2. Gold MH, McGuire M, Mustoe TA, et al. International Advisory Panel on Scar Management.. Updated international clinical recommendations on scar management: part 2--algorithms for scar prevention and treatment. *Dermatol Surg.* 2014 Aug;40(8):825-31
3. Further guidelines by Iwagwa & more (but Mustoe is most widely understood and used in clinical practice)

Ideal scar & assessment

An 'ideal' scar is one that matures rapidly without undue contraction, widening or formation of excessive collagen.

SCAR ASSESSMENT SCALES
1. Vancouver burn scar assessment scale (Sullivan et al. *J Burn Care Res* 1990) scores Pigmentation, Height, Pliability and Vascularity. It needs (ideally) 3 examiners for a reliable result.
2. Clinical Assessment Score, combines a visual analog score with colour, contour, distortion and texture

Of course, there are more scar assessment scales than you can remember, but by and large they use the same (above mentioned) information with different emphasis on different points.

Management of HT / keloid scar

History and examination as above

Prevention

Tension free closure

Avoid micro-movement e.g. taping

Avoid excessive macro-movement e.g. movement across joint

Avoid/minimise absorbable sutures in

Aim for early wound healing by avoiding infection

Site specific precautions e.g. ear clips

General considerations of management

- Trial of non-operative management
- Use of combination therapy
- Warn of patient dissatisfaction

Management options for HT scars

1. Symptomatic e.g. NSAIDS for pain, anti-histamines for itching
2. Compression therapy

   At least 15 mmHg pressure accelerates scar maturation. (Ref: Van der Kerckhone et al.)
3. Silicone gel sheeting

   Silicone dressing leads to more rapid improvement in hypertrophic scar maturation (Ref: Majan et al., RCT vs untreated patients)

   Silicone gel sheeting leads to decreased thickness, pain, itching (Ref: Li-Tsany et al. RCT)
4. Steroid injection leads to decreased production of cytokines and inhibition of fibroblast production

   Maximum dosage often quoted is 120 mg in adult, 80 mg in a child, 40 mg in less than five-year-old and given as 2.5-40 mg per site.

   Local side effects
   - atrophy of skin and subcutaneous tissue,
   - hypo-pigmentation.

   Systemic side effects
   - menstrual dysfunction,
   - suppression of adrenocortical function,

- development of cataract or glaucoma.

5. Laser

    PDL is effective for intense pruritis (Ref: Allison et al.)

6. Surgical excision & reconstruction with Z- or W- plasty. On face absorbable & non-absorbable sutures are equivalent (Ref: Luck et al.) while on chest non-absorbable sutures reduce the risk of HT scars (Ref: Durkaya et al.)

Management options for keloids

1. Corticosteroid

    Can be used alone or in combination with other modalities
    Evidence:

    - Kiil et al. Surgery + Adcortyl, vs Adcortyl alone → 1/3rd recur at 1year (both groups) → Half recur at 5 year (both groups).
    - Steroids alone → 82% patients report improvement in symptoms
    - Too few RCTs in combination treatment

2. Cryotherapy, alone or with Adcortyl

    Problem with pain and hypo-pigmentation

3. Radiotherapy

    With surgery has up to 98% success rate
    Given as <20Gy dose over several fractions
    CI: In young due to concern of malignant transformation later in life

4. Anti-tumors

    - 5-FU (intra-lesional) → 50% response (Ref: Uppal et al.)
    - Bleomycin (Ref: Naeini et al.)
    - IFN-gamma (Ref: Brocker et al.)

General & Misc. topics

General & Miscellaneous

APPROACH TO PATIENT - HISTORY

When did the problem start

How did it start

What is its prognosis (self limiting, progressive, cancer)

Who else is involved in its management (MDT, rheumatologist, dermatologist)

Has any treatment / management been done so far

Did that work? Any complications from the treatment

What is the current problem

How is affecting the patient in activities of daily life, at work and socially

What are patient's concerns

What are their expectations ("What can I do to help you")

APPROACH TO PATIENT - EXAMINATION

[Remember Gillies' principles]

What is missing. How much, what layers

Potential donor sites

APPROACH TO PATIENT - TREATMENT

(individualise to each condition)

EXPECTED CLINICAL QUESTIONS

Diagnosis

Management

Complications

Extravasation injury

CORE KNOWLEDGE
Types of extravasation agents

APPROACH TO PATIENT - HISTORY
Patient details
Age
What is the primary condition that the patient is being treated for
Other medical issues

What was going through?
How long since? At what rate?
When was it last seen to be okay?
Is the venflon still in? If yes then ask the person contacting you to stop the infusion, withdraw what they can with a 10ml syringe, apply compression bandage and elevate limb. (At this stage you should be able to triage the urgency of the situation).

APPROACH TO PATIENT - EXAMINATION

Look:
Location
Size of swelling

Feel:
Is it a subcutaneous extravasation only, or can it be deeper to the deep fascia [be wary of a compartment syndrome]
Capillary refill of overlying skin
Neuro-vascular status of the rest of the limb
Feel compartments

APPROACH TO PATIENT -MANAGEMENT
Do attempt to withdraw with a 10ml syringe, if cannula is still attached

Decision
The practice varies considerably. The following is a summary from my year long experience in a paediatric tertiary care hospital, where every extravasation in the hospital was required to be seen by plastic surgery!

Agent

The main determinant of the potential for injury is the agent that extravasated i.e. n/saline, dextrose, medicine, antibiotics, chemotherapy agents.

Normal saline will be re-absorbed from subcutaneous tissue over several hours (quicker, if it is elevated and a compression bandage applied).

The strength of dextrose determines its potential for damage. <10% dextrose is relatively safe if it extravasates in subcutaneous tissue but 10% or more strength needs to be washed out (see below).

Chemotherapeutic agents vary in their potential to cause tissue damage. They are classified into dessicants, vesicants, irritants according to the mechanism of their skin damage (Ref: ESMO guidelines).

Volume

The volume extravasated is relevant, as it determines the amount of local swelling and pressure effects on the overlying skin.

Management algorithm

Immediate first aid, stop further infusion, keep cannula in & attempt aspiration with a 10ml syringe.

If normal saline or <10% dextrose AND overlying skin viable
then simple compression bandage → elevate observe.

If anything else but not a chemo-therapeutic agent
Infiltrate local anaesthetic → Gault's "watering can" technique i.e. multiple punctures in the skin (depending on the size of swelling), compress to allow any extravasating fluid out, then washout with n/saline through the holes made earlier → compression bandage, elevate and observe. Use aseptic technique and consider antibiotics.

If chemotherapeutic agent has extravasated
Infiltrate with local anaesthetic → hyaluronidase injection subcutaneous and massage for five minutes → then use the watering can technique → compression bandage, elevate and observe.

The observation of the extravasation site can be undertaken at the patient observation time by nursing staff or once a day by a plastics surgery team member for next one week (or until the skin is not considered to be at risk).

Do consider antibiotic cover after a washout. Although it is an aseptic bedside procedure (like iv cannulation) but due to multiple punctures involved, has a risk of causing cellulitis. It can be difficult to say if any skin redness in the aftermath of a wash out is tissue reaction to extravasation or true cellulitis.

RECOMMENDED PAPER

1. Pérez Fidalgo JA, García Fabregat L, Cervantes A, Margulies A, Vidall C, Roila F; ESMO Guidelines Working Group. Management of chemotherapy extravasation: ESMO-EONS Clinical Practice Guidelines. Ann Oncol. 2012 Oct;23 Suppl 7:vii167-73. [https://annonc.oxfordjournals.org/content/23/suppl_7/vii167.full.pdf+html]

Necrotising fasciitis

It is a rapidly progressing and potentially fatal uni- or poly-microbial infection that spreads along deep fascia causing its necrosis, followed by thrombosis of the perforators to skin and skin necrosis.

Clinical picture

1. Skin changes that lag behind fascial destruction
2. Systemic effects e.g. shock, tachycardia, hypotension. Patient can deteriorate fast. Notice any trend in the Vital Signs!
3. Rapid progression and deterioration - within hours, or sooner. hence the importance of a thorough second review even if a patient "looks fine" at first
4. Markers of infection. Temprature, WBC, CRP (may lag the clinical picture by 24-36 hours)
5. Markers of anaerobic metabolism. Lactate, metabolic acidosis (nees blood gases asap)
6. Modification of the "typical signs" by stuttering antibiotic use or immune compromise (e.g. DM)
7. Nec. Fasc. can be mimicked by any rapid swelling causing blistering, e.g. Strep infection

Operative decision is clinical and emergent. The consent should include (but not limited to) these additional points,
1. risk of death
2. several theatre trips (for debridement, dressing changes, & later reconstruction)
3. long term ITU stay
4. large areas of tissue defects that will eventually need reconstruction

While awaiting urgent surgery, do pay attention to fluid resuscitation, placing long lines (by anaesthetist), broad spectrum antibiotics and send several microbiology specimens per op.

The best surgical technique employs more than one senior surgeon to allow rapid assessment and excision of tissues. A commonly used dressing is jelonet and betadine soaked gauze.

The theatre trips (after the index operation) are as per clinical needs, possibly daily until both the wound and the patient "numbers" (vitals, fluid & inotrope requirements, blood tests) improve.

In between theatre trips, manage the patient's fluids and nutrition like that of a major burn.

Reconstructive phase can begin only when all the diseased tissue has been excised and the patient has been stable for several days. The most common reconstruction modality is by staged SSG.

Perineal recon.

CORE KNOWLEDGE
Causes

APPROACH TO PATIENT - HISTORY

Medical history
PMHx, Meds, Allergies
Current functional level
Who is at home

Oncological history
[e.g. follow the TNM pattern]
Diagnosis
Tumour site & size
Nodal involvement
any Mets (and relevant investigations)

Oncological plan by MDT
Intent of resection (curative / palliative)
Extent of resection
Operative approach (& positioning)
Any colostomy/ileostomy planned and its site
Chemotherapy plan
Radiotherapy (neo-adjuvant pr adjuvant, EBRT or brachytherapy)
Named MacMillan nurse for the patient

Surgical history
"Other" surgical operations to abdomen / legs etc [Make sure your potential donor sites are intact]

APPROACH TO PATIENT - EXAMINATION
Most of the patients will be pre-op cancer excision. A combined review with the oncologic surgeon will be most valuable so that the extent of resection, resulting defect, potential donor sites, per-op positioning can be decided and appropriate patient counselling done.

APPROACH TO PATIENT - TREATMENT

Vaginal reconstruction

Acquired vaginal defects have been classified by Cordeiro et al. (PRS 2002) as partial or circumferential. Partial defects may be due to bladder or rectal CA while circumferential defects may be due to cervical CA or any advanced cancer.

The following are Cordeiro's recommendations for reconstruction (Ref: Cordeiro et al.)

Partial defects

Location	Antero-lateral
Common cause	Bladder CA
Reconstructive option	Singapore flap
	Modified Singapore flap

Location	Posterior wall
Common cause	Rectal CA
Reconstructive option	VRAM

Circumferential defects

Location	Upper 2/3rd
Common cause	Cervical CA
Reconstructive option	Rolled rectus / colon

Location	Complete
Common cause	Advanced cancer (any of the above)
Reconstructive option	Bilateral pedicled gracilis

SINGAPORE FLAP

Bilateral fasciocutaneous flaps of inguinal crease tissue based on posterior labial artery and tunnelled under the labia majora. (Described by Wee & Joseph, PRS 1989)

MODIFIED SINGAPORE FLAP

Woods et al. (1992) modified the design by incising through the labia majora to allow easier inset.

ROLLED RECTUS ABDOMINIS

Pedicled muscle only flap where the muscle's ends are sutured together to form a ring. (Tobin and Day, PRS 1988)

GRACILIS

McCraw et al. PRS 1976

Vulvar reconstruction

The history and examination broadly follow the above principles.
The possible reconstructive options are:
- SSG
- Medial thigh (fasciocutaneous) flap
- Gracilis myocutaneous V-Y advancement flap
- "Lotus petal" flap. Mentioned by Niranjan (Seminars in Plastic Surgery, 2006) lotus petal concept is an extension of perforator flaps for perineal reconstruction in general. The idea being that as long as there is a perforating vessel available, some customised flap can be based on it for rotation or transposition. Due to the rich nature blood supply of the perineum, a number of flaps of varying dimensions are possible around the introitus that can be rotated or transposed as desired.

Male perineal reconstruction

Mostly after open or laparoscopic abdomino-perineal resection of low rectal CAs.

EXPECTED CLINICAL QUESTIONS

- Management of patient
- Practicalities of management (positioning the colostomy, side of VRAM to use, theatre positioning etc.)
- Lotus petal concept

RECOMMENDED PAPERS

1. Cordeiro PG, Pusic AL, Disa JJ. A Classification System and Reconstructive Algorithm for Acquired Vaginal Defects. *Plast Recontr Surg.* 2002;110(4): 1058-65

2. Wee JTK, Joseph VT. A new technique of vaginal reconstruction using neurovascular pudendal-thigh flaps: a preliminary report. *Plast Recontr Surg.* 1989;83(4):701-9

3. Woods JE, Alter G, Meland B, Podratz K. Experience with vaginal reconstruction utilizing the modified Singapore flap. *Plast Reconstr Surg.* 1992 Aug;90(2):270-4

4. McCraw JB, Massey FM, Shanklin KD, Horton CE. Vaginal reconstruction with gracilis myocutaneous flaps. *Plast Reconstr Surg.* 1976 Aug;58(2): 176-83.

5. Niranjan N. Perforator Flaps for Perineal Reconstructions. *Seminars in Plastic Surgery.* 2006 May;20(2):133–44.

6. Friedman J, Dinh T, Potochny J. Reconstruction of the perineum. *Semin Surg Oncol.* 2000 Oct-Nov;19(3):282-93.

Pressure sores

CORE KNOWLEDGE
Waterlow score
Other scoring systems
Theory of pressure sore formation
Principles of management
Flap options for common pressure sore sites

APPROACH TO PATIENT - HISTORY
General
Age, gender, where do u normally live
Underlying medical condition. What is happening with it (who is looking after
it, GP/specialist. Prognosis)
PMHX, Meds, Allergies

Specific
How long has this been there for
Who has looked after it, GP/district nurse?
Is it getting better or worse
[Look around for adjuncts- cushions, wheelchair, etc]

Functional status
Ask carers about nursing support, whether living in home or in residential care.
Continence

APPROACH TO PATIENT - EXAMINATION
Look
Grade
Size, site
Base
Edge (epithelising or overhanging)
Surrounding skin- ? Infection/ maceration

Feel (from the surface, or *gentle* probing with a microbiology swab)
Warmth, tenderness of surrounding skin
Undermining
Exposed bone
Distal n/vasc. status (if on a limb)

Move

Adjacent joint [Is the "trochanteric" sore going all the way in to the hip joint?]

Ask:

for recent bloods and wound cultures. Hb, inflammatory markers, trace elements.

APPROACH TO PATIENT - MANAGEMENT

Medical optimisation & selective operation

1. Pressure relief. 2hourly turning, daily review of pressure areas, pressure relieving mattress /wheelchair cushions
2. Good nursing care. Above, plus preventing incontinence (reduce/stop laxatives, treat UTIs), appropriate bowel/bladder management(catheterise judiciously), absorbant pads, mop up incontinence asap.
3. Resolve infection/edema. Bedside sharp debridement of obviously necrotic material or a hydrocolloid gel for slough that cannot be debrided easily. Consider absorbant alginate dressing if predominantly exudative wound, and appropriate non-adherent dressing when the base is clean.
4. Adequate nutrition. Identify need based on caloric requirement, serum albumin and trace elements. Involve dietitian early.

Decision to operate depends on (in addition to PMHx, anaesthetic concerns):

- an assessment of impact of all of the above measures (commonly with an ongoing *improvement* in Waterlow Scale) and
- whether patient is in an anabolic state, as determined by correction of trace element deficiency, improvement in albumin (easily available though not the most reliable) and steady weight gain.

It is only in this favourable situation where the wounds can be expected to heal after surgery. Otherwise, it will be a disastrous situation if both the pressure sore and the donor site fail to heal.

The choice of any operation takes in to account,

1. Site of pressure sore
2. State of local tissues
3. Any previous surgery for the pressure sore. If there has been previous surgery, consider readvancing, else use an option that least interferes with a second operation.

EXPECTED CLINICAL QUESTIONS

- Theory of pressure sore formation
- Tissue pressure (and Starling equilibrium)
- Iceberg phenomenon
- Waterlow score and its components (unless you use a different system)
- Other scoring systems (briefly)
- Multidisciplinary approach

RECOMMENDED PAPERS

1. Bauer J, Phillips LG. MOC-PSSM CME Article: Pressure Sores. *Plast Reconstr Surg.* 2008 Jan;121(MOC-PS CME Coll):1–10.
2. Larson JD, Altman AM, Bentz ML, Larson DL. Pressure Ulcers and Perineal Reconstruction. *Plast Reconstr Surg.* 2014 Jan;133(1):39e – 48e.
3. EPUAP Grading tool [cited 2016 Jun 15]. Available from: http://www.epuap.org/wp-content/uploads/2011/03/EPUAP-Grading-tool.pdf
4. Pressure ulcer treatment: Quick reference guide. [cited 2016 Jun 15]. Available from: http://www.epuap.org/guidelines/Final_Quick_Treatment.pdf
5. Waterlow score card (front). [cited 2016 Jun 15]. Available from: http://www.judy-waterlow.co.uk/downloads/Waterlow%20Score%20Card-front.pdf
6. Waterlow score card (back). [cited 2016 Jun 15]. Available from: http://www.judy-waterlow.co.uk/downloads/Waterlow%20Score%20Card-back.pdf
7. Braden score [cited 2016 Jun 15]. Available from: http://www.bradenscale.com/images/bradenscale.pdf

Pressure sore theory

"Soft tissue injury from unrelieved pressure over a bony prominence".

PATHOPHYSIOLOGY

1. Tissue ischiemia, occurs when external pressure exceeds the capillary pressure (about 30mm Hg)
2. Location, relates to patient position, supine (buttocks, sacrum, heels), sitting (ischium).
3. Severity, related to pressure. Higher pressure causes ulceration sooner
4. Tip of iceberg phenomenon, that damage in deeper tissues usually far exceeds that visible on the skin

Infection and edema make it worse

RISK FACTORS
Increasing age, male

Poor nutrition, decreased sensations

Friction, shear, moisture, immobility

Long term steroid use (e.g. for COPD, IBD)

Major illness

GRADING
EPUAP

I	Non-blanching erythema
II	Partial thickness dermis loss
III	Through dermis & subcutaneous tissue visible
IV	Exposed bone, tendon or muscle

WATERLOW SCORE
Described by Judy Waterlow in 1985, it is a prognostic score to assess progression of pressure sores. It takes in to account,

1. Age
2. Gender
3. BMI
4. Skin type
5. Mobility
6. Continence
7. Malnutrition screening tool (MST 2005 revision)

as well as "special risk scores" for
8. tissue malnutrition (which is different from MST above)
9. neurological deficit
10. long term steroid or cytotoxic medication use
11. major trauma or major surgery

A set of scores is assigned for each category. A total score of 10+ places the patient "at risk", 15+ at high risk and 20+ at very high risk of developing pressure ulcers.

An "improving" Waterlow score is a good indication to consider surgery (if at all).

BRADEN SCORE

This is another commonly used scoring system that takes in to account,

1. Mobility
2. Level of physical activity
3. Nutrition
4. Sensation
5. Moisture
6. Friction & shear

LASER

LASER a device which produces monochromatic, collimated, coherent and high intensity light in the visible and near-visible spectrum. The word LASER is also the acronym for the principle on which this device works i.e. **L**ight **A**mplification by **S**timulated **E**mission of **R**adiation. Similar devices working in the *M*icrowave spectrum are called MASERS. In common usage, all caps are almost never used and the word 'laser' is used as a noun.

Principle

Light Emission by Stimulated Emission of Radiation

When an electron in an atom receives external energy it absorbs it and is said to enter an energised or "excited" ‼ state. (Classical physics talks about occupying a higher orbit, but that is old school). When the application of energy is stopped, the electron needs to return to its stable lowest energy state ("ground state"), and it does so by emitting the excess energy as a photon.

The *amount* of energy emitted as a photon can only have certain discrete values known as quanta (sing.=quantum) and is governed by the laws of quantum mechanics.

The *method* of emission of this energy can be
A. Spontaneous emission (Ref: Figure), i.e. after a short period (few nano seconds) the electron emits the quantum of energy by itself and resumes its resting state
B. Stimulated emission (Ref: Figure) where a passing by photon stimulates the electron to release its excess energy as a photon (and return to ground state). i.e. one photon stimulates the release of another. In this case, both the photons have exactly the same energy (and are "in phase" i.e. their crests and troughs are in sync).

Figure: Spontaneous emission. An 'excited' electron is ready to return to its ground state. It does so spontaneously by emitting a photon. There is no co-ordination between different electrons and the photons emitted are non-coherent (i.e. at random times and in random directions).

Figure: Stimulated emission. An incident photon stimulates the excited electron

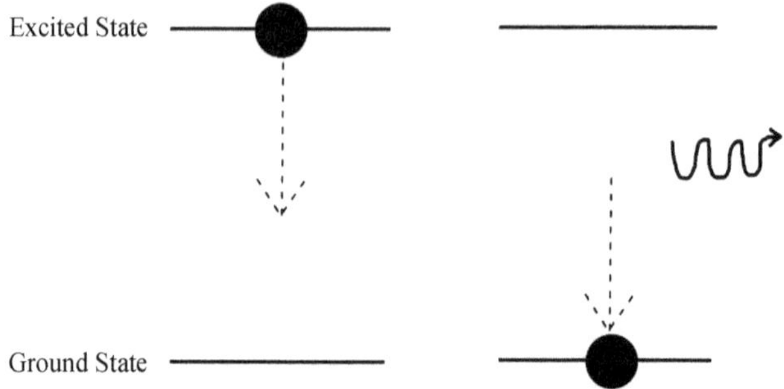

to return to its resting state. The resulting photon is identical to the one that started the process.

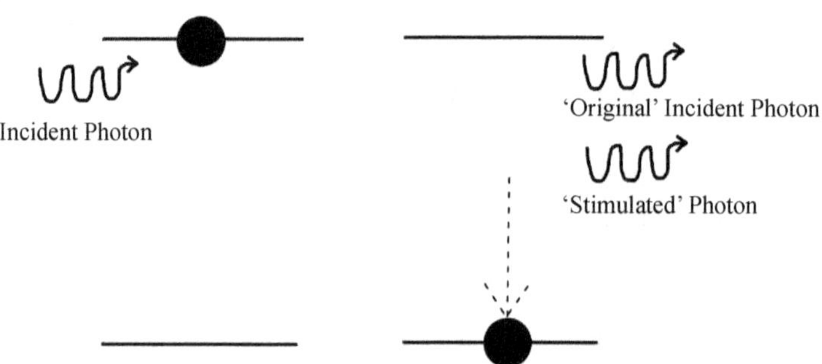

If there are only a few excited electrons, the process of stimulated emission quickly stops. The lasing process can only begin when the number of excited electrons are more than the resting electrons (*population inversion*).

A *dopant* is a small impurity in the lasing medium that helps to provide extra electrons. An energy source (*pump*) keeps the number of excited electrons topped up. The lasing medium has reflective mirrors on both ends that bounce the photons back and forth, helping to stimulate production of more photons. (One mirror may even be partially reflective to keep the process in check).

All these photons are identical in that,
1. they have the same energy (i.e. wavelength) making the laser *mono-chromatic*
2. they are coherent (i.e. in phase) so do not disperse, making the laser beam *collimated*

Aside: Q-switching

'Q-switch' is an electronic or mechanical device that can interrupt the laser excitation process

The whole process of providing energy to the electrons, population inversion and laser production takes a certain amount of time which limits how fast a laser can be switched on or off. A *Q-switch** (i.e. altering the Quality factor) is an electrical or mechanical method to decrease the quality of the lasing medium. Once a 'low quality' system reaches its lasing capability, the Quality of the medium is switched to be better for lasing. This effectively supersaturates the lasing medium and increases the power of the laser considerably.

The quality factor can be changed much faster as compared to the sequence of laser production. By allowing the lasing medium to stay supersaturated, and changing the Q-factor allows the laser to be turned on and off very quickly (in the order of nano seconds).

Instrument

Figure: Lasing set up

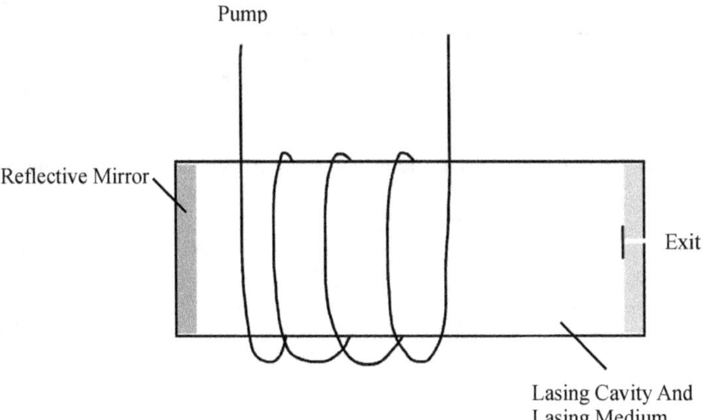

Mechanism of action in medical science

Chromophore
The pigment that is the target for a given laser wavelength.

Selective photothermolysis (Anderson and Parish)
The energy from a given laser wavelength is preferentially absorbed by a specific chromophore, causing it to heat up rapidly and disintegrate.

Clinical parameters used in choosing a laser

1. **Wavelength**. Varies by chromophore being targeted e.g. haemoglobin absorbs at 595 nm therefore PDL (585nm) is used for vascular lesions, port wine stain etc (Fig: Spectrum of light. Table: Common laser wavelengths)

Figure: Spectrum of light

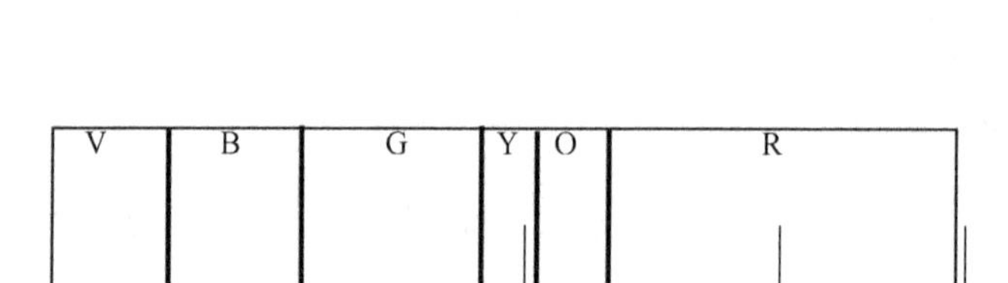

Figure: Relationship of longer wavelength laser with visible light spectrum

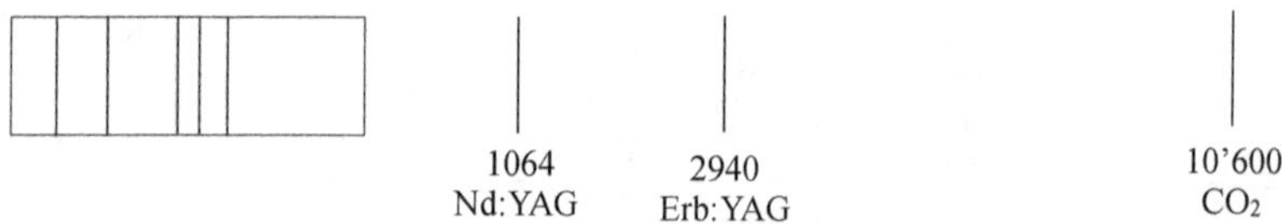

Table: Common laser wavelengths

Wavelength (nm)	Laser
585	PDL
694	Q-switched ruby
755	Alexandrite
1064 (532)	Nd:YAG (Q-switched Nd:YAG)
2940	Erb:YAG
10600	CO_2

2. **Fluence** (=Energy density, J/cm^2), is the energy delivered by the laser, which leads to heat generation, which causes clinical effect. Fluence depends on
   A. Energy
   B. Spot size

   Too little fluence means that the laser energy is absorbed but tissue is not heated enough. Too much fluence generates excessive heat and can cause collateral damage to adjacent structures and increase risk of scarring.

3. **Pulse duration,** determines how long the tissue is exposed to the laser (and hence heats up as a result). Then if the laser is removed, the heat now stored in the tissue [more in the chromophore and less in the adjacent tissue] is dissipated. The rate of energy dissipation is proportional to the amount of energy stored as a result of being targeted by the laser. The time it takes for half the energy to be dissipated is called thermal relaxation time ($T_{1/2}$).

   The aim is to keep the pulse duration shorter than the $T_{1/2}$ to allow heat to escape and prevent collateral damage. $T_{1/2}$ varies with the size of different chromophores - being less for tattoo pigments and more for hair follicles. Hence the pulse duration for lasers targeting tattoos is nano/pico seconds, while those targeting hair is in microseconds.

4. +/- **Surface cooling**.

RECOMMENDED PAPERS

1. Anderson RR, Parish JA. Selective photothermolysis: precise microsurgery by selective absorption of pulsed radiation. *Science.* 1983;220(4596):524-7
2. Nelson AA, Lask GP. Principles and Practice of Cutaneous Laser and Light Therapy. *Clin Plast Surg.* 2011 Jul;38(3):427–36.

3. Farkas JP, Hoopman JE, Kenkel JM. Five Parameters You Must Understand to Master Control of Your Laser/Light-Based Devices. *Aesthetic Surgery J.* 2013 Sep 1;33(7):1059–64.

4. Bernstein E. Laser Tattoo Removal. *Seminars in Plastic Surgery.* 2007 Aug; 21(3):175–92.

Topical negative pressure therapy (TNP)

Acknowledgment: Many thanks to Dr Wardah Bajwa for her help in writing this chapter and searching for the references.

Described originally by Argenta & Morykwas, it is the application of sub-atmospheric pressure in a closed system to improve wound healing.

OBJECTIVES
- Promote healing
- Improve vascularity, e.g. in preparation for an eventual skin graft
- Management of excessive fluid exudate
- Temporising / preparatory step before definitive reconstructive surgery e.g. open lower limb fractures

MECHANISMS OF ACTION
1. Improved wound perfusion, up to 125mmHg (Ref: Morykwas)
2. Decreased bacterial load & toxin levels, by removal of exudate from tissues
3. Decreased edema, by removal of fluid which in turn helps in nutrient diffusion to the wound bed
4. Mechanical stress. Both macro- and micro- stresses on the tissues activate the signal transduction pathways causing cellular recruitment, activation & differentiation
5. Granulation tissue formation. Morykwas (in a porcine model) showed 63% and 103% increase in granulation tissue formation using continuous or intermittent TNP respectively.

INDICATIONS
1. Acute traumatic wounds, (after adequate debridement of course) as a closed dressing system.
2. Chronic wounds, to attempt granulation tissue formation to make it a graftable bed. [TNP works best as part of holistic patient management e.g. infection control, nutrition, medical optimisation etc. Do consider malignancy in the differential diagnosis].
3. Wound bed preparation
4. Fixation of skin grafts, to prevent shearing in the initial phase
5. Dehisced surgical incisions, to promote healing by second intent
6. Acute surgical wounds. There is some evidence to suggest that acute surgical wounds heal better with a TNP applied along the incision line

CONTRAINDICATIONS

1. Grossly infected / dirty wounds
2. Necrotic tissue
3. Active bleeding (or risk of). e.g. *do not* apply over blood vessels
4. Deranged clotting profile
5. Malignancy
6. Exposed organs

CHOICE OF INTERFACE

- Polyurethane foam (PU) - black in colour & softer, "traditional" foam
- Poly vinyl alcohol foam (PVA) - white and stiffer, so requires higher pressures
- Biguanide impregnated gauze (Kerlex™), which comes as a 10cm wide, long roll and can conform to the wound bed.

These foams/gauze cannot be applied directly to skin graft, where an additional layer of non-adherent dressing is used (e.g. paraffin gauze like Jelonet™/ Bactigras™, or silicone dressing like Mepital™). Similarly, applying TNP directly on a viscus is not a good idea.

DRAINAGE

The wound and its foam dressing are sealed with adhesive tapes. A hole in this dressing over the foam allows a silicone tubing to connect to the negative pressure generation machine.

PRESSURE AND TYPE OF SUCTION

On the basis of clinical studies, 125mmHg with an intermittent suction cycle (5 minutes on and 2 minutes off) is quoted as best for wound healing. However, higher pressures and intermittent suction are painful for the patient (esp. when the suction turns back on). [For use as a dressing only (as opposed to its use for generation of granulation tissue), 80mmHg continuous pressure appear to be adequate].

COMPLICATIONS

- Pain
- Hemorrhage / Haematoma
- Frank pus
- Toxic shock
- Contact dermatitis (from dressing adhesive)
- Pressure necrosis from the silicone tubing, [esp. if patient is lying on it e.g. in sacral pressure sores]

RECOMMENDED PAPERS

1. Morykwas MJ, Argenta LC, Shelton-Brown EI, McGuirt W. Vacuum-assisted closure: a new method for wound control and treatment: animal studies and basic foundation. *Ann Plast Surg.* 1997

2. Morykwas MJ, David LR, Schneider AM, Whang C, Jennings DA, Canty C, Parker D, White WL,Argenta LC. Use of subatmospheric pressure to prevent progression of partial-thickness burns in a swine model. *J Burn Care Rehabil.* 1999;20(1 pt 1):15

3. Lipsky B. A report from the international consensus on diagnosing and treating the infected diabetic foot. *Diabetes Metab Res Rev.* 2004; 20(Suppl 1): 68-77

4. Ubbink DT, van der Oord BM, Sobotka MR, Jacobs MJ. Effects of vacuum compression therapy on skin microcirculation in patients suffering from lower limb ischaemia. *Vasa* 2000;29(1):53-7

5. Ubbink DT, Westerbos SJ, Evans D, Land L, Vermeulen H. Topical negative pressure for treating chronic wounds. *Cochrane Database Syst Rev.* 2008

6. Ubbink DT, Westerbos SJ, Nelson EA, Vermeulen H. A systematic review of

7. topical negative pressure therapy for acute and chronic wounds. *Br J Surg.* 2008 Jun;95(6):685-92

8. Swan MC, Banwell PE. The open abdomen: aetiology, classification and current management strategies. *J Wound Care.* 2005;14(1):7-11

9. Levine SM, Sinno S, Levine JP, Saadeh PB. An evidence-based approach to the surgical management of pressure ulcers. *Ann Plast Surg.* 2012 Oct;69(4): 482-4

10. Bovill E, Banwell PE, Teot L et al. Topical negative pressure wound therapy: a review of its role and guidelines for its use in the management of acute wounds. *Int Wound J.* 2008:5(4):511.

11. Connolly M, Ibrahim ZR, Johnson ON 3rd. Changing paradigms in lower extremity reconstruction in war-related injuries. *Mil Med Res.* 2016 Mar 31;3:9

Workhorse Flaps

RFFF: Radial forearm free flap

Definition

It is...	type C or D, fasciocut. or osseo-fasciocut. flap
by...	Cormack and Lamberty classification
based on...	septocutaneous branches of radial artery in distal forearm
Original description	Yang et al. 1981 Song, 1982, Clinics in plastic surgery
Commonly used as	Free flap for H&N/penile/lower limb reconstruction, Pedicled reverse flow flap for dorsum of hand

Markings

Pedicle marking	Midpoint of antecubital fossa, to Radial pulse at wrist between FCR & BR
Skin territory	Whole forearm skin on volar surface, as far as EPL and ECU tendons

Prep & positioning

Informed consent, GA

Supine, arms abducted on arm table, tourniquet available

Abx, prep, drape, WHO checklist

Raising

Allen's test

Template defect & plan in reverse

Tourniquet up

Raise distal to proximal & deep to the deep fascia

Identify & preserve: Radial artery, FCR, cephalic vein
Start raising: ulnar border, distal to proximal
Id & preserve: PL distally, basilic vein, medial cut. nerve of forearm
Start raising: radial border, distal to proximal, from BR

Id & preserve: superficial branch of radial nerve, lateral cut of forearm, cephalic vein (for anastomosis)

Tourniquet down

Stop and check: clamp radial artery and check vascularity of hand

Isolate flap

Variations

1. Osteo-fasciocutaneous flap
   - 40% of width of radius and length between insertions of PT & BR (nearly 10cm) may be taken
   - Splint in above-elbow cast for 4/52
2. Reverse radial forearm flap
   - Rotation axis: radial pulse at wrist
   - Blood flow: retrograde via ulnar artery
   - Venous drainage: retrograde via venae comitantes

Figure: Penile recon with RFFF. a) Dimensions. Circumference of a circle is pi times its diameter, so for a urethra of 1cm diameter a 3cm wide piece of skin is required. Adjacent to it is a 1cm wide 'transition zone' that is de-epithelised to allow folding on to itself. A 1cm dia. neo-urethra with 1cm of subcutaneous tissue on either side (factoring in post-op edema) make a 3cm dia. cylinder, with a circumference of 9cm.

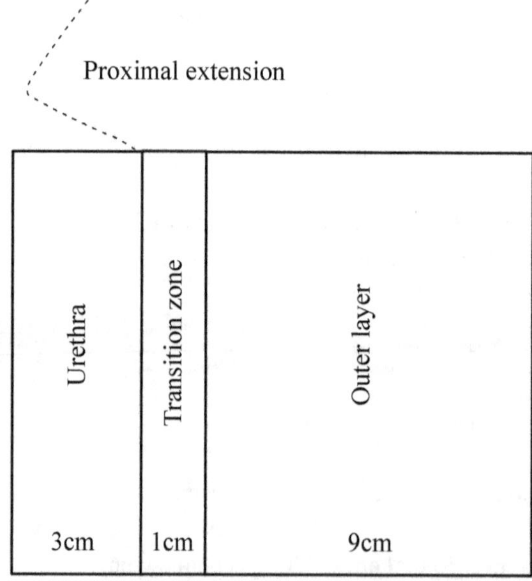

Figure: Penile recon with RFFF (*contd.*) How to fold the RFFF in penile reconstruction. Note the transition zone is de-epithelised before inset.

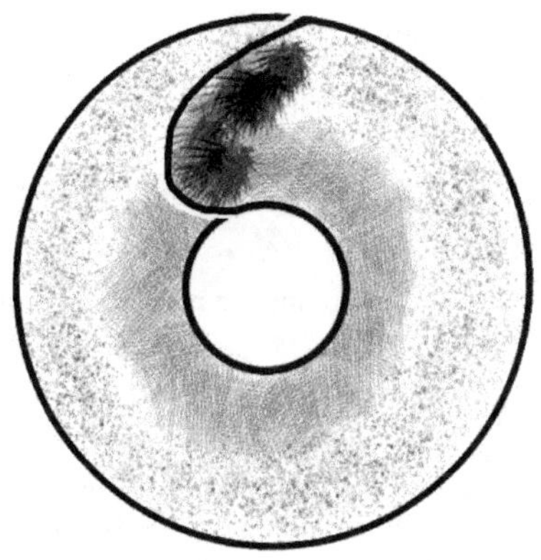

ALT: Anterolateral thigh flap

Definition

It is...	perforator flap*
supplied by...	a myocutaneous, or sometimes a direct cutaneous perforator
based on...	• (>50%) myocutaneous perforators from the descending branch of LCFA (lateral circumflex femoral artery) • (30%) myocut. perf. of *transverse* branch of LCFA • (15%) septocut. perf. of descending branch of LCFA
Original description	Song in 1984, but popularised by Fu Chan Wei
Commonly used as	free flap for H&N and lower limb

* although sometimes referred to as a fascio-cutaneous flap

Markings

Pedicle marking	3cm radius around the midpoint of a line drawn from ASIS to lateral patella
Pedicle length / dia	10-13cm / 2-2.5mm
Skin territory	• Anterolateral thigh skin, centred around the perforator and as an ellipse along the ASIS-patella line. • 8-10cm wide, if closing directly • approx 15x25cm ellipse if donor site is grafted

Prep & positioning

Informed consent, GA
Supine, arms abducted on arm table
Abx, prep, drape, WHO checklist

Raising

Start raising: medial to lateral, subfascially
Id & preserve: all muscular perforators until you know which one to use. Go up to the intermuscular septum between rectus femoris and vastus lateralis
Start raising: lateral to medial, deep to fascia lata, up to the perforator

If no septal perforator found: Do intra-muscular dissection. Ligate all muscular branches (unless you are taking a cuff of muscle) and trace down to main vessels
If septal perforator found: Dissect in intermuscular septum up to LCFA, ligating all else
Id & preserve: Muscular branches of femoral nerve. Rarely, you may encounter transverse and ascending branches of LCFA as well.

Variations

1. Flow through flap. Uses distal end of the descending branch to plug it in to an ischiemic portion of an extremity.
2. Chimeric flap. Uses ascending branch to plug a vascularised fibular graft
3. Cutaneous-only flap. Supra-fascial flap +/- thinned further while preserving subdermal plexus.

Gastrocnemius flap

Definition

It is...	Type 1 muscle flap
by...	Mathes & Nahai classification
based on...	medial or lateral sural artery
Commonly used as	Pedicled flap for local coverage around the knee. Medial gastroc. has a larger size and arc of rotation.

Markings

Pedicle marking	Not necessary to visualise
Skin territory	none

Prep & positioning

Supine with wedge under opposite hip and knee semi-flexed
Tourniquet

Raising

Lazy-S incision centred on midline, between popliteal fossa and midline
Id & preserve: Short saphenous vein and nerve
Incise deep fascia
Separate soleus and medial head of gastroc.
Id & preserve: sural nerve (on deeper surface of gastroc.)
Identify space between the 2 heads of gastroc.
Raise distal to proximal, while taking 1-2cm of tendinous part to help inset
Harvest SSG, mesh and inset
Drain, well padded dressing

Variations

Manoeuvres to increase the flap's reach:
1. Score deep surface
2. Detach from femoral condyle
3. Pass deep to per anserinus (insertion of semitendinosus, gracilis & sartorius)

Groin flap

Definition

It is...	thin fascio-cut. flap
based on...	direct cutaneous branches of superficial circumflex iliac artery
Original description	McGregor & Jackson in 1972
Commonly used as	pedicled flap for upper extremity cover

Markings

Pedicle marking	Starts: 2.5cm below mid-inguinal point Course: from origin to ASIS Branches: given off approx. 1.5cm from origin Superficial branch is in a subcut. plane, 2cm below (& parallel to) inguinal ligament. Deep branch runs on deep fascia (same direction & markings) and penetrates it at lateral border of sartorius (just after crossing lateral femoral cut. nerve)
Skin territory	approx. 10x20cm

Raising

(Consent, GA, prep, drape, WHO checklist, ± Abx) Supine

Start raising: Distal to proximal. Lateral to ASIS, stay superficial to deep fascia

Preserve: SCIA in flap by taking deep fascia with flap at ASIS + take a patch of sartorius fascia

Raise over fascia of iliacus muscle up to origin

Id & preserve: SIEA

Start raising: Medial border

Id & preserve: SIEV & SCIV

Variations

1. Due to multiple branches of femoral artery in the area of the pedicle, a pedicled flap may be raised on 2 arteries and several veins.
2. Superficial circumflex iliac perforator (SCIP) flap, described by Koshima in 2004.

Gracilis flap

Definition

It is...	Type 2 muscle / musculocutaneous flap
by...	Mathes & Nahai classification
based on...	branches from medial circumflex femoral vessels which enter its upper 1/3rd
Original description	Harii & McGraw, 1976 in PRS
Commonly used as	pedicled flap for perineal reconstruction, or free flap for lower limb reconstruction

Markings

Muscle marking	Origin = body & inferior ramus of pubis Insertion = medial upper surface of tibia With the thigh abducted, the most prominent muscle on the medial side is the medial border of adductor longus. The anterior border of gracilis is just behind it.
Pedicle marking	8-10cm below pubic tubercle
Skin territory	3cm anterior and 6-9cm posterior to the line of the muscle, in its proximal 1/3rd

Nerve supply is by Obturator nerve

Prep & positioning

(Consent, GA, prep, drape, WHO checklist, ± Abx)

Supine

Lithotomy position

Feet in stirrups

Break the bottom of the table for easier access

Lithotomy/Colorectal drapes to cover the lower legs

Raising

Incision: over proximal 10cm of the muscle

Start raising: Split fascia over adductor longus and gracilis

Id & retract: Adductor longus. Note that gracilis inserts on proximal tibia, so it moves with flexion-extension of knee, while aductor longus does not.

Id & protect: pedicle & anterior branch of obturator nerve, on top of adductor brevis

+/- Incision: over distal musculo-tendinous portion of the muscle
Identify: gracilis, which now lies between sartorius & semi-membranosus. (It moves when you gently tug the proximal part of the muscle).
Divide the muscle distally (as required), retrieve into the proximal incision (if 2 incision approach is used) and dissect pedicle to desired length.

Variations

1. TUG (Transverse upper gracilis) flap, is a muscle-only flap
2. TMG (Transverse myocutaneous gracilis) flap

TFL: Tensor fascia lata flap

Definition

It is...	Type 1 muscle flap
by...	Mathes & Nahai classification
based on...	ascending branch of LCFA (branch of profunda femoris)
Original description	Hill, 1978, PRS
Commonly used as	pedicled flap for lower abdominal defects

Markings

Muscle marking	Origin = anterior 5cm of outer lip of iliac crest & ASIS Insertion = via iliotibial tract, in to lateral tibial condyle
Pedicle marking	8cm below ASIS (usually divides before entering the muscle)
Skin territory	Superiorly = iliac crest Inferiorly = 15 cm above the knee Antero-posterior = 2 cm on either side of muscle border

Nerve supply is by Inferior branch of superior gluteal nerve (motor) & T12 (sensory to overlying skin)

Raising

(Consent, GA, prep, drape, WHO checklist, ± Abx) Lateral position
Raise: distal to proximal, sub-fascially to elevate fascia lata with it
Id & preserve: pedicle, 8cm below ASIS
+/- preserve: T12, lateral cutaneous nerve of thigh, superior gluteal nerve
Dissect pedicle by medial retraction of rectus femoris

Variations

1. Dissect pedicle proximally up to 10cm, by ligating all other branches of LCFA (while preserving muscular branches of femoral nerve)
2. Osteomyocutanous flap = iliac crest and ASIS at TFL origin may be included.

Free fibula flap

Definition

It is...	Type C or D osseous or osseo-fasciocutaneous flap
by...	Cormack & Lamberty classification
based on...	perforating branches from the peroneal artery
Original description	Taylor, 1975 Hidalgo, 1989 for mandibular defect
Commonly used as	Free flap for head and neck reconstruction

Markings

Bone marking	Usually in its middle 1/3rd, and 20% bigger than the defect
Pedicle marking	multiple perforators at the posterior border, esp. of middle 1/3rd of the fibula
Skin territory	Centre on posterior border of fibula

Prep & positioning

Informed consent, GA

Supine, sand bag under ipsilateral hip, tourniquet

Abx, prep, drape, WHO checklist

Raising

Raise: anterior and proximal

Id & preserve: common peroneal nerve

Raise deep fascia towards posterior intermuscular septum

Id & preserve: septocutaneous branches

Dissect anterior compartment muscles off fibula, to reach inter-osseus membrane. Incise that to reach tibialis posterior

Identify: Osteotomy sites (proximally & distally)

Incise periosteum and elevate it all around.

Gentle traction to expose soleus and FHL posteriorly. (FHL has the peroneal vessels)

Raise: Inferior to superior
Id & protect: anterior tibial vessels. Incise interosseus membrane
Expose: tibialis posterior and divide it, keeping a cuff to protect vascular pedicle and its branches.

Use for recon
Hemostasis, drain, well padded dressing

Postop:
Analgesia, elevate, well hydrate, regular flap obs, check bloods next morning,

Variations
1. Osseos flap only
2. Osseo-cutaneous flap

Definitions

The commonest question you'll hear in training, and in exam is "What is….". An appropriate definition can help you start off that conversation in style and concentrate on decision making.

Wound healing

Wound healing
It is a complex and dynamic process of re-establishing the continuity of a wound by restoration of cellular structure and tissue layers.

Wound healing by primary intent
The process by which a clean cut and well approximated edges heals.

Wound healing by 2nd intent
Wound healing by a process of granulation and re-epithelisation.

Delayed primary healing
Process when an infected wound is allowed to granulate initially before a primary closure.

Foetal wound healing
refers to scarless wound healing in utero due to tissue regeneration. It depends on foetal age, injured tissue and wound length.

Ideal dressing
Simple, inexpensive, absorbent and non-adherent. Provides a moist environment for healing and is antimicrobial.

Pressure ulcer
Soft tissue injury as a result of unrelieved pressure over a bony prominence

Biofilm
Bacterial colonies that adhere to inanimate substances (e.g. plastic, metal, non-viable bone) and secrete a polysaccharide matrix to isolate themselves from surrounding tissues and to protect themselves from host defences.

Scars

Tattoo
A foreign material entered in to the dermis (intentionally) by a needle or as a consequence of trauma, that results in a visible mark in the skin.

Scar

Macroscopic disturbance of normal structure and function of skin architecture resulting from the end product of wound healing.

Ideal scar

Fine, flat, concealed, linear scar lying within a skin crease or at the border of an aesthetic unit or along a resting skin tension line (RSTL).

RSTLs (Resting skin tension lines)

Imaginary lines which lie along the direction of dermal collagen or perpendicular to the long axis of the underlying facial muscles.

Ischaemia

Insufficient supply of oxygen to meet tissue demands.

Reconstructive ladder

Split skin graft

Contains entire epidermis and partial thickness of dermis.

Full thickness skin graft

Contains entire epidermis and full thickness of dermis.

Meshing

The procedure of cutting slits into sheet graft, in order to increase its dimensions prior to insert.

Delay

Any manoeuvre designed to increase blood supply to a flat.

Compartment syndrome

A clinical emergency where soft tissue viability is threatened by increased tissue pressure within a fixed fascial compartment in the body over a prolonged period

Tissue expansion

Increasing the (surface area of) available soft tissue by using its visco-elastic properties and/or new tissue formation.

Stress relaxation

"If *strain* is held constant, the stress decreases the time." i.e. if you stretch tissue by a certain length the amount of force needed to keep the there decreases with time.

Creep
" If stress is held constant, the strain increases with time" i.e. If you keep pulling it, it continues to stretch. Creep is by mechanical (tissues stretching out) or biological (new cell growth).

Topical negative pressure therapy (TNP)
Application of sub-atmospheric pressure to a sealed wound, either
- to act as a temporary dressing,
- to manage excess wound exudate,
- promote wound healing

Replantation
Restoration of an amputated part of an extremity (usually upper extremity).

Flaps
Burrow's triangle
Triangular wedge of skin and soft tissue excised at the end of an incision after local flap transfer, to allow smooth wound closure.

Arc of rotation
Extent of reach of a flap when it is moved about its point of rotation.

Transposition
Rearrangement or shuffle, i.e. the tissue is moved from one place and something else takes its place

Rotation
Movement of the whole so that it is facing a different direction.

Bilobed flap
Transposition flap consisting of two smaller flaps designed at right angle to each other. The primary flap is transposed into the defect whereas the secondary flap closes the primary flap's donor site. (The secondary flap's donor is closed directly).

Dog ear
Three-dimensional excess of soft tissue at the end of a closed wound.

Rhombus
A parallelogram, all of whose sides have the same length. [A rectangle is a special case where all the angles are 90 degrees].

Rhomboid

A parallelogram, whose adjacent sides are of unequal length (and does not have a right angle in it).

Z-plasty

A technique in which two triangular flaps are interdigitated to achieve a gain in length, or change in direction of scar.

Skin cancers

Regression

Partial or total disappearance of melanoma, presumably by a cell or cytokine mediated host response.

Breslow Thickness

The vertical distance between granular layer of epidermis and the deepest melanoma cells, measured by an ocular micro-meter and reported within one 10th of a millimetre.

Spitz nevus

Melanocytic lesion which under light microscopy resembles a melanoma but whose clinical behaviour lies on a spectrum from completely benign ("typical Spitz nevus") to frankly malignant ("Spitzoid melanoma").

Actinic Keratosis

Common pre-malignant lesions on sun exposed skin due to cumulative sun exposure, esp. on Fitzpatrick I & II skin types.

DFSP (Dermatofibrosarcoma protuberans)

Rare soft tissue sarcoma which is locally aggressive but has low malignant potential

Merkel Cell CA

Rare but aggressive tumour of neuroendocrine origin.

Sebaceous CA

Mixed adnexal tumor with a variable site of origin, histologic grade and clinical presentation. Typically on lower eyelid of a woman in her 70s where it can be clinical confused with a BCC

AFX

Spindle cell tumour, either on head and neck of sun exposed individuals in their 70s, or trunk and extremities of younger patients.

Angiosarcoma
Uncommon, aggressive and usually fatal neoplasm of vascular endothelium.

SLNB
A process for surgical staging of clinically node negative cancers, by intra-operative lymphatic mapping and biopsy of sentinel node.

Sentinel node
First node/set of nodes, to which a melanoma drains.

Congenital

Vascular anomaly
A generic term for a set of congenital vascular abnormalities. Most commonly these are either a vascular malformation or a haemangioma.

Vascular malformation
Congenital abnormality consisting of haphazard collection of (microscopically normal looking) vascular elements within skin and subcutaneous tissues (although they can exist in other tissues as well).

Hemangioma
The commonest tumour of infancy which typically appears soon after birth, rapidly increases in size out of proportion to the child and slowly regresses over a period of years.

Hypospadias
A congenital abnormality of male external genitalia characterised by triad of
1.   abnormally positioned ventral meatus,
2.   dorsal preputial hooding, and
3.   a variable degree of ventral curvature ("chordee")

Syndactyly
It is a congenital condition with variable fusion of soft tissue and skeletal elements of adjacent digits.
1.   complete syndactyly: where the webspace extends to include the finger tip
2.   incomplete syndactyly: when the webspace occurs anywhere between normal site and fingertip

A.   simple syndactyly: where skin and soft tissue connections only between adjacent digits
B.   complex syndactyly: + skeletal anomalies

C. complex complicated: via excessively phalange Isak interposed within the abnormal web space

Deprivational Amblyopia
Lack of development of optic pathway in early life due to insufficient stimulus (either due to strabismus, obstruction in visual field).

Lymphoedema
Accumulation of protein rich fluid in interstitial space secondary to lymphatic dysfunction.

Prosthesis
A device that is designed to replace, as much as possible, the function and appearance of missing limb or body part

Distraction osteogenensis
Generation of viable bone by gradual movement of osteotomised bone fragments.

Pharyngeal arches
Mesodermal condensations in the sidewalls of the primitive pharynx which give rise to many of the structures in head and neck.

Encephalocele
Herniation of intra-cranial contents through a cranial defect.

Meningocele
Herniation of CSF + meninges

Meningoencephalocele
Herniation of CSF + meninges + brain

Craniofacial clefts
Anomalies of face and cranium with deficiency or excess of tissues that cleave anatomical planes in a linear fashion (Ref: Mathes' plastic surgery)

Craniofacial microsomia
A spectrum of malformations primarily involving structures derived from 1st and 2nd branchial arches.

Craniosynostosis
Pathologic partial / complete *absence* of one of more cranial sutures. (Note that it is not "premature fusion", as only metopic suture fuses normally, other sutures "mature" but never fuse).

Hypertelorism
Clinical finding of increased inter-orbital distance

Inter-orbital distance
Distance between medial walls of orbit (25mm♀, 28mm♂)

Burns

Burns sepsis
A change in burn patient that triggers a concern for infection

Inhalation injury
Damage to respiratory tract by heat/chemical irritants carried in to the airways by respiration.

Hand and peripheral nerve

Neuroma
Results from abnormal nerve regeneration following a peripheral nerve lesion either from a laceration, pressure, stretch or chemical irritation.

Motor unit
All muscle fibres innervated by a single nerve branch.

Neurapraxia
Injury to a peripheral nerve in which its structure is intact but the nerve conduction is temporarily impaired.

Neurotmesis
Injury to a nerve involving axonal disruption within intact supporting structures.

Neurotmesis
Injury where continuity of a nerve is completely disrupted.

Wallerian degeneration
Response of distal stump after complete transaction of an axon. Immediate = Granular disintegration of axonal cytoskeleton + myelin breakdown

- @D1 = Macrophage recruitment → IL-1 → Nerve Growth factor (NGF) → regrowth
- @D3 = Schwann cells organise in to "Bands of Bugner" which are tubes supporting regeneration
- Proximal = Growth cones from myelinated and unmyelinated fibers → neurotropism to distal end + neurotrophism (i.e. survival of axon if the correct distal end is found)

Endoneurium
Covering around an axon and its Schwann cells.

Perineurium
Covering around a group of axons making a fascicle.

Epineurium
Protective covering round multiple fascicles ("inter-fascicular") or surrounding the periphery of a nerve ("extra-fascicular").

Martin Gruber anastomoses
Connection between motor fibres of median nerve to ulnar nerve in the forearm. They are destined for either median nerve innervated muscles (thenars), or ulnar nerve nerve innervated muscles (interossei). In CTC, in presence of Martin-Gruber anatomoses, thenar muscles are not wasted and NCS show paradox of normal latencies proximally and increased distal latencies.

Richie-Cannieux anastomoses
Communications in palm between recurrent branch of median nerve and deep branch of nerve, so that ulnar nerve innervates the thenar muscles.

Stener lesion
Intra-operative finding in complete UCL tears of thumb MCPj, where adductor aponeurosis is interposed between the UCL and its insertion.

Rheumatoid arthritis
Peripheral symmetric polyarthritis of small joints (usually hands and feet) that spreads to involve larger joints.

Genetics

Syndrome
Multiple malformations occurring in embryologically non-contiguous areas.

Malformations
A morphologic defect in an organ/area of body due to an intrinsically abnormal development process e.g. polydactyly, cleft lip, congenital heart anomaly.

Deformation
Likely due to mechanical forces e.g. positional plagiocephaly.

Disruption
Rare anomaly due to breakdown of normal fetal development process.

Penetrance
Proportion of individuals carrying a particular variation of a gene (called an allele, or genotype) that *also* express the associated trait (phenotype).

Expressivity
The extent of variation in phenotype, for a given genotype.

Gene
Basic unit of heredity

Allele
One member of a pair or series of different form of a gene. (Diploid organism e.g. humans have paired chromosomes and of both chromosomes carry the same copy of a gene, the organism is called "homozygous" for that gene).

Dominant
A phenotype that will be expressed when at least one of its alleles are present.